Imperatives for Action and Impact of Humanitarian Crises Affecting Children

Editor

DANIELLE LARAQUE-ARENA

PEDIATRIC CLINICS OF NORTH AMERICA

www.pediatric.theclinics.com

Consulting Editor
TINA L. CHENG

October 2026 • Volume 73 • Number 5

ELSEVIER

1818 Market Street • Suite 3323 • Philadelphia, Pennsylvania, 19103-2899

http://www.theclinics.com

THE PEDIATRIC CLINICS OF NORTH AMERICA Volume 73, Number 5
October 2026 ISSN 0031-3955, ISBN-13: 978-0-443-42887-6

Editor: Kerry Holland
Developmental Editor: Anirban Mukherjee

Publishing Office: The *Pediatric Clinics of North America* (ISSN 0031-3955) is published bimonthly by Elsevier Inc., 1818 Market Street, Suite 3323, Philadelphia, PA 19103, United States. Periodicals postage paid at New York, NY and additional mailing offices. USA POSTMASTER: Send address changes to *Pediatric Clinics of North America*, Elsevier Customer Service Department, 3251 Riverport Lane, Maryland Heights, MO 63043, USA. Months of issue are February, April, June, August, October, and December. Subscription prices are $311.00 per year (US individuals), $391.00 per year (Canadian individuals), $467.00 per year (international individuals), $100.00 per year (US students and residents), $100.00 per year (Canadian students and residents), and $165.00 per year (international residents and students). For institutional access pricing please contact Customer Service via the contact information below. To receive students/resident rare, orders must be accompanied by name of affiliated institution, date of term, and the signature of program/residency coordinator on institution letterhead. Orders will be billed at individual rate until proof of status is received. Foreign air speed delivery is included in all *Clinics* subscription prices. All prices are subject to change without notice. Orders, claims, and journal inquiries: Please visit our Support Hub page https://service.elsevier.com for assistance.

Reprints. For copies of 100 or more, of articles in this publication, please contact the Commercial Reprints Department, Elsevier Inc., 360 Park Avenue South, New York, NY 10010-1710. Tel.: 212-633-3874; Fax: 212-633-3820; E-mail: reprints@elsevier.com.

The Pediatric Clinics of North America is also published in Spanish by McGraw-Hill Inter-americana Editores S.A., Mexico City, Mexico; in Portuguese by Riechmann and Affonso Editores, Rua Comandante Coelho 1085, CEP 21250, Rio de Janeiro, Brazil; and in Greek by Althayia SA, Athens, Greece.

The Pediatric Clinics of North America is covered in *MEDLINE/PubMed (Index Medicus), Excerpta Medica, Current Contents, Current Contents/Clinical Medicine, Science Citation Index, ASCA, ISI/BIOMED*, and *BIOSIS*.

PROGRAM OBJECTIVE

The goal of the *Pediatric Clinics of North America* is to keep practicing physicians and residents up to date with current clinical practice in pediatrics by providing timely articles reviewing the state-of-the-art in patient care.

TARGET AUDIENCE

All practicing pediatricians, physicians, and healthcare professionals who provide patient care to pediatric patients.

LEARNING OBJECTIVES

Upon completion of this activity, participants will be able to:

1. Review disease outbreaks that are increasing in frequency and complexity and disproportionately affect children in humanitarian settings with disrupted health systems.
2. Discuss how implementation science can strengthen child and adolescent mental health services in humanitarian settings.
3. Recognize firearm violence as a pediatric public health emergency requiring coordinated clinical, community, and policy responses.

ACCREDITATIONS

Physician Credit

The Elsevier Office of Continuing Medical Education (EOCME) is accredited by the Accreditation Council for Continuing Medical Education (ACCME) to provide continuing medical education for physicians.

The EOCME designates this journal-based activity for a maximum of 16 *AMA PRA Category 1 Credit*(s)™. Physicians should claim only the credit commensurate with the extent of their participation in the activity.

All other healthcare professionals requesting continuing education credit for this journal-based activity will be issued a certificate of participation.

ABP Maintenance of Certification Credit

Successful completion of this CME activity, which includes participation in the activity and individual assessment of and feedback to the learner, enables the learner to earn up to 16 MOC points in the American Board of Pediatrics' (ABP) Maintenance of Certification (MOC) program. It is the CME activity provider's responsibility to submit learner completion information to ACCME for the purpose of granting ABP MOC credit.

DISCLOSURE OF RELEVANT FINANCIAL RELATIONSHIPS

The EOCME assesses conflict of interest with its instructors, faculty, planners, and other individuals who are in a position to control the content of CME activities. All relevant conflicts of interest that are identified are thoroughly vetted by EOCME for fair balance, scientific objectivity, and patient care recommendations. EOCME is committed to providing its learners with CME activities that promote improvements or quality in healthcare and not a specific proprietary business or a commercial interest.

The authors and editors listed below have identified no financial relationships or relationships to products or devices they have with ineligible companies related to the content of this CME activity: Yusra Ahmed, MPF; Errol R. Alden, MD, FAAP; Yuriy Antipkin, MD; Christine Apio, MSc, MA; Maria Beg, MPH; Theresa S. Betancourt, ScD, MA; Tania Bosqui, DClinPsych, MSc; Charles Branas, PhD; Ruth A. Etzel, MD, PhD; Jeffrey Goldhagen, MD, MPH; Marsha Rae Griffin, MD; Tameir Holder, MPH; Olivia Isenberg-Landes, MPH; Sarah K.G. Jensen, PhD; Milissa Jones, MD, MPH, LTC, MC, USA, FAAP; Mariia Kiselova, MD; J. Bart Klika, MSW, PhD; Eugene Kongnyuy, MD, PhD; Ugomma Korie, MPH; Olivia Landes, MPH; Danielle Laraque-Arena, MD, FAAP, FCOPP; Sunwoo Lee, MPH; Bruce Lesley, MA; Yvonne (Bonnie) Maldonado, MD; Daniel Martinez-Garcia, MD, MPH; Fernando Sanchez Mendoza, MD; Melissa Merrick, PhD; Shernise Mohammed-Ali, HBSc; Maryam Elisabeth Montrichard, MD, MPH; Chetan Sree Muppavarapu, MPH; Rachel Novick, MPH; Jordan O'Brien, MPH; Martin Ottolini, MD, MEd, Col (Ret), USAF, MC, FAAP; Bruce D. Perry, MD, PhD; Annalicia Pickering, MD; Sonali Rajan, EdD, MS; Owen Robinson, MPP; Vanessa Rouzier, MD; Bruce K. Rubin, MEngr, MD, MBA, FRCPC; Eric A. Russell, MD; Jose Ignacio Santos, MD, MS; Nabiha Subzwari, MPH; Jonathan Sury, MPH, CPH; Oleksandr Volosovets, MD; Paul H. Wise, MD, MPH; Janine Young, MD

The planning committee and staff listed below have identified no financial relationships or relationships to products or devices they have with ineligible companies related to the content of this CME activity:
Kerry Holland; Shyamala Kavikumaran; Michelle Littlejohn; Patrick J. Manley; Anirban Mukherjee

UNAPPROVED/OFF-LABEL USE DISCLOSURE

The EOCME requires CME faculty to disclose to the participants:

1. When products or procedures being discussed are off-label, unlabelled, experimental, and/or investigational (not US Food and Drug Administration [FDA] approved); and
2. Any limitations on the information presented, such as data that are preliminary or that represent ongoing research, interim analyses, and/or unsupported opinions. Faculty may discuss information about pharmaceutical agents that is outside of FDA-approved labelling. This information is intended solely for CME and is not intended to promote off-label use of these medications. If you have any questions, contact the medical affairs department of the manufacturer for the most recent prescribing information.

TO ENROLL

To enroll in the *Pediatric Clinics of North America* Continuing Medical Education program, call customer service at 1-800-654-2452 or sign up online at https://www.pediatric.theclinics.com/cme/home. The CME program is available to subscribers for an additional annual fee of USD 313.00.

METHOD OF PARTICIPATION

In order to claim credit, participants must complete the following:

1. Complete enrolment as indicated above.
2. Read the activity.
3. Complete the CME Test and Evaluation. Participants must achieve a score of 70% on the test. All CME Tests and Evaluations must be completed online.

In order to claim MOC points, participants must complete the following:

1. Complete steps listed above for claiming CME credit
2. Provide your specialty board ID#, birth date (MM/DD), and attestation.
3. Online MOC submission is only available for the American Board of pediatrics' (ABP) Maintenance of Certification (MOC) program

CME INQUIRIES/SPECIAL NEEDS

For all CME inquiries or special needs, please contact elsevierCME@elsevier.com.

Contributors

CONSULTING EDITOR

TINA L. CHENG, MD, MPH
BK Rachford Professor and Chair of Pediatrics, University of Cincinnati, Director, Cincinnati Children's Research Foundation, Chief Medical Officer, Cincinnati Children's Hospital Medical Center, Cincinnati, Ohio, USA

EDITOR

DANIELLE LARAQUE-ARENA, MD, FAAP, FCOPP
Professor of Clinical Epidemiology and Pediatrics, Department of Epidemiology at the Mailman School of Public Health, and Department of Pediatrics at the Vagelos College of Physicians & Surgeons, Columbia University, New York; President Emerita, SUNY Upstate Medical University, Syracuse, New York, USA

AUTHORS

YUSRA AHMED, MPH
Student, Department of Population and Family Health, Mailman School of Public Health, Columbia University, New York, New York, USA

ERROL R. ALDEN, MD, FAAP
Col. USA, Ret.; Past President, International Pediatric Association; Past CEO American Academy of Pediatrics

YURIY ANTIPKIN, MD
Professor and Director, All-Ukrainian Center for Motherhood and Childhood of the National Academy of Medical Sciences of Ukraine, Academician, National Academy of Medical Sciences of Ukraine, Kyiv, Ukraine

CHRISTINE APIO, MSc, MA
Gender-Based Violence in Emergencies Specialist, Humanitarian Response Division, United Nations Population Fund, Geneva, Switzerland

MARIA BEG, MPH
Student, Department of Population and Family Health, Mailman School of Public Health, Columbia University, New York, New York, USA

THERESA S. BETANCOURT, ScD, MA
Salem Professor in Global Practice, Director, Research Program on Children and Adversity, Boston College School of Social Work, Chestnut Hill, Massachusetts, USA

TANIA BOSQUI, DClinPsych, MSc
Associate Professor, Department of Psychology, American University of Beirut, Beirut, Lebanon; Adjunct Assistant Professor, Trinity Centre for Global Health, Trinity College Dublin, Dublin, Republic of Ireland

CHARLES BRANAS, PhD
Professor and Chair, Department of Epidemiology, Columbia University Mailman School of Public Health, New York, NY, USA

RUTH A. ETZEL, MD, PhD
Adjunct Professor, Department of Pediatrics, Georgetown University, Washington, DC, USA

JEFFREY GOLDHAGEN, MD, MPH
Professor of Pediatrics and Chief, Division of Community and Societal Pediatrics, University of Florida College of Medicine-Jacksonville, University of Florida, Jacksonville, Florida, USA; President, International Society for Social Pediatrics and Child Health, Geneva, Switzerland

MARSHA RAE GRIFFIN, MD
President, Community for Children, Inc., Washington, DC, USA

TAMEIR HOLDER, MPH
Doctor of Public Health Candidate, Department of Epidemiology, Mailman School of Public Health, Columbia University, New York, New York, USA

SARAH K.G. JENSEN, PhD
Assistant Professor, Department of Pediatrics, Women and Infants Hospital of Rhode Island, Providence, Rhode Island, USA

MILISSA JONES, MD, MPH, LTC, MC, USA, FAAP
Associate Professor, Department of Pediatrics, Pediatric Clinical Trials Unit, School of Medicine, Uniformed Services University of the Health Sciences, Bethesda, Maryland, USA

MARIIA KISELOVA, MD
Professor and Head of the Department, Faculty of Postgraduate Education (FPE) Department of Pediatrics and Neonatology, Danylo Halytsky Lviv National Medical University Lviv, Ukraine

J. BART KLIKA, MSW, PhD
Chief Research Officer, Prevent Child Abuse America, Chicago, Illinois, USA

EUGENE KONGNYUY, MD, PhD
Deputy Director, Humanitarian Response Division, United Nations Population Fund, Geneva, Switzerland

UGOMMA KORIE, MPH
Alumna, Department of Health Policy and Management, Mailman School of Public Health, Columbia University, New York, New York, USA

OLIVIA LANDES, MPH
Program Coordinator, Columbia Scientific Union for the Reduction of Gun Violence, Department of Epidemiology, Mailman School of Public Health, Columbia University, New York, New York, USA

DANIELLE LARAQUE-ARENA, MD, FAAP, FCOPP
Professor of Clinical Epidemiology and Pediatrics, Department of Epidemiology at the Mailman School of Public Health, and Department of Pediatrics at the Vagelos College of Physicians & Surgeons, Columbia University, New York; President Emerita, SUNY Upstate Medical University, Syracuse, New York, USA

SUNWOO LEE, MPH
Student, Department of Sociomedical Sciences, Mailman School of Public Health, Columbia University, New York, New York, USA

BRUCE LESLEY, MA
Professor and Chair Emeritus of Pediatrics, Professor of Biomedical Engineering, Virginia Commonwealth University Richmond, Virginia, USA

YVONNE (BONNIE) MALDONADO, MD
Taube Endowed Professor of Global Health and Infectious Diseases Vice Provost for Faculty Advancement, Stanford University Stanford, CA, USA

DANIEL MARTINEZ-GARCIA, MD, MPH
PhD Candidate, Faculty of Medicine, School of Global Health, Geneva Centre of Humanitarian Studies, University of Geneva, Project Leader - Paediatrician, Test, Avoid and Cure TB in Children (TACTIC) Project, Medical Department, Médecins Sans Frontières, Operational Center Geneva (OCG), Geneva, Switzerland

FERNANDO SANCHEZ MENDOZA, MD, MPH
Professor Emeritus, Division of Academic General Pediatrics, Department of Pediatrics, Stanford University School of Medicine, Palo Alto, California, USA

MELISSA T. MERRICK, PhD
President and CEO, Prevent Child Abuse America, Chicago, Illinois, USA

SHERNISE MOHAMMED-ALI, HBSc, MPH
Graduate Student, Columbia Scientific Union for the Reduction of Gun Violence, Department of Epidemiology, Mailman School of Public Health, Columbia University, New York, New York, USA

MARYAM ELISABETH MONTRICHARD, MD, MPH
Global Health Consultant, Fleming Island, Florida, USA

CHETAN SREE MUPPAVARAPU, MPH
Student, Department of Epidemiology, Mailman School of Public Health, Columbia University, New York, New York, USA

RACHEL NOVICK, MPH
Student, Department of Epidemiology, Mailman School of Public Health, Columbia University, New York, New York, USA

JORDAN O'BRIEN, MPH
Student, Department of Epidemiology, Mailman School of Public Health, Columbia University, New York, New York, USA

MARTIN OTTOLINI, MD, MEd, COL (Ret), USAF, MC, FAAP
Professor of Pediatrics, Director, Capstone Student Research Program, Office of the Dean, F. Edward Hebert School of Medicine, Uniformed Services University of the Health Sciences, Bethesda, Maryland, USA

BRUCE D. PERRY, MD, PhD
Professor (Adjunct), School of Allied Health, Human Services and Sport, La Trobe University, Melbourne, Victoria, Australia; Principal, Neurosequential Network, Houston, Texas, USA

ANNALICIA PICKERING, MD
Clinical Assistant Professor, Department of Pediatrics, Faculty Fellow, Center for Innovation in Global Health, Member, Maternal Child Health Research Institute, Stanford University School of Medicine, Palo Alto, California, USA

SONALI RAJAN, EdD, MS
Professor of Health Promotion and Education, Columbia Scientific Union for the Reduction of Gun Violence, Department of Health Studies and Applied Educational Psychology, Teachers College, Adjunct Professor of Epidemiology, Mailman School of Public Health, Columbia University, New York, New York, USA

OWEN ROBINSON, MPP
Executive Director, Co-Founder, International Cardiac Alliance, Burlington, Vermont, USA

VANESSA ROUZIER, MD
Assistant Professor of Pediatrics in Medicine, Center for Global Health, Weill Cornell Medicine, New York, New York, USA; Research Site Leader, Clinical Trials Unit, GHESKIO Centers, Port-au-Prince, Haiti

BRUCE K. RUBIN, MEngr, MD, MBA, FRCPC
Professor and Chair Emeritus, Department of Pediatrics, Virginia Commonwealth University, Richmond, Virginia, USA; Visiting Professor, Danylo Halytsky Lviv National Medical University, Kyiv, Ukraine; Professor of Biomedical Engineering

ERIC A. RUSSELL, MD
Associate Professor of Pediatrics, Division of Pediatric Emergency Medicine, Baylor College of Medicine, Houston, Texas, USA

JOSE IGNACIO SANTOS, MD, MS
Professor of Pediatrics, Experimental Research Unit, National Autonomous University of Mexico, Mexico City, Mexico

NABIHA SUBZWARI, MPH
Student, Department of Epidemiology, Mailman School of Public Health, Columbia University, New York, New York, USA

JONATHAN SURY, MPH, CPH
Senior Staff Associate III, National Center for Disaster Preparedness, Columbia Climate School, Columbia University, Doctoral Candidate, Heilbrunn Department of Population and Family Health, Mailman School of Public Health, Columbia University, New York, New York, USA

OLEKSANDR VOLOSOVETS, MD
Head, Department of Pediatrics 2, Bogomolets National Medical University, Kyiv, Ukraine

PAUL H. WISE, MD, MPH
Richard E. Berman Professor of Child Health and Society, Professor of Pediatrics, Professor of Health Policy, Senior Fellow, Freeman Spogli Institute for International Studies, Stanford University, Palo Alto, California, USA

JANINE YOUNG, MD
Professor of Pediatrics, Division of Academic General Pediatrics, University of California San Diego School of Medicine, San Diego, California, USA

Contents

PEDIATRIC CLINICS OF NORTH AMERICA

FORTHCOMING ISSUES

December 2026
Health of Youth in the Carceral System
Elizabeth Barnert, David Keller and Michael DeBaun, *Editors*

February 2027
Child Healthcare Financing: A Primer, Part I
Angelo P. Giardino, Alison Galbraith, Jeffrey B. Anderson, and Renee Turchi, *Editors*

April 2027
Advances in Pediatric Imaging
Jonathan R. Dillman, Brian Coley, and Andrew T. Trout, *Editors*

RECENT ISSUES

August 2026
Advances in Pediatric Dermatology
Kalyani Marathe, *Editor*

June 2026
Climate Change and Children
Maya Ragavan and Abby Nerlinger, *Editors*

April 2026
Perioperative Management and Optimization of the Pediatric Patient with Complex Medical Needs
Moises Auron and Mirna Giordano, *Editors*

Foreword

Humanitarian Crises: Hope in our Next-Generation Leadership

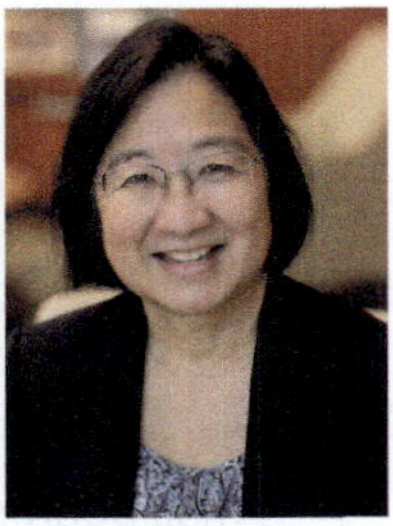

Tina L. Cheng, MD, MPH
Consulting Editor

When we commissioned this issue in late 2024, we did not predict the continued relevance of this topic today. A humanitarian crisis is often defined as an event or series of events that threatens the health, safety, security, or well-being of a large group of people over a wide area, often overwhelming local capacity. These crises may be due to natural disasters, such as earthquakes or floods; man-made emergencies, such as armed conflicts or plane crashes; or complex emergencies that may combine natural and man-made elements, such as food insecurity or displaced populations. No matter the cause, these crises are frequently preventable or capable of being mitigated. The consequences often fall disproportionately on children.

This issue is well timed, as the American Academy of Pediatrics recently published a policy statement on "The Effects of Armed Conflict on Children and Adolescents."[1] It notes that one in five children and adolescents resides in armed conflict zones, with millions displaced because of conflict. It emphasizes that pediatric professionals play critical roles in addressing the challenges faced by children in these settings and from these settings. The policy statement outlines strategic interventions, including access to physical and mental health care services, safeguarding education, safe spaces for children and families, and providing bereavement and psychosocial support. Specific recommendations are outlined related to state, federal, and global policies; strengthening systems; trauma-informed care; and promoting research.

Amid the humanitarian crises that exist today it is easy to lose hope. What gives me hope is our young people, the children we care for and their next-generation leadership. A friend recently made me aware of the results of a 2025 World Economic Forum survey of young global leaders.[2] When asked about the most important leadership skills for a world in transformation, what were their top responses? The most important leadership skills they mentioned were a moral compass and empathy. They also mentioned vision and storytelling, resilience and tolerance for failure,

Pediatr Clin N Am 73 (2026) xv–xvi
https://doi.org/10.1016/j.pcl.2026.05.012 pediatric.theclinics.com

foresight and future preparedness, and the ability to engage a wide and varied set of stakeholders. Those are wise ideas that we need to implement today. Over 80% of the young global leaders agreed that current leaders are not incentivized to emphasize long-term results over short-term gains. This issue of *Pediatric Clinics of North America* strengthens our ability to be resilient; to advocate, communicate, and message effectively; to widen our set of stakeholders; and to think long term. I look forward to a world focusing on what our young global leaders prioritize: a moral compass and empathy.

Tina L. Cheng, MD, MPH
Children's Hospital Medical Center
University of Cincinnati
Cincinnati Children's Research Foundation
3333 Burnet Avenue, MLC 3016
Cincinnati, OH 45229-3026, USA

E-mail address:
Tina.cheng@cchmc.org

REFERENCES

1. Shenoda S, Kadir A, Pitterman S, et al, Section on International Child Health. The effects of armed conflict on children. Pediatrics 2018;142(6):e20182585. https://doi.org/10.1542/peds.2018-2585.
2. World Economic Forum and the Forum of Young Global Leaders. Next generation leadership for a world in transformation: driving dialogue and action. 2026. Available at: https://reports.weforum.org/docs/GFC_White_Paper_on_New_Leadership_Models_for_Future_Generations_2026.pdf. Accessed May 17, 2026.

Preface

Imperatives for Action and Impact of Humanitarian Crises Affecting Children

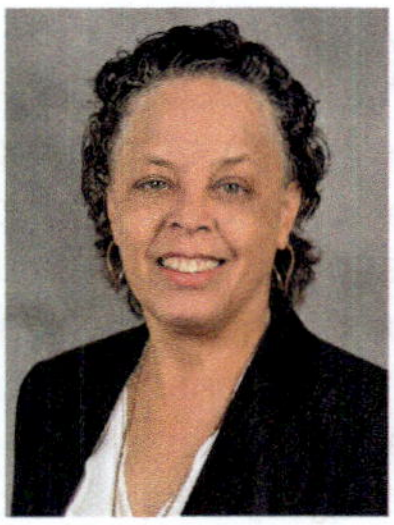

Danielle Laraque-Arena, MD, FAAP, FCOPP
Editor

Humanitarian crises affecting children exist worldwide and in the twenty-first century are ever present and present existential threats to our humanity. Humanitarian crises transcend national borders and require multilateral responses. Understanding the inherently political nature of global health problems and that health itself has been politicized is essential in framing the nature of crises and how we respond to crises. Awareness that politization affects the setting of priorities, funding, and the supply of core resources provides needed context. Recognition that violence is represented not only by physical harm but also by sexual and psychological harm and underlying oppressive and protracted injustices is critical to the framing of challenges met in responding to crises. Whether such crises are due to "natural disasters," "human-induced" emergencies, or chronic and complex humanitarian emergencies, recognition and robust responses must lead to sustainable, lasting solutions. Undergirding these ideas are the rules and principles of international humanitarian law (IHL). While the world has not evolved to resolve conflicts peacefully, IHL establishes that even wars have limits and should provide protection to people affected by armed conflicts. Bolstered by numerous conventions, charters, treaties, and regulations, the world community continues to provide guardrails and ethical pathways to protect the most vulnerable. A challenge noted by the International Committee of the Red Cross is the interplay of IHL and human rights.[1] Maintaining the highest standards and thresholds to protect children is the focus of this compendium. Guidance from the 17 Sustainable Development Goals established by the United Nations in 2015 with objectives that address poverty and protection of the planet set a target date of 2030, from which we can measure progress.[2]

A core tenet in our discourse is that understanding humanitarian crises lies in the framework of the Convention on the Rights of the Child.[3] Given that armed conflicts

Pediatr Clin N Am 73 (2026) xvii–xxi
https://doi.org/10.1016/j.pcl.2026.05.008
0031-3955/26/© 2026 Published by Elsevier Inc.

have represented the majority of crises affecting children in the twentieth and twenty-first centuries, we discuss various precepts, such as the doctrine of proportionality.[4] Over the past 50 years, the number of civilian casualties has steadily increased. Currently, not only are civilians the majority of victims, but also children are overwhelming represented in the number of deaths with the unapologetic use of psychological trauma and famine as weapons of war. Furthermore, the killing, injuring, maiming, abduction, rape, abuse, or neglect of children is never justified, nor is the withholding of humanitarian assistance to any side or explicit targeting of civilians.

We recognize that this compendium, the first of its kind for the *Pediatric Clinics of North America*, cannot be all encompassing in its analysis. What we aim to do is to center our discussions on three building blocks: child rights; responding to gender-based violence; and support for the preservation of the health of communities and the cultures that envelop children even in the face of chaos. Child health professionals (CHPs) in medicine, nursing, psychology, public health, social work, and related fields have a vital role to play in raising awareness of the scope of crises affecting children. CHPs should understand the need not only for immediate responses to acute events (eg, physical and mental health support) but also that the responses (eg, coordination, multilateral financial support) must be sustained over multiple years of recovery to be effective in reducing the long-term impact of such crises on overall health. Understanding that *without sustained, child-centered investments* as noted in the article reporting on the Sudanese humanitarian crisis, long-term harm to maternal and child health across the life course will be the outcome. There must be support for the rebuilding of necessary vital health infrastructures in partnership with local governments. We urge dialogue, effective communication, and respect for culture and for each other in calling out injustices as we tackle the myriad of health and public health issues that exist at baseline and are exacerbated in moments of crisis. Knowledge and adherence to humanitarian principles must guide our fierce advocacy in full partnership with the voices of children and families worldwide. We signal the need for representation and voices of our public health trainees. In the article "*Humanitarian Crises: Trainee Perspectives*," by Subzwari and colleagues, article 16 of this compendium, students echo the need for a *courageous curriculum* that equips higher education students with the analytical skills to drive transformative work and to effect sustained efforts in response to humanitarian crises, and thereby advance health equity, eliminating health disparities. Necessary is humility to establish both the causes and the solutions to worldwide challenges.

In preparing this compendium, we held two videoconferences with the authors. The goal of these virtual meetings was to thank all the authors, many of whom are still living and working in precarious situations around the world. Another goal was to share perspectives to bring about a cohesive and comprehensive view of what is possible in response to the ever-growing number of crises faced worldwide. On July 16, 2025, the first of these conferences reaffirmed the commitment to continue the discourse that will drive action from the global community. Vanessa Rouzier, Haitian American pediatrician and infectious disease physician who for years has been immersed in the response to the chronic and complex humanitarian crises in Haiti, expressed it well. She said, "small steps" make a difference," "staying alive," and "every life matters." She stresses a call-to-action that is built on hope. In addition, the tracing of the historical and current context of the complex humanitarian crisis in Haiti points to lessons learned regarding the negative impact of embargoes, sanctions, and lack of long-term investments on health care infrastructure with resulting increases in child mortality and worsening of child well-being. The risk of violence, as in other countries, has posed immense challenges to the health care system and the survival of children.

The compendium begins with the discussion of the epidemiology of humanitarian crises, an understudied area. We do this deliberately to detail the tools that support timely and accurate reporting of the scale of crises that lead to effective responses during acute and chronic phases of humanitarian and public health crises. The prioritization of the welfare of children, the most vulnerable among us, must center our quest for the eventual elimination of these crises. Acute and sustained responses to address the multitudes of health impacts to children, women and girls, their families and communities, we contend, are the only ways to forge hopeful futures for children worldwide. The scientific and technological advances of the twenty-first century provide both useful and dangerous tools (eg, AI [artificial intelligence], drones). How we use these tools in support of humanity requires intergovernmental collaborations, within country action, leadership by the health community, and a global human rights framework.

In 2025 to 2026, we face unprecedented challenges to global stability. While prevention of the escalation of conflicts to the point of crisis is one of the lessons we must garner, equally important is our immediate response to current crises. Where possible, we underscore the historical origins of conflicts and the impact of colonialism and systems of oppression on the lives of children. We emphasize how sexual violence, starvation, and the propagation of infectious diseases are used to effect maximum harm and terror. Given that several of the authors are in the United States, the compendium addresses humanitarian crises within the borders of the United States as well as global crises affecting children. An eye on equity and application of sound public health measures are emphasized.[5,6]

The compendium of articles in this *Pediatrics Clinics of North America* is entitled the "Imperatives for Action and Impact of Humanitarian Crises Affecting Children." Beginning with a framing of child rights and the necessary global response from humanitarian voices, the discourse is anchored on the concepts of global organizational capacity, clinical capabilities, and advocacy. The compendium is organized into three sections: *Global Organizational Response Capability in Humanitarian Crises: What the Pediatric Health Professional Should Know; Impact of Humanitarian Crises on Child Health; and The Urgency of Action: Case Studies in the Twenty-First Century.* This issue not only hopes to bring renewed awareness of the human scale of crises globally affecting children but also puts forth a call-to-action by pediatric clinicians and the world community to reduce the unimaginable scale of harm to children. We must heed the reality that some humanitarian disasters have been generally ignored and reverse this course.[7] Preparedness and transnational collaboration involving both nonmilitary and military responses are crucial. Careful consideration of the legal, ethical, and operational implications inherent in using armed forces in civilian contexts is needed when responding to both natural and human-induced humanitarian disasters. As reflected in the article by Jones and Ottolini, military humanitarian operations involve a complex balance of what capabilities are brought to bear and severe limitations in gaining local trust and legitimacy. The Geneva Convention and Principles of Humanitarian Aid apply, but inherent tensions are discussed when attempting to mitigate suffering while engaged in armed conflicts.

While it is not the focus of the compendium, available technologies of the twenty-first century can assist us to better respond and prevent humanitarian crises. The modalities include not only building awareness and competence during interpandemic and crisis periods but also collaborative efforts among domain experts and visualization experts that support epidemiologic modeling to disseminate timely vital information and predictive modeling to avert new challenges. These challenges will certainly include climate-associated disasters and complex emergencies. Technological advances must be matched by a worldwide commitment to apply lessons learned to forge paths that heal deep-seated conflicts.[8–10]

On a personal note, as I put together the series of articles based on epidemiologic perspectives and recruited authors on the topic of humanitarian crises affecting children, my thoughts went back to my own childhood experience of leaving my native land of Haiti in 1962 and fleeing dictatorship. I reflect now on the opportunities and challenges my family faced in a new country. Uncertainty, threat of violence, interruption of education, economic difficulties, food insecurity, and potential loss of culture and real loss of family and friends were just part of that journey. In humanitarian crises, all these difficulties are compounded by immense threats to life, the brutality of war, sexual violence, internal and external migration across unfamiliar lands, interruption of the normal developmental and educational processes necessary for children to thrive, and the impact of long-lasting psychological trauma. Drawing from the vast experience of the article authors, the compendium shares some insights on how humanitarian crises affect children, and the role of humanitarian actors in mitigating negative effects of these crises, while we collectively strive for a more peaceful world. CHPs and their many allies have a vital role to play. We can and must face the challenges ahead. Working for peace and justice is not a useless endeavor. It offers the only hope for our world.

DISCLOSURES

The author has no conflicts of interest to disclose.

Danielle Laraque-Arena, MD, FAAP, FCOPP
Department of Epidemiology and Pediatrics
Mailman School of Public Health and
Vagelos College of Physicians & Surgeons
Columbia University
New York, NY, USA

E-mail address:
dl3365@cumc.columbia.edu

REFERENCES

1. Melzer N, Kuster E. International humanitarian law: a comprehensive introduction. Cambridge University Press: International Committee of the Red Cross (ICRC); 2016. p. 10.
2. United Nations Department of Economic and Social Affairs Sustainable Development. Available at: www.sdgs.un.org/goals. Accessed February 11, 2026.
3. Convention on the Rights of the Child. Human Rights Program, Department of Canadian Heritage. Minister of Supply and Services, Canada 1991. Available at: https://www.ohchr.org/sites/default/files/Documents/ProfessionalInterest/crc.pdf. Accessed May 19, 2026.
4. Sullivan ET. The doctrine of proportionality in a time of war. Minn J International Law 2007;135. Available at: https://scholarship.law.umn.edu/mjil/135. Accessed May 19, 2026.
5. Schneider L. Twenty years after Hurricane Katrina, what are its legacy and lessons. JAMA 2025;334(12):1049–50.
6. Gee RE. From Katrina to COVID-19: hard-learned lessons and resilience. AJPH 2020;110(10):1502–3.

7. Goldhagen J, Elkrail SE, Affan A. Responding to the humanitarian crisis in Sudan. BMJ Paediatr Open 2024;l8(1):1–2.
8. Smith J, Roberts B, Knight A, et al. A systematic literature review of the quality of evidence for injury and rehabilitation interventions in humanitarian crises. Int J Public Health 2015;60:865–72. https://doi.org/10.1007/s00038-015-0723-6.
9. Smith J, El-Solh S, Hanball L, et al. Realising health justice in Palestine: beyond humanitarian voices. Confl Health 2025;19:7. https://doi.org/10.1186/s13031-024-00634-0.
10. Young H. Public nutrition in emergencies: an overview of debates, dilemmas and decision-making. Disasters 1999;23(4):277–91.

Professional Reflection

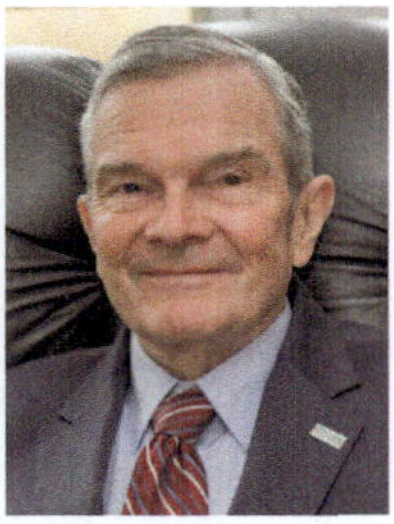

Errol R. Alden, MD, FAAP

Parents, teachers, caretakers, and communities once again face perilous times affecting our children's futures. Over one-fourth of the world's children are displaced by either human-made conflicts and/or natural disasters. Parents are being overwhelmed by anti-vaccine and other health misinformation. The burden for pediatric professionals and parents is enormous.

This compendium, with its impressive list of authors, lays out the history as well as today's challenges facing our children and those responsible for caring for them. It closes with case studies illustrating possible solutions addressing and alleviating many of these issues.

At this time of unparalleled crises facing the world's children, this compendium is a must-read for all those responsible for our children and for those who wish to advocate and contribute to improving their lives and future.

Errol R. Alden, MD, FAAP
Col M.C. Ret
Past President
International Pediatric Association

E-mail address:
ealden41@aol.com

Pediatr Clin N Am 73 (2026) xxiii
https://doi.org/10.1016/j.pcl.2026.05.013
0031-3955/26/© 2026 Published by Elsevier Inc.
pediatric.theclinics.com

Global Organizational Response Capability in Humanitarian Crises: What the Pediatric Health Professional Should Know

Global Epidemiology of Humanitarian Crises Affecting Children

Danielle Laraque-Arena, MD

KEYWORDS

• Epidemiology • Crisis affected • Humanitarian crisis • Crude mortality rate • Famine • Gender-based violence

KEY POINTS

- Epidemiology teaches us that timely, quality data acquisition and dissemination is needed to respond to global humanitarian obligations. Our children around the world are disproportionately affected by humanitarian crises. They cannot wait for international law and actors to catch up to evident realities. Child health/pediatric clinicians, educators, and researchers and their allies must play a pivotal role in mitigating harm to children affected by humanitarian crises (HC).
- The epidemiology of HC must address priority areas such as water and sanitation, nutrition and food security, maternal and child health, mental health as well as knowledge gaps in areas such as neonatal health, child protection, noncommunicable diseases, sexual and reproductive health, ethics and health systems preparation, and sustainability.
- Timely and robust epidemiologic research is essential to support effective interventions addressing the impact of HC. New technologies and the application of epidemiologic modeling can provide tools to appraise the impact of HC and useful predictions to avert predicted adverse health outcomes.
- The precepts of child rights must be applied to understand the context of HC, provide insights into public health interventions, and focus on the collective trauma of such crises in addition to and in contrast to the impact of individual trauma.
- Understanding resilience can inform our approach to health promotion in the context of HC. Supportive supervision is essential to the work of public child health professionals, enabling evidence-based actionable steps and allowing contextualization and adaptation to circumstances.
- Epidemiologic research should pose questions specific to the context of HC when questions cannot be answered in nonemergency settings. Preparedness and management of HC should be guided by such research.

Mailman School of Public Health, Department of Epidemiology and Vagelos College of Physicians & Surgeons, Department of Pediatrics, Columbia University, 722 West 168th Street, New York, NY 10032, USA
E-mail address: dl3365@cumc.columbia.edu

Pediatr Clin N Am 73 (2026) 891–915
https://doi.org/10.1016/j.pcl.2026.04.003 pediatric.theclinics.com

Abbreviations	
CDC	Centers for Disease Control and Prevention
CHE	complex humanitarian emergencies; CHWD, Child Health and Wellbeing Dashboards
CMR	crude mortality rate
COI	conflicts of interest
CRC	Convention on the Rights of the Child
DP	Doctrine of Proportionality
FEWS NET	Famine Early Warning Systems Network
FRC	Famine Review Committee
GAVI	Global Alliance for Vaccines and Immunizations
GBV	gender-based violence
HC	humanitarian crises
IASC	Inter-Agency Standing Committee
ICVAC	International Classification of Violence Against Children
IDP	internally displaced person
IPC	Integrated Food Security Phase Classification
IRC	International Rescue Committee
LMIC	low and middle-income countries
MUAC	mid-upper arm circumference
SD	standard deviation
SRH	sexual and reproductive health
UNHCR	The United Nations High Commissioner for Refugees
UNICEF	UN International Children's Emergency Fund
USAID	United States Agency for International Development
WASH	water, sanitation and hygiene
WFH	weight-for-height
WFP	World Food Programme
WHO	World Health Organization

OVERVIEW

A review of the epidemiology of humanitarian crises (HC) entails an assessment of the extent of the humanitarian assistance needed globally.[1–3] The latest Lancet Commission report estimates that in 2026, 239 million people require humanitarian assistance.[4] The International Rescue Committee (IRC)[5,6] has stated that the current extent of the HC is evidence of "systematic failure" in 4 dimensions: a failure of states, diplomacy, laws, and humanitarian operations. The IRC concludes that states do not protect their citizens, nor do they uphold international law. The IRC further identifies hunger as a weapon of war and intentional targeting of civilians as a tool of control, resulting in death and/or disability of the affected populations.

Crisis affected populations include the resident population, internally displaced persons (IDPs), refugees, and returnees.[7,8] Refugees can be grouped by countries of asylum, country of origin, asylum seekers, IDPs, and other people in need of international protection. The IRC Watchlist lists 20 countries—10% of the global population, that account for 89% of those in need: 80% are individuals who have fled across borders and 76% are internally displaced.[9–11] The United Nations High Commissioner for Refugees[8] (UNHCR) reports that 123.2 million persons were forcibly displaced (2024). The UN International Children's Emergency Fund (UNICEF) Displacement information reports that at the end of 2024, 48.8 million children were displaced by conflict or violence and 4.4 million were displaced due to disasters.[12,13] Between 2010 and 2024, the global number of displaced children had tripled from its base number of 17 million. According to UNHCR, more than 2.3 million children were born as refugees from 2018 to 2024 alone, the equivalent of 337,800 children per year. The most notably

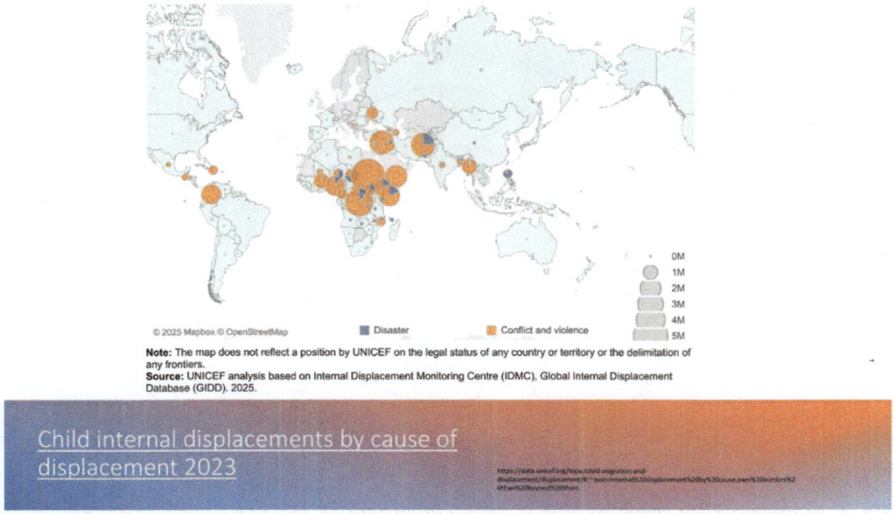

Fig. 1. Child Internal Displacement 2023. Map lines delineate study areas and do not necessarily depict accepted national boundaries. (Source Displacement, June 2025. UNICEF. Available in: https://data.unicef.org/topic/child-migration-and-displacement/displacement.)

besieged places around the world are Sudan, Myanmar, the Gaza Strip, the Democratic Republic of the Congo, and Afghanistan. Nonetheless, many more countries are affected (**Fig. 1**).

Definitions and Metrics

The World Health Organization (WHO) in collaboration with the Inter-Agency Standing Committee (IASC) has defined HC as "Any circumstance where humanitarian needs are sufficiently large and complex to require significant external assistance and resources, and where a multi-sectoral response is needed, with the engagement of a wide range of international actors."[14] HC fall into 3 distinct categories, natural disasters, human-induced disasters, and complex humanitarian emergencies (CHEs) (**Box 1**). Various frameworks for understanding the impact of such crises have been put forth.[7,15–17] Two examples are noted in **Figs. 2** and **3** displaying the epidemiologic profile of incidence and mortality of CHE and the impact for crisis-affected populations.[7,17] Application of sound infectious disease epidemiology has identified 3 pathogens (*Streptococcus pneumoniae*, *Haemophilus influenzae* alone as causing >50% of all pneumonia deaths, and rotavirus as the primary cause of severe childhood diarrheal disease). These 3 pathogens are implicated globally and in CHE-related mortality and provide inferential evidence of how

Box 1
Types of humanitarian crises

- Natural disasters (eg. earthquakes, tsunamis, tornadoes, hurricanes, etc.)
- Human-induced emergencies (eg radiation, war, internal conflicts, small arms)
- Chronic and complex emergencies (political and social context, public health infrastructure challenges, acute on chronic exacerbation of infectious disease epidemics)

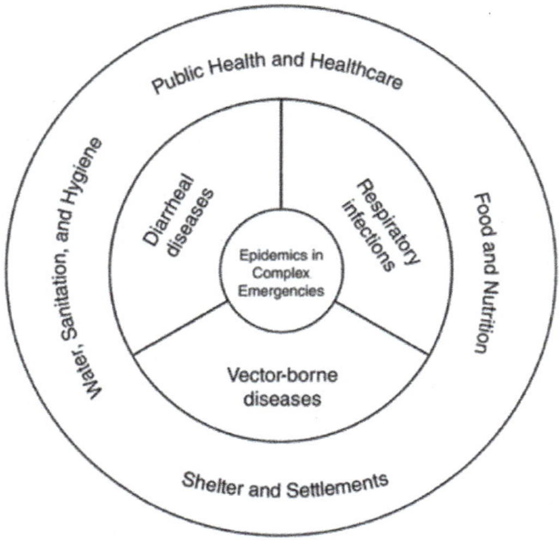

Fig. 2. Framework for complex humanitarian emergencies. (*Source* Gonzalez PA, Fernandez JC, Gan RK, Camporro AF, Martinez JAC. The epidemiologic profile of incidence and mortality from epidemics in complex humanitarian emergencies from 1990 to 2022 – A scoping review. Trop Med Int Health. 2024;29:343–353. DOI: 10.111/tmi.13982.[17])

to prevent illness in CHE. Global Alliance for Vaccines and Immunizations (GAVI) and other organizations have been called upon to apply the case of universal vaccination in CHE.[18,19] Cited frameworks have centered the most important contributors of morbidity and mortality as the deterioration of public health infrastructures

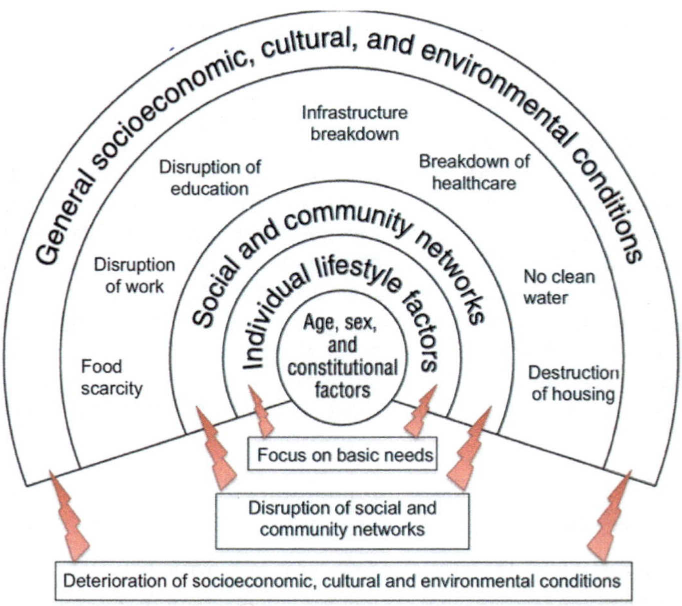

Fig. 3. Framework for crisis-affected population. (*Source* Zenner D. Crisis-Affected Populations and Tuberculosis. 2017. Microbiol Spectrum 5(1):TNM17–0031-2016. Doi: 10.1128/microbiolspec. TNM17–0031-2016.[7])

and the emergence and re-emergence of infectious diarrheal and respiratory diseases.

Crisis-affected populations may be categorized in the literature as follows.[7,8] Notably, refugees are those that have crossed international borders due to fear of persecution and determination that returning to their home of origin is unsafe.

- Refugees by country of asylum
- Refugees by country of origin
- Asylum seekers
- Internally displaced persons
- UN Refugee Relief and Works for Palestinian Refugees (UNRWA) Palestine refugees noted given the special status of the Palestine in the UN as a nonmember observer status.
- Other people in need of international protection usually represented by individuals who have been forcibly displaced
- International migrants: persons living in a country or areas other than their country of birth
- Stateless individuals
- Refugees returning home

These various categorizations are noted to reflect the complexity of migrations—either voluntary or forced. Understanding the flow of individuals, their journeys, their "legal" status, and their ability or inability to access needed services as guided by international law and the maintenance of their human rights is essential to understanding the actions needed to protect children and their families.

Among natural disasters, a pandemic is defined as a circumstance where an infectious disease is widespread throughout a whole country or worldwide. A public health crisis, a term also used in the context of discussions of HC, is a significant event that threatens health and well-being, often requiring urgent governmental or societal response.[20] In addition to its basic definition, HCs are categorized according to levels of severity (1, 2, 3) depending on the level of public health response required.[14] Levels 2 and 3 have moderate and severe effects on public health and require regional or global WHO responses. Types of disasters include, for example, hurricanes, earthquakes, and tsunamis, while human-induced disasters consist of emergencies such as radiation exposure, wars, and conflicts. Chronic and complex emergencies usually have an overlay of multiple crises in the context of economic, social, and political upheavals with erosion of critical infrastructures necessary to respond to basic human needs such as safe shelter, food, clean water, and suitable clothing.

What is Epidemiology?

It is reasonable to begin our discourse of the epidemiology of global HC affecting children with basic and evolving definitions of epidemiology that help frame the epidemiologic process.[21–23] Epidemiology as a discipline evolved about a century ago in response to the need to understand the emergence and control of diseases and health events. The definition provided in Lilienfeld's seminal article has been used as a starting point to analyze the evolution and broadening of the concepts contained in the field of epidemiology.[22] This grounding definition is "Epidemiology is a method of reasoning about disease that deals with biological inference derived from observations of disease phenomena in population groups." Subsequent definitions discussed in a review of gray literature and published literature from 1978 to 2017 identified 102 definitions.[21] These definitions highlighted 20 terms and concepts related to epidemiology that are useful in understanding the power of epidemiology in both identifying and responding to public health crises. The most common terms include the words: population, study, disease, health, distribution, and control. These terms have been retained over time.

Definitions of epidemiology have been cited as important to identify the task inherent in epidemiologically driven responses. A revised definition published by Evans is perhaps most useful. That is, "Epidemiology is the quantitative analysis of the circumstances under which disease processes, including trauma, occur in population groups, the factors affecting their incidence, distribution, and the host responses, and the use of this knowledge in prevention and control."[23] Since the work of Lillenfield and Evans there has been an explosion of specific disciplines of epidemiology including, for example, pharmacoepidemiology, molecular epidemiology, and genetic epidemiology. Most recently, spatial epidemiology has been developed to analyze geographic distribution of health outcomes and is a required public health course in some schools of public health. Spatial representation and estimation by population density serve to highlight the most affected countries and the causes of death.[8] This field integrates epidemiology, geography, and statistics to better examine the components of the definition as noted by Evans. Notably it assesses disease incidence, mortality, environmental, demographic, behavioral, socioeconomic, and genetic factors. It has been useful in the discourse of health disparities and in better understanding access to health care services. Key tools include disease mapping, examining the relationship between environmental, social factors, and health outcomes, detection of clusters of diseases, outbreaks, and in the assessment of risk. Current trainees and researchers and the public in general are very familiar with geographic information used for spatial modeling and integration of data. Another term that reflects the evolution of our thinking is the understanding that epidemiology is a science and facilitates the understanding of disease transmission, control, and treatment. In the field of human medicine surveillance is particularly relevant to the identification of new pathogens (eg, HIV, SARS-Co-2). Syndromic surveillance is particularly useful to the recognition and treatment of new diseases, especially of infectious etiology.

Other Considerations

The field of epidemiology is related to many other fields useful in the discussion of HC. These fields include ethics, philosophy, and epistemology, integrating complex societal factors when analyzing and responding to HC. Other developments have been the integration of the concepts of epidemiology in subspecialties such as cancer epidemiology, cardiovascular epidemiology, obesity epidemiology, nutritional epidemiology, psychiatric epidemiology, reproductive epidemiology, and many others that are distinct in focus. With increased awareness of the impact of social policy on health other definitions have emerged. Nancy Krieger in her book *Epidemiology and the people's health: theory and context* expands the definition of epidemiology to encompass not only the distribution but also the social determinants of health.[24] She evokes an ecological perspective that is a wholistic approach to the various proximal and distal policies and structures that impact health. This approach is particularly relevant when discussing the global epidemiology of HC in countries with very different social and economic systems.

Despite these advances, there does not appear to be a distinct humanitarian epidemiology discipline. Nor is there formal training in field epidemiology.[25] Addressing the evidence gap in humanitarian health can be framed by addressing the types of research and posing relevant research questions, as detailed by Kohrt and colleagues[15] *Methodological* research can ask the key questions regarding protection of the rights of research participants, ethical guidelines, use of research methods adapted to humanitarian circumstances, and the identification of the needs of the populations affected by the crisis. *Descriptive epidemiology* can examine causes, stressors, particular burdens for neonatal mortality, and public health information that can better leverage the determination of mortality and morbidity. *Discovery* can identify new technologies (eg, use of mobile text messages), treatments (eg, vaccines), and strategies (eg, credible messengers, families, community health workers) that support valid evidence and evaluations of interventions. The scope of interventions can include intervention research, implementation research and health system research—critical to delivering the full definition of epidemiology—to better assess the most effective mental and psychosocial interventions addressing conflict-affected children.[26] Attention to cultural adaptations can be addressed in implementation research; and health system research can assess the best balance between emergency service delivery and long-term systems strengthening to address the collective trauma of HC.[15]

An evidence review of the research on health interventions in HC clarifies how the epidemiology of HC, their impact, and responses might be organized (**Fig. 4**).[27] This article identified specific areas to frame the understanding of the scope of the problems precipitated by HC, both direct and indirect. Additionally, as suggested by the definitions noted above, this quantitative analysis of the circumstances under which disease processes and trauma occur in populations is linked to the analysis of factors that may impact on incidence, distribution, and host response to the crisis. Comparisons are critical in understanding the impact of the crisis, so baseline, pre-event, event, and post-event incidences are essential to the assessment and determination that a crisis indeed is occurring. The categories in the assessment of HC themes include

- The measured impact of the disruption of water, sanitation and hygiene (WASH)
- Incidence of communicable diseases and their control; evoking the role of immunizations and vaccines in disease control with baseline measures being critical to the assessment of the impact of the crisis
- Nutrition with baseline population data on access to food, incidence of malnutrition pre-event, and subsequent rates of malnutrition and famine
- Occurrence of sexual and reproductive health (SRH), including gender-based violence (GBV) during the acute crisis

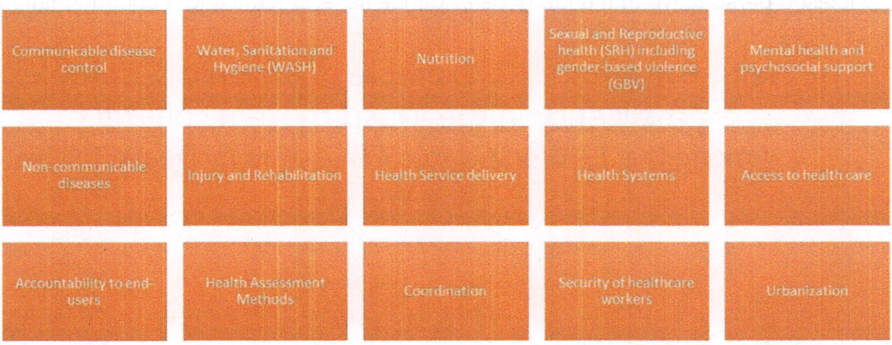

Fig. 4. Compendium themes of humanitarian interventions. (Blanchet K, Sistenich V, Ramesh A, Frison S, Warren E, Smith J, Hossain M, Knight A, Lewis C, Post N, Woodward A, Ruby A, Dahab M, Pantuliano S, Roberts B. London School of Hygiene and Tropical Medicine, Harvard School of Public Health and the Overseas Development Institute (ODI). An Evidence review of research on health interventions in humanitarian crises. Executive Summary. https://www.elrha.org/docs/document/elrha-hher2-executivesummary.pdf.)

- Mental health and psychosocial impact of crises and support systems available pre- and post-event
- The impact on the identification and management of noncommunicable diseases due to the breakdown of health systems, access to health care, health care delivery, health assessments, health care coordination, and the security of health care workers in war and conflict zones.
- Injury incidence pre-event, event, and post-event with implications for rehabilitation. Studies have reported traumatic injuries, crush injuries to extremities, axial injuries, other musculoskeletal injuries, open head injuries, compartment syndromes, and nonmusculoskeletal injuries. Additionally, burns, spinal injuries, and children requiring amputations, surgical outcomes, and long-term disabilities are among the injury statistics needed in assessing the impact of HC.
- The differential impact of urbanization on diseases and control/response methods.

Response Considerations

As noted, the evidence review of known interventions addressing HC is depicted in 15 thematic areas (see **Fig. 4**).[27] The response to HC is a critical aspect of the definition of epidemiology given the aim of restoring public health. Determination of mortality, morbidity, and an approach to vulnerable populations such as children is germane. Rapid response is necessary with field assessments and surveys. Ongoing monitoring of evidence-based surveillance is essential to not ignore vulnerable populations (eg, women and girls, ethnic minorities).

History informs us that wars have increasingly involved greater segments of the civilian population, affecting children and women disproportionately.[28] In World War I 5% of the casualties were reported to be civilian; in World War II 50% were civilians; in the Vietnam War 80% of casualties were civilian. Current conflicts that are representative of the disproportionate impact borne by civilians are: the internal civil war in Sudan, the decades long Palestine-Israeli crisis, reignited following the attack of October 7, 2023, and exacerbated by the devastation in the Gaza Strip, and the complex, multilayered emergencies in Haiti (**Fig. 5**).

Given the inherent sociopolitical context of responses, as noted by Holmsten (2023) it is wise to identify "Who is doing What and Where."[29] The credibility, scientific rigor, nonbiased perspective that undergirds evidence assessments and recommendations

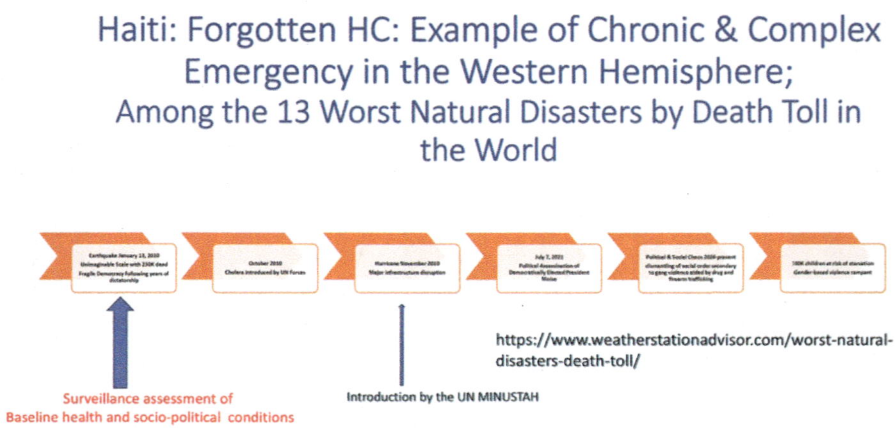

Fig. 5. Complex humanitarian crisis timeline, Haiti 2025.[95]

is contingent on the Who is involved. Not only collaborative but true partnerships allow situation analysis, needs assessments, development of cogent proposals, quality activity data acquisition, delineation of the surveillance data, and the generation of internal reports shared to communicate effectively and honestly with the public and policy makers. Addressing both misinformation and disinformation is contingent upon evidence-based judgments. Who is determinant of these parameters and how information is presented. Humanitarian actors must not only be collaborative but respectful of culture, cognizant of the power dynamics and how this influences public and policy discourses and actions on behalf of children and families. The what refers to what is discussed and what is ignored. And the Where is related to focus—and calling out of the often-forgotten places.

Adherence to the precepts of community-based participatory research and the idea of "participatory epidemiology"[30] is accentuated in the work of Colombo and colleagues in a series of publications.[31–34] The investigators review knowledge gaps and how to make sense of the data that are available when meeting the challenging circumstances of HC and the variability of data across crises. The role of clinicians and key informants in providing key insights to contextualize quantitative data is underscored. Specific methods are highlighted such as SMART (Specific, Measurable, Achievable/Acceptable/Ambitious, Realistic/Relevant, Time-bound) methodology for nutrition and mortality assessments,[35] local/regional District Health Information for routine data management, maternal death, and perinatal surveillance and response as well as emergency disease surveillance systems. The lack of financial and human resources is signaled as a limitation to the use of complex data systems, functionality, coverage, and completeness. Team-based approaches that integrate clinicians in the assessment of the quality of data signals the need of triangulation of data that are plausible, data that are reliable, and the use of other sources and methods. This triangulation is essential in meeting the data challenges posed by HC. The need for so-called barefoot epidemiologists, who can collaborate with anthropologists, demographers, and sociologists, is featured to better understand place-specific priorities. The need for trained humanitarian epidemiologists is argued to be necessary as core to the teaching of public health.[25,32] That training should emphasize not only context, but knowledge and preferences by wealth and gender in understanding the history of exclusion of the needs of the most vulnerable populations especially in low and middle-income countries (LMICs).[30] Intentional focus on rural, often neglected population areas, inclusion of the ignored "minorities" but also inclusion of large majorities (notably women and girls) must be part of the re-conceptualization of epidemiology.

A framework that establishes minimum standards for response has been developed and revised over time. The Sphere Humanitarian Charter and Minimum Standards outline: Minimum Standards in Water Supply and Sanitation, Nutrition, Food Aid, Shelter and Site Planning, and Minimum Standards in Health Services.[36] New threats posed by modern-day crises that include malnutrition, famine, and re-emergence of previously controlled infectious diseases—negating the advances of the past 50 years—have invoked the utility of predictive modeling. Predictive modeling can document the threat of resurgence of, for example, infectious diseases such as measles and polio, due to waning immunization, vaccine hesitancy, and refusal and the influence of complex political/social circumstances.[37–39] The data can allow us to better prepare for the impact of climate change in ways not envisioned in the past.[40,41] The predictions must compel us to act in preventive mode to change the adverse consequences of increasingly complex crises. Understanding data input to estimate impact of HC can begin to convey to the public the importance of quality data and the complexity of acquiring these data.

Data-informed Immediate Response to Humanitarian Crises Affecting Children

Rapid assessment aims to achieve multiple measurable objectives[42]:

- Determination of the magnitude of the emergency
- Identification of existing and potential public health problems. In considering the impact of HC on children early, the role of the child health professional is particularly crucial. Baseline immunization rates with levels that have achieved herd immunity for the population is such an example. The organizational capacity of established health systems to attend to infants, children, adolescents, and young adults will mitigate harm. As experienced with COVID-19, networks of health care delivery were crucial in expediting the administration of immunizations according to the evidence-based recommended schedules as well as the newly developed COVID-19 vaccine. This required not only the involvement of pediatric offices, but also urgent centers and other local response settings such as ambulance corps with existing trained professionals. Necessary assessments are of pre-response to endemic diseases, baseline mortality rates, morbidity incidence rates, nutritional status, sources of health care, and anticipation of the impact of disruption of health services. The principles of emergency management must be applied.[43]
- Availability of nutritional assessment for all infants and children with attention to children with special care needs is indispensable. Pediatric health professionals are well placed to integrate their ongoing relationships with families to the assessment of acute needs.
- Determination of need for external response.
- Consideration of the health system requirements in the face of the crisis.

Measurement Consideration

Five epidemiologic areas are most commonly used, relevant, and useful to assess HC.[44] These include:

1. Mortality (first, crude mortality rates (CMRs), then disaggregated by age and gender).
2. Incidence of the most important diseases or conditions (morbidity).
3. Nutritional status, also disaggregated by age with specific considerations for those less than 5 years.
4. Activities data, such as immunizations performed, and
5. Functioning of the vital sectors for food, water, sanitation, shelter (cooking) fuel, and electricity.

Mortality

With respect to mortality rates, baseline comparisons are critical to assessing the impact of a crisis. In a humanitarian emergency and crisis, the CMR is greater than the baseline, pre-event CMR. In general, the Centers for Disease Control and Prevention (CDC) define a humanitarian threshold as 1 death per 10,000 per day. Public health crises are noted at CMR greater than 1 per 10,000 per day for all ages; greater than 2 per 10,000 per day greater than 5 years or a CMR above what would be expected based on the baseline population. Different definitions are applicable in higher income settings.[44]

Data Dashboard of Key Indicators

Capturing morbidity and related metrics of child well-being can be complicated. The UNICEF data and analytics provide a snapshot of child well-being indicators.[2,45] The framework for selection of these indicators is set by UN Convention on the Rights of the Child (CRC), the international legal framework adopted in 1989.[46]

Based on the CRC framework, 4 domain areas are selected to include *survival, protection, development, and participation* plus the cross-cutting domain of contextual and policy factors.[45] The standard age categories for children and adolescents as recommended by the WHO are used. At least one indicator is chosen for each domain, and thresholds are established to assess progress of individual countries. Country-specific performance against these thresholds is assessed taking into consideration global and regional targets of the Sustainable Development Goal targets.[15] The Child Health and Wellbeing Dashboards (CHWD) were launched on May 4, 2022. While it is noted that progress has been made in child survival in the past decades, current threats include the threats of climate change, conflict and other humanitarian disasters, disease outbreaks, and inequities in social, education, and health services accessibility.[45] Surveillance of the CHWD indicators specific to individual countries can be used to measure the impact of HC, both short term and long term.[47]

Epidemiologic Modeling and the Importance of Predictions in Crisis Management

Epidemiologic modeling has evolved as a distinct discipline to use available data to predict likely health outcomes. Sensitivity analysis permits the examination of the impact at various intervention thresholds. The types of modeling (eg, compartmental or agent-based) place emphasis on both scenario-based and predictive analyses used in planning management of HC.[48] The best illustrations of this are the models predicting the spread of infectious diseases such as measles and polio as a result of the disruptions created by HC and/or dismantling of public health infrastructures. These disruptions may include lack of access to quality surveillance data, erosion of immunization/vaccine coverage, and complicated migration patterns. The story of Israel-Gaza resulting in the spread of infectious diseases such as scabies, varicella, hepatitis A, respiratory infections, diarrheal disease, and the first polio case in Deir al-Balah in an unvaccinated child is exemplary.[37,49] Modeling of the possibility of re-emergence of vaccine-eliminated infectious diseases in the United States—namely measles, rubella, diphtheria, polio, and the globally eradicated smallpox—given the current level of vaccination rates, predicts measles may become endemic. The model predicts that 51.2 million measles cases will occur in a 25 year period, 9.9 million rubella cases, 4.3 million polio cases, 197 diphtheria cases, 10.3 million hospitalizations, and 159,200 deaths.[38]

Nutritional Status and Case Examples

The third epidemiologic area emphasized in the assessment of the impact of HC is nutritional status. Nutritional assessment consists of measuring height/length, weight, with weight/height as the primary measure, and/or mid-upper arm circumference (MUAC) for children 65 to 110 cm tall (a proxy for 6–59 months). The definition of severe malnutrition is low weight-for-height (WFH) or wasting WFH less than 2 standard deviations (SD) below the Center for Health Statistics/CDC/WHO median, or a Z-score less than 2SD from the M50 manya low MUAC (<12.5 cm).[28,50] Many lessons were learned from the experience of Biafra, Bangladesh, and Ethiopia. Differences between acute food crisis and famine were learned in support of accurate surveillance and the following are defined.[29,51–53]

1. Acute food insecurity with 20% of a population suffering from extreme food shortages. Surveillance assessment includes understanding what children are eating, how much is being eaten, what is being done to get food (e.g. stealing, long lines),

and food diversity. The global metric for food insecurity is the Integrated Food Security Phase Classification (IPC) system (**Fig. 6**).[53]

2. Malnutrition with 30% of children under the age of 5 years experiencing acute malnutrition. The best measure is weight/height, but in its absence MUAC is a secondary and acceptable measure. The risks and early signs of malnutrition include disruption in feeding, disruption in primary care and other health care services, and disruption of WASH. Assessing the lack of diversity of food is essential for children. Associated diarrheal diseases are exacerbated in the presence of malnutrition. Nutritional status and food security assessments both acute and long-term are reflected in data reporting on prevalence of wasting, stunting, and underweight children with the inherent implications for child development.
3. Famine: Reasonable evidence is that 2 of 3 thresholds have been reached: starvation, acute malnutrition, and mortality (>2 deaths/10,000/day). However,

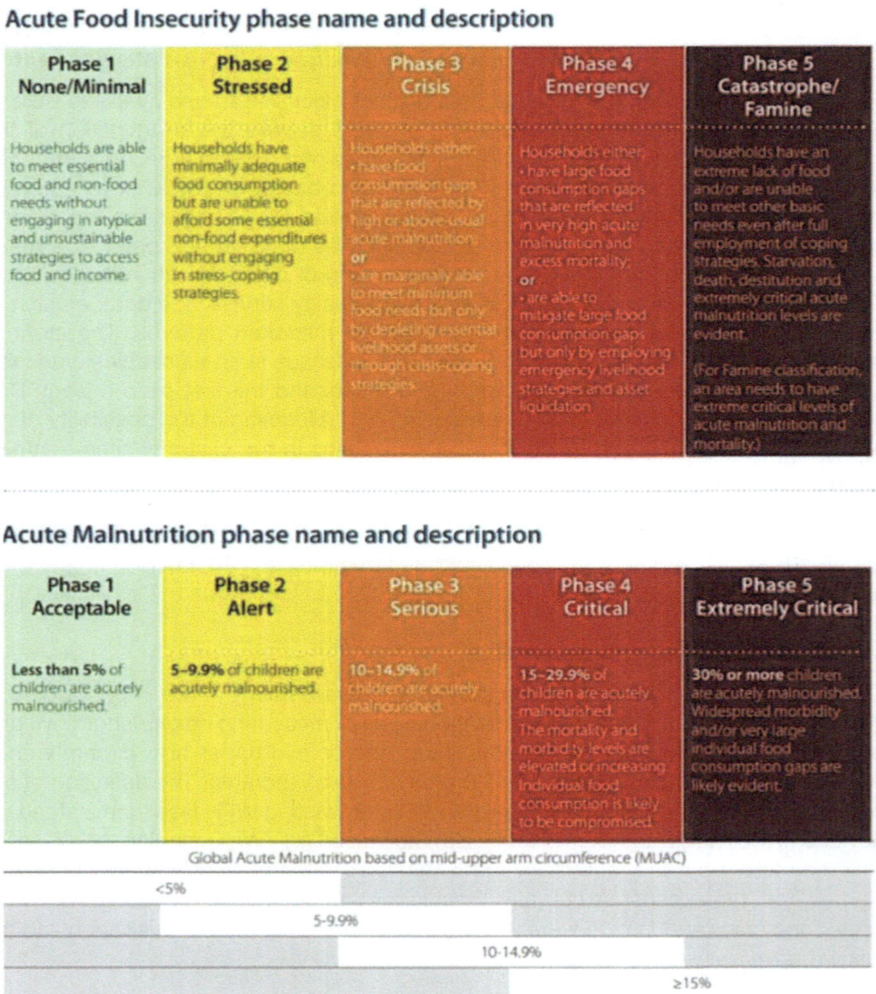

Fig. 6. Integrated Food Security Phase Classification (IPC) system (Used with permission from the Integrated Food Security Phase Classification).[53]

establishing that mortality is due to acute malnutrition is difficult since malnutrition itself places an infant or child at increased risk for infection and recovery from trauma is problematic in the face of malnutrition. Epigenetic effects of famine are another nuance needed in the assessment of the impact of HC. Important in this declaration is the recognition that severely malnourished children must have specialized therapeutic feeding to avert refeeding syndrome, providing basic foods is not sufficient.[54,55] Pregnant individuals also require special assistance from trained health personnel. Long-term effects of those who are famine exposed prenatally are being documented.[56,57]

Four famines are current in South Sudan, Somalia, Yemen, and North-East Nigeria as reported in 2023.[29,58] The Gaza Strip has recently been added to the group with the Declaration of Famine now occurring in northern Gaza and expected to expand to southern Gaza.[53,59] Important to averting famine in areas of conflict, natural, or "human-induced" disasters is an understanding of how to recognize the early warning signs in the wake of crises. We need not wait for a declaration of famine—that declaration is a confirmation of failure of states to govern, hence is inherently political.[54] Accordingly, states are reluctant to make these declarations. The federal government and UN agencies are the usual actors making such a declaration.[60] The majority of declarations of famine occur in the context of conflicts, predominantly noninternational conflicts.

The research methodology examining 2 case studies—Tigray-war, Ethiopia (2020–2022) and South Sudan (from the start of the civil war 2013 to present) is salient.[29] This analysis examined not only the complexities of the declaration of famine but also key conclusions on how political tensions among actors, social media, and political pressure affect such declarations and how to formulate the foundation of a process that heeds technical and political restraints, and applies the Early Warning Systems. The issues of ethics as well as positionality are discussed by the authors of the analysis of Ethiopia and South Sudan where famine was declared in the former region and not in another—under similar circumstances. After extensive analyses, the authors of the report indicated potential criteria for a newer process:

- Determine what level of governmental approval and involvement is feasible and strong consideration for decreasing the involvement of government's involvement due to potential conflicts of interest (COIs)
- Consideration of whether a declaration of famine and relief might occur without governmental approval incurs challenges to sovereignty. This consideration would imply the involvement of a neutral organization(s) as well as a priori agreement to the participation of the international community. Again, COI even among those agencies charged with response to crises remain a challenge.

Disruption of Other Activities: Immunizations/Vaccines

The impact of HCs on infectious diseases, their prevention and elimination, is best exemplified by the analysis of the role of measles and the emergence of polio in the Gaza Strip.[38,39,49] Content areas for better understanding epidemiology, research methods, ethical considerations, and tackling misinformation and disinformation with clarity are displayed in **Fig. 7**.

Functioning of Vital Sectors

In HC the functioning of vital sectors is totally disrupted. These sectors include areas of sanitation facilities, morgues, fuel, and electricity as previously cited. Other vital systems include health systems, educational institutions, information technology

A Understanding and Acceptance

Areas of Focus for Public Understanding & Acceptance	Activities
Epidemiology	CDC data stratified data based on age, race, gender, pregnancy status, geographic area; surveillance, contact tracing, vaccine distribution data
Research	Vaccine development and safety translation pathway: • Safety and Efficacy Data • RCT designed with an equity lens • Vaccine Hesitancy Scale – stratified data, child and adult
Ethics	Access Special Populations considerations (pregnant women, children) Racial, ethnic, cultural biases
Clarity & Credibility of public health messages	Public deliberation, Toolkits, Resources, Transparency, Sharing of complex data and mechanisms of action of vaccines, e.g. immunological response

B Deployment Strategies

Areas of Focus for Vaccine Deployment	Activities
Epidemiology	CDC **data stratified** data based on age, race, gender, pregnancy status, geographic area; surveillance, contact tracing, vaccine distribution data
Deployment framework: Public health principles of herd immunity No Missed opportunities/no wrong door for vaccination Location of deployment (pediatric experience of medical home) Urgency of deployment Prioritization of deployment Effectiveness of deployment WHO, COVAX, FPM	• Effective community sensitive messages • Selection of deployment sites • Prioritization of targets of vaccination and timing of such decisions based on supply • Data of tracking of effectiveness of distribution strategy • Strategy of messaging of vaccine choice • Continuous and dynamic evaluation • Maintenance of cold chain and supply • **WHO operational plan COVID-19 partners platform -#10 pillar- mass vaccination ; WHO and COVAX proportional allocation–augmented by Fair Priority Model (FPM)-** emphasizing special situations of need
Ethics	Equity in distribution of vaccines Consider needs of all and special populations (e.g. women and children)
Clarity & Credibility of public health messages	Public deliberation, Toolkits, Resources, Transparency, Sharing of complex data and mechanisms of action of vaccines, e.g. immunological response

Fig. 7. Frameworks for public acceptance and deployment of vaccines. (*A*) Understanding and acceptance. (*B*) Deployment strategies. (*Adapted in part from* Czabanowska K and Kuhlmann E. Int J Health Plann Mgmt. 2021;36(S1):14-19.)

infrastructure, social media, news outlets, water sources, and transportation. The various frameworks for identifying the sectors most affected are noted in **Figs. 2** and **3**.[7,17]

Sexual Violence Against Children

Sexual violence against children is not always cited as a defining category of HC but the scale of global GBV and its capacity to destroy physical, emotional, and long-term child well-being merits emphasis. This type of assault falls in the category of protection as set by the UN child health and well-being dashboard. The International Classification of Violence Against Children (ICVAC)[61] lists the inclusion 1 categories of violence as follows:

1. Violent killing of a child
2. Physical violence against a child
3. Sexual violence against a child

4. Psychological violence against a child
5. Neglect of a child
6. Other acts of violence against a child not elsewhere classified

Child marriage, trafficking in children, child labor, and the recruitment of children in armed forces and groups are not included among the categories and subcategories of the ICVAC, but merit mention. Reported in some settings (eg, Haiti) are restavèks (child slaves).[62]

Immediate and Long-term Consequences of Humanitarian Crises

As noted in the evidence review 15 categories of intervention themes have been identified[27] (see **Fig. 4**). The 15 categories are grouped by those that address early recovery and forced displacement health topics: communicable disease control, WASH, nutrition, SRH, including GBV; mental health and psychosocial support; noncommunicable disease; injury and physical rehabilitation; health services, and health systems. The contextual factors are also noted in the article inclusive of access to services, assessment methods, coordination, accountability, urbanization, and health worker security.

The increasing observation that both health and nonhealth professionals, namely journalists and international humanitarian staff workers, seeking to provide aid and/ or report on HC have been killed in alarming numbers is relevant to our discussions of how epidemiology and its many methods face serious challenges.[54,63] Additionally, the power of radio to engage the public and harness health response interventions has been documented. A free press is one of the humanitarian actors essential to the dissemination of quality data.[64]

Lastly, the topic of worker resilience in the face of enormous hardships for all affected by crises—moral injury and brain drain—merits mention. The recent reports globally, in headlines such as this "permanent USAID cuts slam humanitarian programs worldwide: We are being pushed off a cliff," February 27, 2025[65,66] echo sentiments of those laid off due to the cuts in international aid. The repercussions for health professionals globally and programs that they administer are already being felt.[67] Moral injury "can occur when someone engages in, fails to prevent, or witnesses acts that conflict with their values or beliefs." As reported by many, health professionals worldwide are feeling the pain of "watching your life's work be destroyed."[68] Compounding the emotional consequences of joblessness and moral injury is the resulting brain drain affecting public health—especially in the field of epidemiology. Supportive supervision may be key to improving the well-being of practitioners and integrating the themes they view as essential to their work (e.g. contextualization/ adaption to circumstances, evidence-based advocacy).[69]

CONTEXT FOR APPRAISING EPIDEMIOLOGY OF HUMANITARIAN CRISES AFFECTING CHILDREN

International Law and Human Rights

In addressing HC affecting children, it is relevant to review core concepts of international humanitarian law and human rights as codified in declarations, conventions, treaties, and regulations. Pertinent to these reviews is an examination of the Doctrine of Proportionality (DP) based on the concept of a "just war."[70]

We begin with a review of the establishment of the UN which was spurred by a World War II postwar vision to set forth a new world order that presumably would avert another world war. The formation of the UN, initiated by Woodrow Wilson's idea of the League of Nations, was composed of a series of charters, and then the agreement of the founding nations in 1942 as the Declaration of the UN. The Charter of the UN (considered a treaty) is the founding document. It was signed on June 26, 1945, in San Francisco, at the conclusion of the UN Conference on International Organization and came into force on October 24, 1945.[71,72] While it is beyond the scope of this article to review a detailed history or functioning of the UN, a few key provisions and declarations are relevant to the determination of the assessment of when an HC is occurring and the core epidemiologic components that must be surveilled.[72]

- The UN Covenants on Human Rights and other major human rights treaties are proposed as a "new customary law or recognized general principles of law with respect to some of the rights expressed."[72,73]
- The Declaration on Principles of International Law, drawn by consensus of the member nations, elaborates the major principles of international law in the UN Charter, in particular the use of force, dispute settlement, nonintervention in domestic affairs, self-determination, duties of cooperation and observance of obligations, and "sovereign equality."[72] Currently, there are 193 member countries, with 2 nonmembers: the Holy See (Vatican) as a permanent observer and by resolution A/RES/67/19 of November 29, 2012, the General Assembly accorded non-Member Observer State status to Palestine.[74,75]

While neither the UN nor its agencies were conceived of as legislative bodies, the union of these nations was envisioned to provide harmonization of actions at the world stage for issues of mutual importance. Some of these actions may be codified in the traditional processes of treaties and customary law.

The UN declarations and humanitarian actors provide the framework and epidemiologic data to measure the occurrence, impact, and necessary response to HC. Many data sources and data acquisition methods and analyses derive from these UN agencies and their commitment to data quality globally. Data quality becomes central in circumstances of social and political upheaval. A noncomprehensive list of germane agencies and declarations is below.

Humanitarian Declarations: Core Elements Undergirding Assessment of Humanitarian Crises Response

- UN Universal Declaration of Human Rights[76] proclaims "a common standard of achievement for all peoples and all nations". There are 30 articles that register the basic rights, prohibited actions, and equal treatment and due processes to be accorded to every human being.
- The UN Convention on the Rights of the Child[46] has 54 articles addressing the rights of children (those <18 years of age), unless, under the law applicable to the child, majority is obtained earlier. The use of this framework in research has proved useful.[77,78] The precept of this convention establishes the rights of all children. These rights are relevant in times of war and conflict and apply to the preservation of those rights for children caught on all sides of any conflict. That includes, for example, the right to survival (Article 6), nonseparation from parents (Article 9), freedom of religion (Article 14), protection from all forms of physical or mental violence (Article 19), receipt of appropriate protection and humanitarian assistance (Article 22), and all the rights set forth by the convention and other international human rights.
- UN Convention on the Prevention and Punishment of the Crime of Genocide, adopted December 9, 1948.[79] Accompanied by 19 articles the convention establishes that genocide is "a crime under international law, contrary to the spirit and aims of the UN."

- UN Declaration of Famine as noted previously follows established metrics of food insecurity, malnutrition, and mortality related to starvation. The 2 agencies most involved in assessing the occurrence of famine as set by the IPC are the Famine Review Committee (FRC) or the United States Agency for International Development (USAID) Famine Early Warning System.[53] The FRC is a specialized committee consisting of a panel of technical experts in the areas of food security, livelihoods, nutrition, and health and is activated to provide independent review of IPC analyses.[80] Since its inception, the FRC has conducted Famine Reviews in various contexts, including for Ethiopia, the Gaza Strip, Somalia, South Sudan, Sudan, and Yemen. The USAID established the Famine Early Warning Systems Network (*FEWS NET*) in 1985 in response to the famines in East and West Africa and the need for earlier warning of potential food security crises. Both the FRC and the FEWS NET, for example, have confirmed that the Gaza strip has reached phase 5 of the classification system that defines famine (see **Fig. 6**).[81]

Humanitarian Actors

These international organizations are cited because of their role in responding to HC. Given the inherent political context of HC, this incomplete listing is not an endorsement or assessment of the effectiveness of these organizations to fundamentally change the conditions that aggravate the occurrence of HC or fair and just responses to such crises. As pointed out by some authors, the basis for international, collective response must be rooted in the creation of infrastructures necessary for sustainable economic programs and lead to affected-country rebuilding and leadership with the only condition for the involvement of foreign assistance is a measure of tangible results.[82] A comprehensive introduction is referenced by Melzer (2016)[83]

- *UNICEF*, originally the *UN International Children's Emergency Fund*, officially *UN Children's Fund* since 1953, is an agency of the UN responsible for providing humanitarian and developmental aid to children worldwide.[84]
- The WHO, founded in 1948, is the UN agency that is organized to connect nations, partners, and people "to promote health, keep the world safe and serve the vulnerable – so everyone, everywhere can attain the highest level of health."[42,85] The WHO is stated to organize to lead global efforts to expand universal health coverage. Among its stated functions is to direct and coordinate the world's response to health emergencies by using science-based policies and programs. Recently, the United States has pulled out of the WHO.[86] The impact of recalling and reassignment of US government personnel has had immediate impact on the ability of the WHO to respond effectively to HC and the full impact will need to be assessed.
- Created by United Nations General Assembly resolution 46/182 in 1991, the IASC is the longest-standing and highest-level humanitarian coordination forum of the UN system. It brings together the executive heads of 19 organizations and consortia to formulate policy, set strategic priorities, and mobilize resources in response to HCs.[87]
- The World Bank Group is a family of 5 international organizations that make leveraged loans to LMICs. It is the largest and best-known development bank in the world and an observer at the UN Development Group. With 189 member countries, the World Bank Group stated purpose is to fight poverty through sustainable solutions.[88]

- UN High Commission for Refugees[12] is a refugee agency that works to ensure the rights of those who seek asylum and assist in finding safe refuge for those who have fled violence, persecution, or war at home.
- The World Food Programme (WFP)[89] is an international organization within the UN, the branch related to food assistance. It is governed by the WFP Executive Board, which consists of 36 Member States and provides intergovernmental support, direction, and supervision of activities.
- *GAVI*, officially *Gavi, the Vaccine Alliance* (previously the *GAVI Alliance*, and before that the *Global Alliance for Vaccines and Immunization*) is a public–private global health partnership with the goal of increasing access to immunization in LMICs. It is the largest organization distributing donations of money toward vaccines; from 1990 to 2016, more than a third of donor money for immunization was channeled through Gavi. In the advent of the COVID-19 pandemic, a WHO deployment framework for mass vaccination in collaboration with COVAX and a Fair Priority Model was devised (**Fig. 7**).[90]

Doctrine of Proportionality in a Time of War

The DP in a Time of War has a long history based on the concept of a "just war."[70] This doctrine has heightened relevance due to the increasing number of armed conflicts around the world. Relevant are the continued efforts of international law and human rights organizations to establish the boundaries of action of a civil society and our ultimate attainment of global peace. Wars and internal conflicts currently being waged are noted geographically,[91] inclusive of Russia-Ukraine, Gaza-Israel Middle East, Myanmar, Haiti, and Sudan to name a few and numerous countries throughout the globe.

Dating back to the time of Cicero, extending to St. Augustine and St. Thomas Aquinas, the "just war" guardrails indicated that attacking a sovereign had to be motivated for good or the avoidance of evil. They argued that going to war was justified only if "all human understanding and natural reason,"[70] that is, all judicial processes and peaceful means had been exhausted in resolving a conflict. Prerequisites to a just war have been listed by other philosophers, laying down the constraints on nations who might choose to wage war out of expediency. These parameters were challenged by the Bush President policy on preemptive strike in a national policy to combat terrorism on the presupposition of deterrence and expressed imminent threat. From these perspectives and historical milestones the concept of proportional response can be understood.

The doctrine of proportionality states that "(1) any sovereign undertaking a war should measure its response in proportion to claimed wrong, and (2) the means used to carry out that war should be proportionate to the desired goal."[70] The measured response has been detailed over the years and in one analysis is composed of several steps with the aim of having the good outweighing the magnitude of potential harm to achieve the given objective. These analyses underscored that the loss of many lives or great deal of property being destroyed would tip the balance away from the good.[70] The Geneva Convention of 1864 marks the first international use of the concept of proportionality, and in its deliberations addressed "the way that wounded soldiers were treated"[70] and provision of safe harbor to families. This notion bears particular significance given that current wars disproportionately kill children.

Establishment of the DP is linked to the development of the parameter for establishing genocide under international law. Over decades, the concept of DP has continued to evolve but not until the UN Charter were limits identified to prohibit the threat of or use of forces, except in cases of self-defense or collective defense. Three components in the determination of genocide are generally agreed upon:

- Culpability: that is the event is human induced
- Attacks are aimed at a particular group—by ethnicity, national origin, religion, and so on
- The actions aim to systematically destroy all structures, making survival impossible
- The DP is ignored

The legal framework of genocide is beyond the scope of this article, but is a peremptory norm of international law, an international legal obligation that is accepted and recognized by the States of the international community. In the twenty-first century, there are recognized ongoing genocides inclusive of the Rohingya genocide (2016, who live in Rakhine state in northwestern Myanmar); Yazidi genocide (2014–2017), Darfur Sudan (2003–2005), South Sudan, DR Congo; with the latest declaration on September 16, 2025, the UN Independent International Commission of Inquiry on the Occupied Palestinian Territory, including East Jerusalem, and Israel, reported that Israel had committed genocide.[92–94]

SUMMARY

This article draws from the extant literature and current realities regarding HC. The overview provides data informed classification of HCs and definitions of epidemiology as a basis for assessing the magnitude and scope of the problems faced by children linked to actionable crisis response. The use of spatial representation and visualization methods, epidemiologic quantitative and qualitative methods, with the triangulation of contextual elements can be used to understand the possible venues to mitigate both the direct and indirect impact of HCs affecting children. Remaining challenges include tackling misinformation and disinformation regarding HCs, access to quality data, implementing the various epidemiologically driven interventions and grounding global response on the precepts of international law, human rights, and child rights.

DISCLOSURE

The author has no financial disclosures or conflicts of interest to disclose.

REFERENCES

1. UNICEF Data Profiles. Migration and Displacement Country Profiles - UNICEF DATA.
2. UNICEF Data and Analytics. Child Health and Well-being Dashboard _ New 2023 | Tableau Public. Profile - unicefdata | Tableau Public.
3. UNICEF – child internal displacements by cause of displacement 2023. Fichier cree le : 7/8/2025 9:25:59 PM. Available at: https://data.unicef.org/topic/child-migration-and-displacement/displacement/#:~:text=Internal%20displacement%20by%20cause,own%20borders%20than%20beyond%20them.
4. Spiegel P, Martinez E, Abrahim O, et al. Johns Hopkins Center for Humanitarian Health-Lancet Commission on health, conflict, and forced displacement: health in a world of crises and impunity; www.thelancet.com, Vol 407, May 23,2026.
5. The International Rescue Committee. Available at: www.rescue.org.
6. Miliband D. KEYNOTE REMARKS BY DAVID MILIBAND (IRC) source: proceedings of the Annual Meeting (American Society of International Law), 2021, Vol.

115 (2021), pp. 3-7 published by: Cambridge University Press on behalf of the American Society of International Law Stable URL. Available at: https://www.jstor.org/stable/10.2307/27131263.

7. Zenner D. Crisis-Affected populations and tuberculosis. Microbiol Spectr 2017; 5(1):TNM17-0031-2016.
8. Ratnayake R, Abdelmagid N, Doolye C. What do we know (or could know) about estimating population sizes of internally displaced people. Journal of Migration and Health 2022;6:100120.
9. IRC watchlist of 20 countries. Available at: https://www.rescue.org/sites/default/files/document/6423/ircwatchlist2022reportfinal.pdf.
10. Global Humanitarian Overview 2022 Report. Available at: https://reliefweb.int/report/world/global-humanitarian-overview-2022.
11. IRC Emergency Watchlist 2025: "A World out of Balance", Sudan, occupied Palestinian territory and Myanmar top of Humanitarian Crisis Ranking- Urgent Action Possible and Needed. IRC 2025 Emergency Watchlist - Sudan | ReliefWeb.
12. The United Nations. High commissioner for refugees. 2025. Available at: https://www.unhcr.org/refugee-statistics/data-summaries.
13. The United Nations. High Commissioner for Refugees (UNHCR, 2021). 2025. Available at: https://data.unicef.org/topic/child-migration-and-displacement/displacement/#:~:text=Internal%20displacement%20by%20cause,own%20borders%20than%20beyond%20them.
14. Core Commitments for Children. CCC/SCOPE/Humanitarian UNICEF. 2025. Available at: https://www.corecommitments.unicef.org/ccc-1-1; https://www.corecommitments.unicef.org/level-3-and-level-2-emergencies.
15. Kohrt BA, Mistry AS, Anand N, et al. Health research in humanitarian crises: an urgent global imperative. BMJ Glob Health 2019;4:001870.
16. Warsame A, Blanchet K, Checchi F. Towards systematic evaluation of epidemic responses during humanitarian crises: a scoping review of existing public health frameworks. BJM Global Health 2020;5:e002109.
17. Gonzalez PA, Fernandez JC, Gan RK, et al. The epidemiological profile of incidence and mortality from epidemics in complex humanitarian emergencies from 1990 to 2022 – a scoping review. Trop Med Int Health 2024;29:343–53.
18. Close RM, Pearson C, Cohn J. Vaccine-preventable disease and the underutilization of immunizations in complex humanitarian emergencies. Vaccine 2016; 34:4649–55.
19. Laraque D. Global child health: reaching the tipping point for all children. Acad Pediatr 2011;11(3):226–33.
20. United Nations. Human rights office of the high commissioner. Available at: https://www.ohchr.org/en/ohchr_homepage.
21. Frérot M, Lefebvre A, Aho S, et al. What is epidemiology? changing definitions of epidemiology 1978-2017. PLoS One 2018;13(12):e0208442.
22. Lilienfeld DE. Definitions of epidemiology. Am J Epidemiol 1978;107(2):87–90. PMID:341693.
23. Evans AS. Re:" definitions of epidemiology". Am J Epidemiol 1979;109(3): 379–81. PMID:453174.
24. Krieger N. Epidemiology and the People's Health: Theory and Context. 1 es. Oxford: OUP USA; 2013. p. 400.
25. Ratnayake R. Training in epidemiology and disease control for humanitarian emergencies. J Epidemiol Community Health 2010;1–2. https://doi.org/10.1136/jech.2010.125963.

26. Laraque-Arena D. Operating principles and competencies for engagement in Global/Local settings. Pediatr Clin Am 2021;68:351–6.
27. Blanchet K, Sistenich V, Ramesh A, et al. London School of Hygiene and Tropical Medicine, Harvard School of Public Health and the Overseas Development Institute (ODI). An Evidence review of research on health interventions in humanitarian crises. Executive Summary. file:///C:/Users/arena/Downloads/1820194_Hossain.pdf.
28. Burkle FM. The epidemiology of war and conflict in handbook of bioterrorism and disaster medicine. In: Antosia RE, Cahill JD, editors. Handbook of bioterrorism and disaster medicine. Boston: Springer; 2006.
29. Holmsten B. Famine declarations in conflict situations. Goteborgs Universitet; 2023. Available at: gupea.ub.gu.se.
30. Catley A. Participatory epidemiology: reviewing experiences with contexts and actions. Prev Vet Med 2020;180:105026.
31. Colombo S, Checchi F. Decision-making in humanitarian crises: politics, and not only evidence, is the problem. Epidemiol Prev 2018;42(3–4):214–25.
32. Colombo S, Richiardi L, Canova C. On behalf of the board of the Italian Association of Epidemiology. Epidemiol Prev 2024;48(3):254–9.
33. Colombo S, Altare C. Making sense of shaky data in humanitarian crises. Front Public Health 2025;13:1602366.
34. Colombo S, Terracini B. Estimating and interpreting mortality data in conflicts: challenges, controversies, and significance. Epidemiol Prev 2025;49(1):84–90, gennaio-febbraio.
35. The SMART Project. Measuring mortality, nutrition and food security in crisis situation. The SMART methodology Version 1 2006;1–109. Available at: www.smartmethodology.org.
36. Sphere handbook. Available at: https://spherestandards.org/handbook-2018/.
37. McGee F, Sin MA, Chen M, et al. Preparedness for visualization in the next pandemic. IEEE Computer Graphics and Applications 2025;95–100. Available at: https://creativecommons.org/licenses/by/4.0/.
38. Kiang MV, Bubar KM, Maldonado Y, et al. Modeling reemergence of vaccine-eliminated infectious diseases under declining vaccination in the US. JAMA 2025;333(24):2176–87.
39. Orenstein WA. The role of measles elimination in development of a National Immunization Program. Pediatr Infect Dis J 2006;25(12):1093–100.
40. Williams H, Downes E. Development of a course on complex humanitarian emergencies: preparation for the impact of climate change. J Nurs Scholarsh 2017; 49(6):661–9.
41. Quinn JM, Krylyuk V, Romaniuk O, et al. Epidemiological humanitarian aid: data for evidenced-based decision making in disaster and conflict medicine. Prehospital Disaster Med 2017;32(Supplement 1):S88–9.
42. World Health Organization. (WHO, 2019) epidemiological data analysis for the early warning alert and response network (EWARN) in humanitarian emergencies. A quick reference handbook. 2025. Available at: https://iris.who.int/items/93fd7323-e90d-4685-9d9a-f7bd4f8a8ae5.EMROPUB_2019_EN_22341.pdf(530.51KB.
43. Sigua JA, Caymaz E, Castro-Delgado R. Emergency medical care provided by humanitarian organizations in response to sudden onset disasters in Southeast Asia: a scoping review. Disaster Medicine and Public Health Preparedness. 19, 2025. e196.
44. Fottrell E, Byass P. Identifying humanitarian crises in population surveillance field sites: simple procedures and ethical imperatives. Public Health 2009;123:151–5.

45. Requejo J, Diaz T, Park L, et al. On behalf of the children in all Policies, Data and Learning Working Group. Child health and wellbeing dashboards: accountability for children's rights. Available at: www.thelancet.com. Accessed May 14, 2023.
46. Convention on the Rights of the Child. Printed by the human rights program department of Canadian heritage. Minister of Supply and Services Canada; 1991. Available at: https://www.ohchr.org/sites/default/files/Documents/ProfessionalInterest/crc.pdf.
47. Bosqui T, Abdulrahim S, Afifi RA, et al. Psychological and social suffering of another generation of Palestinian children living under occupation: an urgent call to advocate. Health & Human Rights Journal 2024;26(2):147–50.
48. Aylett-Bullock J, Gilman T, Hall I, et al. Epidemiological modelling in refugee and internally displaced people settlements: challenges and ways forward. BMJ Glob Health 2022;7:e007822.
49. Grotto I, Agha H, Al-Halaweh A, et al. Public health, war and cross-border challenges: the recent cVDPV2 polio outbreak in Gaza. Health policy. The Lancet.com eClinical Medicine 2025;81(81):103136.
50. Hosseinzadeh-Attar MJ, Belay GD, Ardalan A, et al. Assessment of malnutrition and anthropometric measurement among 0-59 months aged children in Amibara and Awash fentale districts, afar national regional state of Ethiopia. Hum Antibodies 2019;27:S43–52.
51. De Waal A. Starvation is a lifelong sentence: gaza's civilians must be protected in accordance with international las. BMJ 2025;390:R1607.
52. Webinar on Genocide and Famine in Gaza/Health information for all (HIFA.ORG). Available at: https://www.hifa.org/dgroups-rss/webinar-genocide-and-famine-gaza.
53. FEWS Net, Famine Early Warning Systems Network. Gaza Food Security Alert. August 22, 2025. Famine is now occurring in northern Gaza and expected to expand to southern Gaza. Available at: https://fews.net/.Downloaded10.13.2025.
54. De Waal A. Famine in Gaza: an example of the global humanitarian crisis. Am J Clin Nutr 2024;119:1383–5.
55. Checchi R, Frison S, Abede WKT, et al. Can we predict the burden of acute malnutrition in crisis-affected countries? Findings from Somalia and South Sudan. BMC Nutr 2022;8(1):92.
56. Li C, O Grada C, Lumey LH. Famine mortality and contributions to later-life type 2 diabetes at the population level: a synthesis of findings from Ukrainian, Dutch and Chinese families. BMJ Glob Health 2024;9:e015355.
57. Moraru A, de Almeida MM, Degryse JM. PALTEM: what parameter should be collected in disaster settings to assess the long-term outcomes of famine? Int J Environ Res Publ Health 2018;15:857. Available at: www.mdpi.com/journal/ijerph.
58. De Waal A. The end of famine? Prospects for the elimination of mass starvation by political action. Polit Geogr 2018;62:184–5.
59. Sutherland C. World leaders react as IPC report confirms famine in Gaza. 2025. Available at: https://time.com/7311728/gaza-famine-ipc-report-world-leaders-reactions/.
60. Jerving S. Tigray 'famine' was 'over politicization', says former WFP official. DevEx; 2023. Available at: https://devex.com/news/tigray-faminewas-overt-politicization-says-former-wfp-officia-104825.
61. The international classification of violence against children. The boundaries of the ICVAC. Available at: https://data.unicef.org/resources/international-classification-of-violence-against-children/file:///C:/Users/arena/Downloads/ICVAC-Report-v39-WEB%20(1).pdf.

62. Dube A, Moffatt M, Davison C, et al. Health outcomes for children in Haiti since the 2010 earthquake: a systematic review. Prehospital Disaster Med 2018; 33(1):77–88.
63. Unesco. Available at: https://www.unesco.org/en/safety-journalists/safety-journalists-crisis.
64. Hugelius K, Adams M, Romo-Murphy E. The power of radio to promote health and resilience in natural disasters: a review. Int J Environ Res Publ Health 2019;16: 2526.
65. World News. Trump's permanent USAID cuts slam humanitarian programs world-wide: "we are being pushed off a cliff.". Available at: https://apnews.com/article/trump-usaid-cut-doge-musk-dbaf0e89d72938caabee8251f7dfb4a7.Downloaded09.
66. Imray G. 2025. Available at: https://www.independent.co.uk/news/world/americas/usaid-donald-trump-south-africa-hiv-ngo-b2706185.html.
67. Fraser S, Global Policy. Consequences and implications for the international development assistance sector from the closure of USAID. 2025. Available at: https://www.globalpolicyjournal.com/blog/20/03/2025/consequences-and-implications-international-development-assistance-sector-closuredownloaded10.
68. Suleta K. Moral injury and brain drain are destroying our public health force. Perspectives. 2025. Available at: https://www.medpagetoday.com/opinion/second-opinions/116457Downloaded10.14.
69. Abujaber N, Ryan M, McBride KA, et al. Implementing supportive supervision in acute humanitarian emergencies: lessons learned from Afghanistan and Ukraine. PLOS Glob Publ Health 2024;4(4):e0002416.
70. Sullivan ET. The doctrine of proportionality in a time of war. Minn J Int Law 2007; 135. Available at: https://scholarship.law.umn.edu/mjil/135.
71. United nations charter. Available at: https://www.un.org/en/about-us/un-charter.
72. Schachter O. United Nations Law. Am J Int Law 1994;88(1):pp1–23.
73. D'Amato A. The concept of human rights in international law. Columbia law review Association, Inc. Available at: https://www.jstor.org/stable/1122161.
74. Declaration of principles of international law. Available at: https://international.vlex.com/vid/res-67-19-resolution-861191788.
75. United Nations non-member States. Available at: https://www.un.org/en/about-us/non-member-states.
76. Universal Declaration of Human Rights. udhr.pdf.
77. Wallace JG, Chernet R, Formica MK, et al. IAACT. Gun violence and the voices of youth on community Safety in the Time of COVID in East Harlem, NY: a youth participatory action research cross sectional study. Injury Epidemiology 2023; 10:34.
78. Malla P, Fray N, Formica M, et al, IAACT. IAACT. Engaging East Harlem, New York you in gun violence prevention research and child rights: a preliminary study. Inj Epidemiol 2023;10(Suppl 1):60.
79. General assembly resolution 260 A (III). Human rights instruments. Universal instrument. Convention on the prevention and punishment of the crime of genocide. 2025. Available at: https://www.ohchr.org/en/instruments-mechanisms/instruments/convention-prevention-and-punishment-crime-genocideDownloaded10.
80. Famine Review Committee (FRC). 2025. Available at: https://www.ipcinfo.org/ipcinfo-website/frc/en/downloaded10.
81. Gaza Strip. Famine confirmed in Gaza Governorate, project to expand/1July-30 September 2025. IP -Integrated Food Security Phase Classification. Available at: https://www.hi-us.org/sn_uploads/document/IPC_Gaza_Strip_Acute_Food_Insecurity_Malnutrition_July_Sept2025_Special_Snapshot.pdf.

82. Laraque F. The Instrumentalization of Revolutionary Thought/A collection of essays and reflections. Boston: Trilingual Press; 2014.
83. Melzer N. (Kuster E) international humanitarian law: a comprehensive introduction. International Committee of the Red Cross (ICRC); 2016.
84. Unicef. Available at: http://unicef.org.
85. Thieren M. Health information systems in humanitarian emergencies. Bull World Health Organ 2005;83:584–9. Ref no. 04-018903.
86. White House. 2025. Available at: https://www.whitehouse.gov/presidential-actions/2025/01/withdrawing-the-united-states-from-the-worldhealth-organization/downloaded10.
87. Interagency Standing Committee. Available at: https://interagencystanding committee.org/the-inter-agency-standing-committee.
88. World Bank. Available at: https://www.worldbank.org/ext/en/home.
89. World food Programme. Available at: https://en.wikipedia.org/wiki/World_Food_ProgrammeDownloaded10.02/254:45PM.
90. GAVI. The vaccine alliance. Available at: https://www.gavi.org/.
91. World population review. 2025. Available at: https://worldpopulationreview.com/country-rankings/countries-currently-at-wardownloaded10.
92. Human Rights Council, Sixtieth session. Legal analysis of the conduct of Israel in Gaza pursuant to the Convention on the Prevention and Punishment of the Crime of Genocide. 16 September 2025. A/HRC/60/CRP.3. English only.
93. Kranz M. Business insider. Available at: https://www.businessinsider.com/genocides-still-going-on-today-bosnia-2017-11.
94. Ohchr. Available at: https://www.ohchr.org/en/press-releases/2025/09/israel-has-committed-genocide-gaza-strip-un-commission-finds.
95. Sillin J. 13 worst natural disasters by death toll in the world. Available at: https://www.weatherstationadvisor.com/worst-natural-disasters-death-toll/Downloaded 08.29.20253:18PM.

SUGGESTED READING

Bloxham L. What is a humanitarian crisis?. 2022. Available at: https://www.concern.org.org.uk/news/what-is-a-humanitarian-crisis.

BSS News. Online portal of Bangladesh Sangbad Sangstha. 100,000 Haitian kids at risk of starving to death. UNICEF; 2023. Downloaded 08.04/2025 10:42AM.

Core strategies to prevent violence against children and A global technical package to prevent violence against children. Available at: http://www.cdc.gov/violence prevention/vacs/.

De Waal A, Hilhorst D, Jansen A, et al. Routledge humanitarian studies series. Milton Park, Abingdon: Routledge 2 Park Avenue Square; 2021. https://doi.org/10.4324/9781003167013.

Knipe DM, Levy O, Fitzgerald KA, et al. Ensuring vaccine safety: comprehensive safety testing is based on experience with prior vaccines. Viewpoint: perspective in insights. 2020. Available at: Sciencemag.org.

NYC Health. NYSDOH and NYCDOHMH wastewater monitoring identifies polio in New York City and urge unvaccinated new yorkers to get vaccinated now. Health. Available at: https://www.health.ny.gov/environmental/wastewater/. Accessed October 13, 2025.

Saito S, Farahani M, Kunda S, et al. Effects of stop-work orders on HIV testing, treatment and programmes for prevention of vertical transmission in four sub-saharan

African countries. J Int AIDS Soc 2025;28:e70034. https://doi.org/10.1002/jia2.70034. Available at: http://onlinelibrary.wiley.com/doi/10.1002/jia2.70034/full.

Science Insider Health. International hunger watchdog faces political attacks over famine Gaza reports. 2025. Available at: https://www.science.org/content/article/international-hunger-watchdog-faces-political-attacks-over-gaza-famine-declaration.

Spiegel PB, Salama P, Maloney S, et al. Quality of malnutrition assessment surveys conducted during famine in Ethiopia. JAMA 2024;292(5):613–8.

Stein F, Remley K, Laraque-Arena D. Pursley. New resources and strategies to advance the AAP's values of diversity, inclusion and health equity. Pediatrics 2018;141(4):e20180177.

UNICEF/Olena Hrom. Nearly 2,000 children killed or injured in Ukraine war: UNICEF. Available at: https://news.un.org/en/story/2024/05/1149661.

Ward H, Toledano MB, Shaddick G, et al. Oxford handbook of epidemiology for clinicians. OUP Oxford; 2012. 2012/05/24/, 417p.

Strengthening Child and Adolescent Mental Health Services and Systems in Humanitarian Settings

The Potential of Implementation Science

Tania Bosqui, DClinPsych, MSc[a,b,*], Sarah K.G. Jensen, PhD[c], Theresa S. Betancourt, ScD, MA[d]

KEYWORDS

- Mental health • Psychosocial support • Systems strengthening
- Implementation science

KEY POINTS

- Evidence for the effectiveness of mental health and psychosocial support for children and adolescents in humanitarian settings does not organically translate into practice.
- Implementation science offers mechanisms with which we can better scale-*out* and scale-*up* evidence-based interventions while maintaining quality and contextual relevance.
- Examples from Rwanda and Lebanon demonstrate the potential for implementation science to move beyond randomized controlled trials to real world impact.

INTRODUCTION

Worldwide, 1 in 4 people live in conflict-affected places, and over half of the world's conflict-affected population is children.[1] Children residing in settings of armed conflict are at risk of adverse mental health and developmental outcomes due to direct exposure to potentially traumatic events, but also indirect exposure through a wide range of daily stressors, including disrupted family environments, interpersonal loss, destruction of routines and structure, fragmented communities, and uncertainty about the

[a] Department of Psychology, American University of Beirut, Beirut, Lebanon; [b] Trinity Centre for Global Health, Trinity College Dublin, Dublin, Republic of Ireland; [c] Department of Pediatrics, Women and Infants Hospital of Rhode Island, Providence, MA, USA; [d] Research Program on Children and Adversity (RPCA), Boston College School of Social Work, Chestnut Hill, MA, USA

* Corresponding author. Department of Psychology, American University of Beirut, Beirut, Lebanon.
E-mail address: tb33@aub.edu.lb

Pediatr Clin N Am 73 (2026) 917–928
https://doi.org/10.1016/j.pcl.2026.04.004 **pediatric.theclinics.com**
0031-3955/26/

Abbreviations	
IASC	Inter-Agency Standing Committee
MHPSS	mental health and psychosocial support
PDSA	plan-do-study-act

future.[2–4] Armed conflict exacerbates every public health issue and has been termed the greatest public health concern for children globally.[5]

The global prevalence of diagnosable mental disorders is 1 in 10 in children and adolescents, making up around one-fifth of all disease-related disability worldwide.[6] Within war-affected populations, prevalence rates of mental disorders are 2 to 3 times higher than the global average.[7] Higher rates tend to be observed in children with more direct or prolonged exposure. For example, in Ukraine, youth in a war-affected region were 4 times more likely to show elevated traumatic stress reactions than those in peaceful regions.[8] In Palestine, prevalence rates of mental disorders in children have been estimated around 35% and have risen to 75% during the second *intifada* (uprising).[9] Though high, these numbers do not reflect subclinical distress, nor indigenous constructs of distress that may be missed by standard screening tools.[10]

MENTAL HEALTH AND PSYCHOSOCIAL SUPPORT

The complex picture of risk and protective factors shaping mental health among children and adolescents in humanitarian settings is critical to inform mental health and psychosocial support (MHPSS) interventions. Drawing on the diathesis-stress model[11] and social ecological theory,[12] addressing risk factors and strengthening protective ones can help shield children from the harms of war, displacement, and political insecurity. MHPSS is defined as any intervention that aims to protect or promote psychosocial well-being or prevent or treat mental health conditions.[13] Given extremely limited human resources to provide such support, particularly during humanitarian emergencies, the Inter-Agency Standing Committee (IASC)[13] developed guidance centered around an intervention pyramid that includes focused specialist and nonspecialist community-based interventions (**Fig. 1**). It is grounded in a

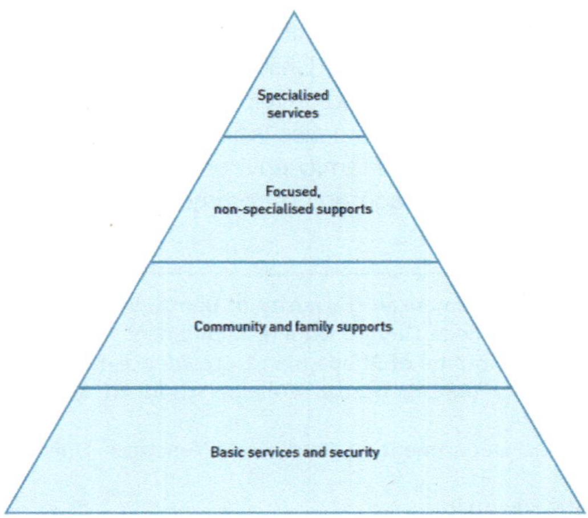

Fig. 1. Mental health and psychosocial support in emergencies intervention pyramid (IASC, 2007). (*Source* Inter-Agency Standing Committee (IASC) (2007). IASC Guidelines on Mental Health and Psychosocial Support in Emergency Settings. Geneva: IASC.)

task-sharing model, widely endorsed by MHPSS providers, in which interventions can be delivered by trained and supervised nonspecialist mental health providers. This can improve the feasibility of implementation, as long as strong systems for training and supervision are enacted and systems for referrals are defined.

Recent reviews of research gaps identified key priorities which includes scaling evidence-based MHPSS with quality and sustainment. This gap limits the use of evidence-based MHPSS in common practice, where actors on the ground need to know what and *how* to deliver MHPSS at every level of the IASC pyramid, across the social ecology of the affected child, and across different humanitarian sectors. An implementation science and systems strengthening approach will be critical in the years ahead to help the field deliver evidence-based MHPSS interventions at scale—with quality—while strengthening sustainable health and social services systems in war-affected settings.[4,14,15]

IMPLEMENTATION SCIENCE IN MENTAL HEALTH AND PSYCHOSOCIAL SUPPORT

Implementation science is the *scientific study of methods to promote the systematic uptake of research findings and other evidence-based practice into routine practice*.[15] It arose from a recognition that evidence generated from research was not routinely integrated into practice, and evidence-informed practice changes were occurring at a glacial pace. A review on research from the US National Institutes of Health found that it took an average of 17 years to translate just 14% of health research into common practice.[16] Implementation science is intended to address services gaps, and support the use of evidence-based interventions at a broader scale, along with strategies to ensure sustainment and quality. It can accelerate the use of evidence-based practices in accessible, sustainable, and high-quality care for those who can most benefit, improving the theory-practice gap and reducing health inequities.[17] Research, especially when blending both effectiveness and implementation questions, can help to identify uptake barriers and facilitators at individual, practitioner, service, and system levels, as well as develop, apply, and test strategies to overcome barriers and improve uptake and scale.[18,19]

In recent years, implementation science leaders have espoused the use of hybrid designs to better overcome time lags that plague the translation of evidence to common practices in health care.[17] Three common hybrid designs have been put forth; (1) hybrid type I designs which involve testing the effects of an intervention while observing and gathering information on the implementation process; (2) hybrid type II designs which involve testing of both intervention effects and implementation strategies; and (3) hybrid type III designs which mainly focus on the testing of an implementation strategy while observing and gathering information on the intervention's impact on relevant outcomes.

While the evidence base for the effectiveness of MHPSS in low- and middle-income countries and conflict-affected settings is steadily growing,[20] evidence for *how* to implement at scale while maintaining quality, is limited. A systematic review identified only 14 studies that included explicit testing of implementation strategies,[21] reflecting a tendency to use type 1 designs and prioritize effectiveness testing over scalability.[22] Despite some more recent type II trials (eg, in Rwanda[23] and Lebanon[24]), a massive evidence-to-practice gap in MHPSS services in humanitarian settings remains.

Pathways to scale for evidence-based MHPSS interventions for war-affected children, youth, and families include scaling-*up* and scaling-*out*. Scaling-up refers to the expansion of service delivery to serve more people in the same population or setting, while scaling-out refers to the adaption of an existing evidence-based intervention to new population or setting, as well as mechanisms to imbed interventions into health systems, policy, regulation, or politics.[19] Existing evidence on scaling-attempts for MHPSS in humanitarian and conflict-affected settings are largely focused on scaling-up and not scaling-out.[21] To have greater impact, scaling-up *and* scaling-out are needed to optimize accessibility, reach, and sustainability of care across settings and populations.

There are multiple existing frameworks to support implementation science efforts including Exploration, Preparation, Implementation, Sustainment (EPIS);[25] Reach, Effectiveness, Adoption, Implementation, and Maintenance (REAIM);[26] Consolidated Framework for Implementation Research (CFIR),[27] Promoting Action on Research Implementation in Health Services (PARIHS),[28] and the roadmap to impact.[29] The EPIS framework has guided several hybrid type II studies in postconflict settings.[30,31] Use of an established implementation science framework can help researchers and practitioners analyze and document the implementation ecology, its features and opportunities, as well as potential strengths and pitfalls at each level, compiling existing knowledge to help identify different pathways to scale.

CHALLENGES TO MENTAL HEALTH AND PSYCHOSOCIAL SUPPORT SCALING

There are multiple structural and systemic barriers facing MHPSS service strengthening in war-affected settings. These include the devastation of infrastructure, lack of skilled and motivated personnel leading to high staff turnover, poor supervision and long-term technical support of nonspecialist and specialist staff leading to burnout and poor quality services, and poor referral mechanisms, as well as major competing priorities for tight resources in other areas of health, and a failure to bridge the humanitarian-peacebuilding-development nexus.[14,21,32–35] These are often compounded by an overall lack of mental health policy and leadership at the national level, resulting in little political will to distribute financial resources, worsened by active political instability and insecurity.[36] Ongoing occupation, attacks on health care facilities and staff, and the control of humanitarian aid, such as in Gaza, make efforts to provide any contextually meaningful mental health support at scale deliberately futile.[37]

On the demand side, limited mental health literacy, practical barriers (such as transport, childcare, and time), and stigma, all contribute to reduced help-seeking.[38] In contexts of collective trauma linked to decades of war, occupation, and political instability, other contributing factors include a mismatch between individual clinic-based specialist care and collective need. For example, in Lebanon, the primary reason for not seeking mental health services is the perception that everyone is experiencing the same thing and that difficulties will get better on their own.[39] While in Gaza, the violation of justice, freedom, and human rights are inextricably linked to mental health and care provision.[40] In current practice, the mismatch between service assumptions, including the pathologization of reactions to oppression, occupation and settler colonialism, and the need for contextually relevant care that responds to collective need, is a core barrier.[41]

Scale-up pathways for contextually relevant mental health interventions are challenging—but not impossible. Troup and colleagues[21] identified core scale-up strategies in humanitarian settings. These include integrating mental health services into primary health care and community-based services using Train-the-Trainer models and task sharing, sustainable supervision models and referral mechanisms. On the demand side, community mobilization and sensitization can be used to improve mental health awareness at the community level, as well as embedding community detection mechanisms at the organizational level, and strengthening wider social ecological environments through working with families and communities, and advocating at the national and international level. Strong examples of such sensitization and awareness can be witnessed in Ukraine where the first Lady, Olena Zelenska, has launched a mental health campaign called *How Are You?* and led an effort to increase access to mental health services during Ukraine's ongoing war.[42] Scale-*out* strategies can include collaboration with government ministries to integrate government approved guidelines into national policy. For example, after the Tsunami in Sri Lanka, a mental health policy was developed by the Ministry of Health with the support of local key actors, the WHO and the International Medical Corps to integrate mental health care into accessible primary care settings.[43]

In using an implementation science framework in the preparation phase, human resources for MHPSS in humanitarian settings might include the selection of trainees based on motivation, experience, and integration within communities, contextually and culturally relevant interventions and training, and refresher trainings and ongoing collaborations with technical experts.[30] Further preparation steps might include proactive community detection and manualizing protocols for MHPSS evidence-based interventions, as well as integrating them into existing systems—from primary care to schools and social protection programs—to address multiple levels of the care continuum.[23,44]

CASE EXAMPLE 1: SUGIRA MURYANGO (STRONG FAMILY) PROGRAM IN RWANDA

An example of moving beyond randomized control trials to implementation science approaches to scaling can be seen in the efforts to scale the Sugira Muryango (SM/Strong Family) program in postgenocide Rwanda. The SM intervention is a strengths-based home visiting intervention designed in postgenocide Rwanda to promote early childhood development and prevent violence by engaging both male and female caregivers in nurturing care relationships with their young children ages 0 to 3. The intervention has been tested in several trials[45,46] and has demonstrated significant effects on improving anxiety and depression in male and female caregivers, while also reducing violence in the home by building skills in parental self-regulation, problem-solving, and conflict resolution along with standard content on play/stimulation, nutrition, and hygiene. The theory of change is shown in **Fig. 2**. To identify and reach

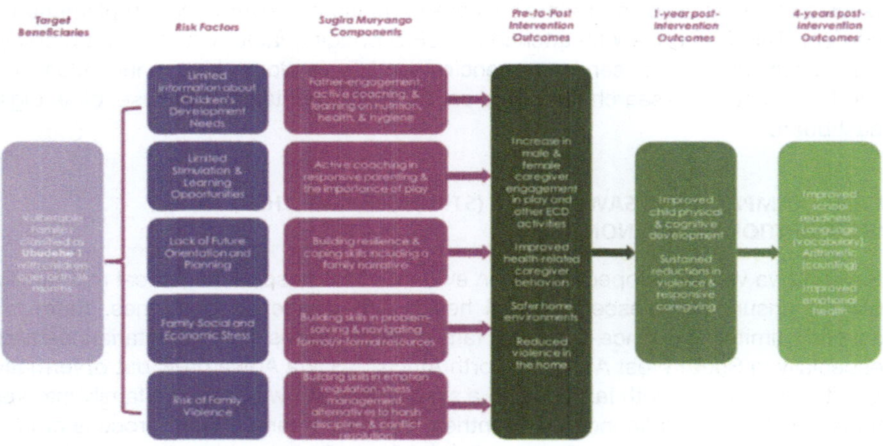

Fig. 2. Theory of change for the Sugira Muryango program. (*Source* Black, C.J et al., (2025), Scaling up home-visiting to promote early childhood development and prevent violence in Rwanda: a hybrid type-2 effectiveness-implementation trial. J Child Psychol Psychiatr, 66: 1484-1499. https://doi.org/10.1111/jcpp.14160.)

vulnerable Rwandan households with a child aged 0 to 3 years, the intervention was integrated with the Rwandan government's Vision Umurenge Poverty Reduction Strategy.[47] In recent years, the SM team has worked closely with the government of Rwanda and the University of Rwanda, testing the PLAY Collaborative strategy to scale the intervention to all households eligible for the social protection program using a Collaborative Team Approach.[23]

The PLAY Collaborative strategy is guided by the EPIS implementation science framework and focuses on accompaniment of government partners to eventually fully own and run the program. Individuals with expertise in delivering the intervention comprises an expert Rwandan Seed Team for training and supervision. The PLAY Collaborative also includes cross-site learning efforts across 3 districts and the signing of a common charter committing all partners to quality improvement including use of plan-do-study-act (PDSA) cycles to identify barriers and enhance facilitators to delivery and sustainment of the evidence-based practice. In the Play Collaborative Scale Hybrid Type II study, PDSA cycle problem solving sessions were held at all levels of government from national to district, sector, and clusters of villages. The PLAY Collaborative implementation science research questions were first about the effectiveness of the intervention when delivered by existing community child protection volunteers[48] as well as understanding issues of burden, incentives, cost, and intervention quality. A digital dashboard tool is currently being co-created with government stakeholders and tested to ensure that data on implementation quality are readily available for government leaders, community-level managers, and Seed Teams. Under the PLAY Collaborative strategy the SM team trained 2608 child protection volunteers (inshuti z'umuryango/IZUs) to deliver SM to more than 20,000 households across 3 Districts. PLAY Collaborative meetings engaged a total of 15,351 GoR officials and local stakeholders (eg village leaders, community health workers, psychologist practitioners) across the implementation ecology. The PLAY Collaborative strategy was designed together to advance GoR strategic goals related to coordination as well as data-driven monitoring and case management across social welfare and child protection systems.

The SM team used EPIS to guide implementation processes, including analysis of recordings and minutes of each PLAY Collaborative meeting, to illuminate implementation barriers by region and share successful solutions to overcoming implementation barriers. This was done with attention to EPIS bridging factors such as partnerships with health and social services agencies, and technology-driven innovations that will be tested in research focusing on the implementation and use of a digital dashboard.[23]

CASE EXAMPLE 2: THE SAWA AQWA (STRONGER TOGETHER) FAMILY INTERVENTION IN LEBANON

Sawa Aqwa was developed based on evidence that despite the critical role families play in ensuring adolescent mental health and protection outcomes, there is a severely limited evidence-base for family interventions in humanitarian settings, especially in South West Asia and North Africa.[49] Sawa Aqwa grew out of formative qualitative research with families and a systematic review of existing family interventions in low-and-middle income countries, through a participatory process of intervention development with Community Advisory Boards comprising adolescents and caregivers across multiple sites, and international and local experts in family interventions and MHPSS in the region. The theory of change is displayed in **Fig. 3**. The aim was to develop a contextualized intervention that addressed the social ecology of

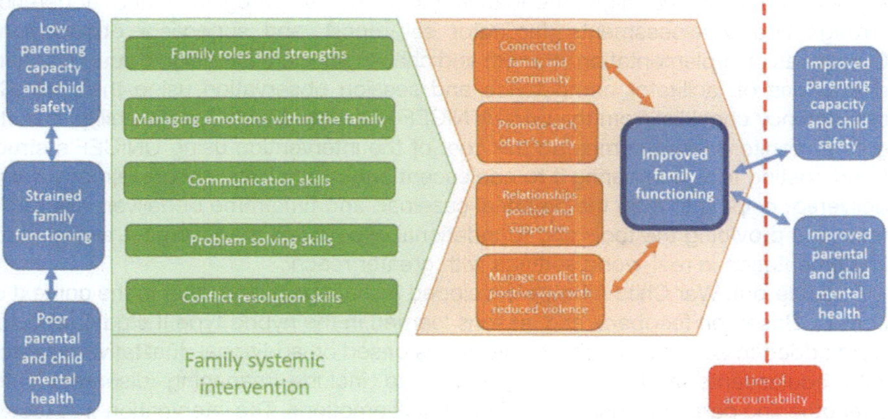

Fig. 3. Theory of change for the Sawa Aqwa (Stronger Together) family-focused psychosocial support intervention. (*Created in* Microsoft Powerpoint.)

adolescents, suitable for non-specialist delivery and wide-scale implementation in Lebanon and other similar contexts.

Sawa Aqwa involves 6 weekly sessions, and one booster session 1 month later. Sessions involve 90-min meeting with the whole family and an additional 30-min for parents only. Sessions include (a) family roles, strengths and goals, (b) joint emotional regulation, (c) communication, (d) problem management, and (3) conflict resolution. A fully powered hybrid Type II effectiveness-implementation randomized control trial with over 350 families demonstrated effectiveness of the intervention for adolescent and mother reported family functioning, caregiver mental health, parenting, and adolescent wellbeing for adolescents who completed the intervention,[24] as well as for optimal implementation in terms of costing, format, training, supervision and maintenance of quality.

Using an integrated implementation framework drawing on both the Roadmap to Impact and EPIS (**Fig. 4**), we focused on quality and feasibility as indicators of successful implementation ultimately leading to greater impact. For quality, the Sawa

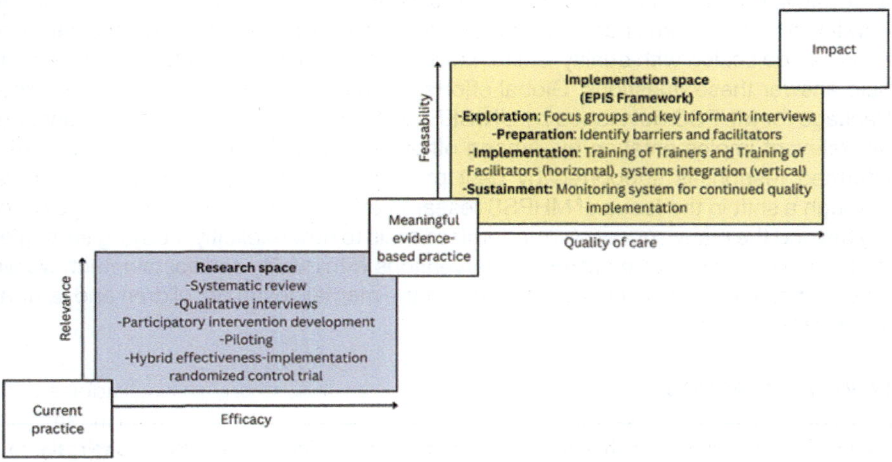

Fig. 4. Integrated implementation framework. (*Created in* Canva.)

Aqwa team identified high attendance (adolescents, caregivers) and adherence through fidelity assessments (facilitator self-report, and supervisor observation). Core areas of implementation strength and challenges were identified through training evaluations of facilitator competence and session observation using the FamACT competency checklist from the WHO/UNICEF EQUIP toolkit.[50] For feasibility, investigators monitored and compared the cost of the intervention using UNICEF's structured costing tool, comparing it to adolescent and group interventions already being delivered, helping to map the potential caseload and timeframe of delivery per facilitator and providing the tools and foundational experience to implement and monitor implementation in real-world settings with greater reach.

To scale-out, War Child Alliance developed the intervention further in the context of Jordan. Based on feedback and lessons learned in the hybrid type II study, modules were added to address specific family needs based on additional qualitative research with adolescents and their caregivers,[51] to include managing disagreements, strengthening parenting, and managing difficult emotions. The intervention was tested in a feasibility trial with 62 families in Jordan, replicating findings from Lebanon. Efforts for both scale-out and scale-up have been made. While scale-up efforts include the continued delivery of the intervention by implementing partners, such as War Child and Terre des Hommes Italia in Jordan and Lebanon—further training of facilitators conducted by Premieres Urgences Internationale to deliver the intervention to families during the war on Lebanon—further scale-out efforts have been made. These include adaptation of the intervention to families in Iraq through GIZ and Green Deserts, the integration of the FamACT competencies into clinical psychology and social work training programs in Lebanon, and integration into a core module of the Diploma in Child and Adolescent Mental Health in Humanitarian Settings in the Middle East and North Africa, a capacity building initiative co-led by Save the Children and the American University of Beirut.

SUMMARY

There is great potential for implementation science to inform the scale-up and scale-out of contextually relevant evidence-based MHPSS services in conflict-affected and humanitarian settings. This can ultimately lead to strengthened and more sustainable MHPSS systems through pathways that consider quality, feasibility, cost, context, accessibility, acceptability and reach. It is time to shift focus from what works to *how* it works, for whom under what circumstances, and how evidence-based interventions can be scaled with quality, sustainability and reach. Implementation science can help answer these questions. Global efforts, such as through the Minimum Services Package for MHPSS developed by UNICEF/WHO can help to support local contextually relevant implementation by, among other things, aiming to deliver faster, better informed responses supported by best practice guidelines, standards, and tools. Through a shift in the focus of MHPSS research efforts in humanitarian settings building beyond the many successful randomized trials to now explicitly studying strategies for scaling evidence-based MHPSS interventions with quality and sustainment, we will be better able to inform decisions to support the mental health of children and families living through turmoil.

INSIGHTS TO ACTION

- Implementation at scale should be informed by evidence for optimal pathways to scale, to maximize reach while maintaining quality.

- In complex humanitarian settings, systemic and structural barriers, and contexts of occupation and ongoing violence, are major challenges.
- Consideration for quality, feasibility, cost, context, accessibility, acceptability and reach are essential for the strengthening and sustainment of mental health systems.

DISCLOSURE

The authors have no financial disclosures or conflicts of interest to disclose.

REFERENCES

1. UNICEF. Every five seconds, a child is displaced, injured, or killed in the Middle East and North Africa's conflicts. 2025. Available at: https://www.unicef.org/press-releases/every-five-seconds-child-displaced-injured-or-killed-middle-east-and-north-africas. Accessed June 10, 2025.
2. Miller KE, Chen A, Koppenol-Gonzalez GV, et al. Supporting parenting among Syrian refugees in Lebanon: a randomized controlled trial of the caregiver support intervention. J Child Psychol Psychiatry 2023;64(1):71–82.
3. Pat-Horenczyk R, Rabinowitz RG, Rice A, et al. The search for risk and protective factors in childhood PTSD: from variables to processes. In: Pat-Horeczyk BD, Ford JD, editors. Treating traumatized children. London, UK: Routledge; 2008. p. 51–72.
4. Kanan G, Leão T. Post-traumatic stress disorder in youth exposed to the Syrian conflict: a systematic review and meta-analysis of prevalence and determinants. J Human Health Psych 2024;29(10):1433–49.
5. Tol WA, Le PD, Harrison SL, et al. Mental health and psychosocial support in humanitarian settings: research priorities for 2021-30. Lancet Glob Health 2023;11(6):e969–75.
6. Kieling C, Buchweitz C, Caye A, et al. Worldwide prevalence and disability from mental disorders across childhood and adolescence: evidence from the Global Burden of Disease study. JAMA Psychiatry 2024;81(4):347–56.
7. Carpiniello B. The mental health costs of armed conflicts-a review of systematic reviews conducted on refugees, asylum-seekers and people living in war zones. Int J Environ Res Public Health 2023;20(4):2840.
8. Osokina O, Silwal S, Bohdanova T, et al. Impact of the Russian invasion on mental health of adolescents in Ukraine. J Am Acad Child Adolesc Psychiatry 2023;62(3):335–43.
9. Khamis V. Post-traumatic stress and psychiatric disorders in Palestinian adolescents following intifada-related injuries. Soc Sci Med 2008;67(8):1199–207.
10. Hassan G, Ventevogel P, Jefee-Bahloul H, et al. Mental health and psychosocial wellbeing of Syrians affected by armed conflict. Epidemiol Psychiatr Sci 2016;25(2):129–41.
11. Zuckerman M. Diathesis-stress models. In: Zuckerman M, editor. Vulnerability to psychopathology: a biosocial model. London: Springer; 1999. p. 3–23.
12. Bronfenbrenner U. Ecological models of human development. In: Readings on the development of children. Oxford: Elsevier; 1993. p. 37–43.
13. Inter-Agency Standing Committee (IASC). Guidelines on Mental Health and Psychosocial Support in emergency settings. Geneva: IASC; 2007.
14. Betancourt TS, Rawlings L, Subrahmanian R. Strengthening adaptive social protection for children in crisis: the role of implementation science. 2025. Available

at: https://blogs.worldbank.org/en/investinpeople/Strengthening-adaptive-social-protection-for-children-in-crisis. Accessed October 4, 2025.
15. Eccles MP, Mittman BS. Welcome to implementation science. Implementation Sci 2006;1:1.
16. Balas EA, Boren SA. Managing clinical knowledge for health care improvement. Yearb Med Inform 2000;(1):65–70.
17. Curran GM. Implementation science made too simple: a teaching tool. Implement Sci Commun 2020;1:27.
18. Proctor EK, Bunger AC, Lengnick-Hall R, et al. Ten years of implementation outcomes research: a scoping review. Implementation Sci 2023;18:31.
19. Aarons GA, Sklar M, Mustanski B, et al. "Scaling-out" evidence-based interventions to new populations or new health care delivery systems. Implementation Sci 2017;12:111.
20. Barbui C, Purgato M, Abdulmalik J, et al. Efficacy of psychosocial interventions for mental health outcomes in low-income and middle-income countries: an umbrella review. Lancet Psychiatry 2020;7(2):162–72.
21. Troup J, Fuhr DC, Woodward A, et al. Barriers and facilitators for scaling up mental health and psychosocial support interventions in low- and middle-income countries for populations affected by humanitarian crises: a systematic review. Int J Ment Health Syst 2021;15(1):5.
22. Massazza A, May CR, Roberts B, et al. Process evaluations of mental health and psychosocial support interventions for populations affected by humanitarian crises. Soc Sci Med 2022;303:114994.
23. Black CJ, Placencio-Castro M, Phend G, et al. Scaling up home-visiting to promote early childhood development and prevent violence in Rwanda: a hybrid type-2 effectiveness-implementation trial. J Child Psychol Psychiatry 2025;66(10):1484–99.
24. Bosqui T, Brown F, Farah S, et al. Findings from the hybrid effectiveness-implementation trial of the Sawa Aqwa (Stronger Together) Family Intervention for at-risk adolescents in Lebanon. J Child Psychol Psychiatry. in press.
25. Moullin JC, Dickson KS, Stadnick NA, et al. Systematic review of the Exploration, Preparation, Implementation, Sustainment (EPIS) framework. Implement Sci 2019;14(1):1.
26. Glasgow RE, Harden SM, Gaglio B, et al. RE-AIM planning and evaluation framework: adapting to new science and practice with a 20-year review. Front Public Health 2019;7:64.
27. Damschroder LJ, Aron DC, Keith RE, et al. Fostering implementation of health services research findings into practice: a consolidated framework for advancing implementation science. Implement Sci 2009;4:50.
28. Bergström A, Ehrenberg A, Eldh AC, et al. The use of the PARIHS framework in implementation research and practice—a citation analysis of the literature. Implement Sci 2020;15(1):68.
29. Jordans MJD, Kohrt BA. The roadmap to impact framework: a model for planning the scaling up of complex mental health interventions. Health Policy Plan 2021;36(3):442–52.
30. Freeman JA, Farrar JC, Placencio-Castro M, et al. Integrating Youth Readiness Intervention and entrepreneurship in Sierra Leone: a hybrid type II Cluster Randomized Trial. J Am Acad Child Adolesc Psychiatry 2024;63(7):708–19.
31. Aarons GA, Hurlburt M, Horwitz SM. Advancing a conceptual model of evidence-based practice implementation in public service sectors. Admin Policy Ment Health 2011;38(1):4–23.

32. Baingana F, Mangen SO. Scaling up of mental health and trauma support among war affected communities in northern Uganda: lessons learned. Intervention 2011;9(3):291–303.
33. Shackman J, Price BK. Mental health capacity building in northern Sierra Leone: lessons learned and issues raised. Intervention 2013;11(3):261–75.
34. Travers Á, Abujaber N, McBride KA, et al. Identifying best practice for the supervision of mental health and psychosocial support in humanitarian emergencies: a Delphi study. Int J Ment Health Syst 2022;16:11.
35. Boothby N, Veatch M, Pentes M. Evaluating treatment of Axis I mental health disorders in Aceh, Indonesia. The Psychiatrist 2011;35(7):248–55.
36. El Masri R, Zreik T, Chaar S, et al. Barriers and enablers to a coordinated MHPSS response in Lebanon: a case study of the MHPSS Taskforce. SSM - Mental Health 2024;6:100354.
37. MSF. Without a ceasefire, healing mental trauma in Gaza is impossible. 2024. Available at: https://www.msf.org/without-ceasefire-healing-mental-trauma-gaza-impossible. Accessed October 24, 2025.
38. Bosqui T, Hanna E, McEwen F, et al. Pretreatment dropout of refugee children seeking mental health care in a humanitarian context: A qualitative study. Int J Mental Health Systems. in press.
39. Karam EG, Karam GE, Farhat C, et al. Determinants of treatment of mental disorders in Lebanon: barriers to treatment and changing patterns of service use. Epidemiol Psychiatr Sci 2019;28(6):655–61.
40. Jabr S, Berger E. Community mental health, psychoanalysis, and freedom: the case of Palestine. Int J Applied Psychoanalytic Studies 2023;20(2):285–301.
41. Roberts T, Miguel EG, Torre C, et al. Reconceptualising the treatment gap for common mental disorders: a fork in the road for global mental health? Br J Psychiatry 2022;221(3):553–7.
42. UNICEF. UNICEF helps 'How Are You?' campaign boost mental health in Ukraine. 2023. Available at: https://www.unicef.org/ukraine/en/press-releases/unicef-helps-how-are-you-campaign-boost-mental-health-ukraine. Accessed September 12, 2025.
43. Budosan B, Mahoney J, Dorego W, et al. Three models of scaling up mental healthcare post-disaster: common challenges. Intervention 2020;18(1):18–27.
44. Sadik S, Abdulrahman S, Bradley M, et al. Integrating mental health into primary health care in Iraq. Ment Health Fam Med 2011;8(1):39–49.
45. Betancourt TS, Jensen SKG, Barnhart DA, et al. Promoting parent-child relationships and preventing violence via home-visiting: a pre-post cluster randomised trial among Rwandan families linked to social protection programmes. BMC Public Health 2020;20:621.
46. Jensen SK, Placencio-Castro M, Murray SM, et al. Effect of a home-visiting parenting program to promote early childhood development and prevent violence: a cluster-randomized trial in Rwanda. BMJ Glob Health 2021;6(1):e003508.
47. Bond L, Farrar J, Borg RC, et al. Alternate delivery platforms and implementation models for bringing evidence-based behavioral interventions to scale for youth facing adversity: a case study in West Africa. Implement Sci Commun 2022;3(1):16.
48. Bond L, Placencio-Castro M, Byansi W, et al. Factors associated with nonspecialist quality of delivery within a family strengthening Intervention in Rwanda: a parallel latent growth model. Prev Sci 2025;26(1):107–21.

49. Bosqui T, Mayya A, Farah S, et al. Parenting and family interventions in lower and middle-income countries for child and adolescent mental health: a systematic review. Compr Psychiatry 2024;132:152483.
50. EQUIP. Ensuring quality in psychological support. 2020. Available at: https://equipcompetency.org/en-gb. Accessed September 1, 2022.
51. Brown FL, Yousef H, Bleile ACE, et al. Nurturing families: a feasibility randomised controlled trial of a whole-family intervention with vulnerable families in Jordan. Glob Ment Health 2024;11:e51.

Humanitarian Pediatrics

Jeffrey Goldhagen, MD, MPH[a,b,*],
Daniel Martinez-Garcia, MD, MPH[c,d]

KEYWORDS

- Humanitarian pediatrics • Humanitarian crisis • Bearing witness • Temoignange
- Child rights

KEY POINTS

- Humanitarian pediatrics is proposed as an essential new evolutionary phase of pediatrics that responds to the complex *polycrises* shaping children's health.
- Humanitarian pediatrics is a child rights–based practice that integrates clinical care, public health, policy, research, and advocacy to address harms of humanitarian crises globally and within the US.
- Grounded in the UN Convention on the Rights of the Child, Geneva Conventions, and humanitarian principles, Humanitarian Pediatrics emphasizes equity, justice, participation, and protection of the humanitarian space.
- Central to its practice is *Témoignage*—bearing witness—through which pediatricians expose structural harms, advance accountability, and influence policy and justice systems.

INTRODUCTION

Since the turn of the century, our knowledge of the impact of global humanitarian crises (**Box 1**) and the social, environmental, commercial, and political determinants of health on children has transformed our understanding of the genesis of child health and wellbeing—demanding a new developmental phase of pediatrics—*humanitarian pediatrics*.

Humanitarian pediatrics inherits the past 75 years of the evolution of Pediatrics and Global Health movements (**Figs. 1** and **2**). It is a transdisciplinary practice that integrates pediatrics, behavioral health, public and humanitarian health, epidemiology, and social, political, and environmental sciences—to address the unique needs and

[a] University of Florida, Jacksonville, FL, USA; [b] International Society for Social Pediatrics and Child Health, Geneva, Switzerland; [c] Test, Avoid and Cure TB in Children (TACTIC) Project, Medical Department, Médecins Sans Frontières, Operational Center Geneva (OCG); [d] Faculty of Medicine, School of Global Health, Geneva Centre of Humanitarian Studies, University of Geneva, Geneva, Switzerland

* Corresponding author. Department of Pediatrics, University of Florida College of Medicine-Jacksonville, 841 Prudential Drive, Suite 1900, Jacksonville, FL 32207.
E-mail address: Jeffrey.goldhagen@jax.ufl.edu

Pediatr Clin N Am 73 (2026) 929–941
https://doi.org/10.1016/j.pcl.2026.05.001 pediatric.theclinics.com

Abbreviations	
CRC	United Nations Convention on the Rights of the Child
ISSOP	International Society for Social Pediatrics and Child Health
SDG	Sustainable Development Goals

rights of children and youth to optimal survival and development. It will help catalyze the transformation of pediatrics from a primarily clinical discipline to one capable of addressing the existential threats, polycrises, and oppression confronting children worldwide.

The needs of children are as unique as the humanitarian crises in which they are engulfed or from which they are fleeing—crises that include the direct impact of armed conflict and violence, forced displacement, environmental and climate-related disasters, political instability, exploitation, and economic collapse—and their indirect effects on the structural determinants of children's health and wellbeing (see **Box 1**). In such crises, children bear a disproportionate burden of morbidity, mortality, and long-term developmental, physical, and psychological trauma. Humanitarian Pediatrics addresses and responds to the needs of children by incorporating clinical medicine, systems development, policy generation, and training and research into a unified discipline.

It is important to note that humanitarian crises seldom occur as single events, but are interconnected as *polycrises*, conditions in which multiple crises occur simultaneously, interact, and compound their effects.[1] Complicating polycrises, children also confront mounting systems of oppression—such as racism, sexism, classism, ableism, colonialism, and xenophobia. These forms of oppression intersect and generate compounded disadvantages for individual and groups of children.

It is also important to note that the 20th century gave rise to the global humanitarian ecosystem with the creation of the International Committee of the Red Crescent and the Geneva Conventions[2] It is this ecosystem of rules that has created a *humanitarian space* that allows for specific protections and care for children in the settings of humanitarian crises. Humanitarian pediatrics also relies heavily on the elements of disaster medicine that include key concepts of disaster preparedness and response; and disciplines relevant to pediatrics—including infectious diseases, tropical medicine, emergency medicine, neonatal care, perinatal care, vaccinology, and outbreak prevention and response.

It is crucial to understand that humanitarian pediatrics is as relevant to children in the United States as it is globally—as multiple humanitarian crises impact tens of millions of American children. In 2023, 13.8 million children in the United States lived in food-insecure households.[3] Nearly 20% of children live in poverty and half are food insecure—50% of school age children are eligible for free or reduced lunch programs.[4] In 2022, 17% of children living in US households, more than 12.1 million children, experienced one or more forms of housing insecurity.[5] Firearms have become the leading cause of death for children and adolescents, with death rates rising sharply over the past decade.[6] The United States incarcerates more children per capita than any country in the world, many of whom are tried in adult courts and incarcerated in adult jails and prisons—and held in solitary confinement.[7]

The treatment of children at the Southern border has risen to the level of torture.[8] Children have been forcibly separated from their parents and subjected to physical and psychological trauma.[9] Now, the same is occurring in cities across the country. Deteriorating child labor laws are resulting in increasing injuries, disruption of schooling, exploitation, and long-term health issues.[10] Housing instability, community

Box 1
Impact of global humanitarian crises

Armed conflicts
- More than 520 million, 20% of the world's children live in active conflict zones—a 60% increase since 2010.[20]
- Globally, 1.6 billion, 65% percent of the global population of children, live in a country affected by armed conflict.[21]

Displacement
- Nearly 50 million children have been recently displaced due to conflict and violence.[22]
- Recent weather-related disasters have led to 40 million internally displaced children in 44 countries.[23]
- Children account for approximately 40% of all forcibly displaced people. In 2025, 8 million children were born into humanitarian crises, including climate disasters and armed conflict.[24]

Climate change
- Increasing heat exposure is worsening acute and chronic health conditions.[25]
- Malnutrition resulting from climate-related crop failures and food insecurity impair children's growth and development.[26]
- Trauma and toxic stress, anxiety, depression, and grief follow climate-related natural disasters.[27]
- Climate-related displacement and migration place children at increased risk for exploitation and trafficking, child labor, early marriage, and interrupted health care.[28]
- Education and development are impacted by school disruptions, physiologic effects of heat exposure, and loss of play spaces.[29]
- The population of street children is increasing in many regions due to rising urbanization, conflict, and economic instability.[30]

Child labor
- Approximately 160 million children are engaged in child labor worldwide.
- Upwards of 55 million of these children are involved in hazardous labor.[31]
- An estimated 100 to 150 million children live on the streets worldwide.[32]

Globalization
- Globalization has had a profoundly negative impact on economic equality and equity contributing to expanded child and intergenerational poverty.
- Global corporations aggressively target children contributing to epidemics of obesity and diabetes, adolescent addiction, lowered rates of breastfeeding, and unnecessary demand for consumer products.[33]
- Global disparities in economic development disproportionately affect children and public health systems.[34]
- Migration in search of economic security displaces children and separates families.[35]
- Globalization's effects on environmental degradation and climate change have fueled global environmental injustice.

Authoritarianism
- The descent of a growing number of countries into authoritarianism, nationalism, and fascism undermines children's health and wellbeing by reshaping the political, social, economic, and structural determinants of child health.[36]
- Oligarchies distort public priorities.
- Nationalism marginalizes migrant, refugee, minority, and Indigenous children.
- Youth are being targeted, forcibly displaced from their homes, deported, separated from their families, and divorced from social and societal systems and structures on which they depend.
- The resulting toxic stress will have a sustained impact on children's life course development, health, and wellbeing.

Health threats
- Pandemics and global health threats result in loss of access to education, nutrition, and routine health care.
- Emerging diseases threaten progress in child survival.

- Vaccine inequities leave millions of children unprotected.
- The breakdown of public health and social systems results in chronic underinvestment in children.
- Cultural and moral crises normalize violence and consumerism, and the disregard for truth erodes the ethical foundations of societies.

violence, poverty, neglect, and isolation are contributing to a growing mental health crisis among US youth, with rapidly increasing rates of anxiety, depression, suicide, and unmet mental health needs.[11]

OPERATIONALIZING HUMANITARIAN PEDIATRICS

Humanitarian Pediatrics is operationalized through child rights–based approaches that are grounded in the UN Convention on the Rights of the Child (CRC)[12] and Geneva Conventions,[2] and guided by the humanitarian principles of equity, social justice, impartiality, neutrality, and interdependence of rights. Education and research will be required to build a professional workforce equipped with the skills and competencies to practice, train, and advance this emerging discipline. The practice of humanitarian pediatrics requires inclusion of communities in developing solutions, using a decolonial lens to empower communities collectively to address the root cause determinants of health and facilitate access to the tools and resources necessary to address them. Ultimately, humanitarian pediatrics aims to create a coherent and robust global capacity to protect child health, mitigate the consequences of polycrises, and fulfill children's fundamental rights to survival and development, even in the most difficult conditions.

Humanitarian pediatrics addresses both the direct harms of polycrises and oppression, and the often-greater indirect impacts resulting from the collapse of health systems and essential services critical to children's optimal survival, development, and wellbeing. Grounded in a child-rights framework, and recognizing the interdependence of rights, Humanitarian Pediatrics extends beyond health care delivery to advance children's protection, promotion, and participation rights, as articulated in the CRC (**Table 1**), and respond to the impact of oppression in shaping children's lived experiences. It further affirms that children require age-appropriate and evidence-based clinical guidelines, protocols, systems, and resources that are frequently

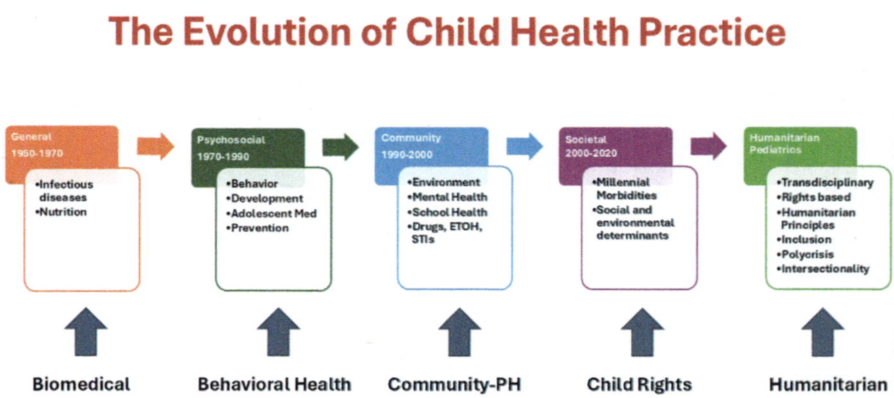

Fig. 1. Evolution of contemporary pediatrics. ETOH, alcohol; STI, sexually transmitted infections.

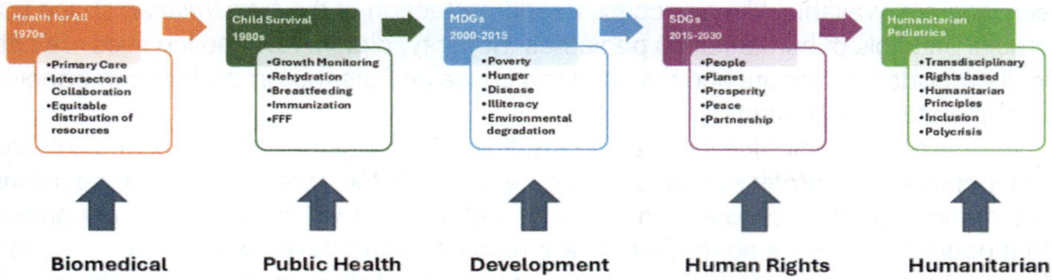

Fig. 2. Evolution of global health movements.

absent from conventional medical and humanitarian responses, as for instance, in armed conflict zones and medical triage circumstances.

By necessity, humanitarian pediatrics also focuses on the material needs of children, including access to care, medicine, and skilled health staff, as well as to housing, food, education, and other protection and promotion rights necessary for optimal survival and development—whether in the United States or global settings. It also encompasses a focus on ensuring the conditions necessary to provide care and social

Table 1
Promotion, protection, and participation rights in the UN Convention on the Rights of the Child

Promotion		**Protection**		**Participation**	
UNCRC Articles #		UNCRC Articles #		UNCRC Articles #	
Parental guidance	5	Nondiscrimination	2	Respect for voice	12
Name, nationality, identity, language, culture	7 8 3	Kidnapping Protection from all forms of violence	11 19	Freedom of expression Freedom of thought, conscience and religion	13 14
Family unification, family environment	9 10 25	Review of treatment in care	20 25	Freedom of association Right to Privacy	15 16
Freedom of thought, conscience and religion	14	Adoption Refugee children	21 22	Access to information	17
Parental responsibilities, state assistance	18	Children with disabilities Child labor	23 32		
Health and health care	24	Drug abuse	33		
Leisure and play	31	Sexual exploitation	34		
Social security and standard of living	26 27	Abduction, sale and trafficking	35		
Education	28 29	Juvenile justice	37 40		
		Armed conflicts	38		
		Rehabilitation of child victims	39		

Reproduced with permission from Steven H. Woolf; The Youth Mental Health Crisis in the United States: Epidemiology, Contributors, and Potential Solutions. Pediatrics November 2025; 156 (5): e2025070849. https://doi.org/10.1542/peds.2025-070849. Copyright© 2025 by the AAP.

services are available. Hence access to and protection of the *humanitarian space* is a crucial principle of humanitarian pediatrics. Security, diplomacy, and logistics are critically important to secure and maintain this space and are thus important components of humanitarian pediatrics.

Humanitarian pediatrics will provide credibility to the global roles pediatricians and other child health professionals play and help secure their presence where decisions are made related to children's health and wellbeing. It will catalyze the recognition that pediatricians have agency—they are respected and have the knowledge, expertise, and experience necessary to advance the rights of children and sustainable development goals (SDGs).[13] It will facilitate the translation of these assets into a currency that is valued by the global institutions and organizations determining the future of children. Unfortunately, when confronted by polycrises and oppression, these institutions and organizations have generally failed to fulfill children's rights as articulated in the CRC—International and human rights laws, courts, conventions, accords, policies, and statements have failed to protect children and advance equity, social justice, and child rights. In the future, pediatricians trained in humanitarian pediatrics will have the knowledge, competencies, and credibility to engage in the development of intersectoral and interdisciplinary strategies to address the current crises impacting children.

HOW TO RESPOND

There is a nascent commitment of pediatricians and pediatric associations to respond to national and global humanitarian polycrises. It is important and urgent to explore and provide strategies to support and sustain this response—on the local, regional, national, and international levels.

Among these strategies is the practice of *Témoignage*, a French term meaning *bearing witness*.[14] At its core, *bearing witness* means refusing silence—naming the harm, while using the authority of pediatricians and Pediatrics to press for accountability, advance their rights, and ultimately to seek peace. With respect to humanitarian crises, children affected by war often lose their rights to safety and their ability to be heard. Children's voices can be amplified by:

- Documenting and sharing stories of children's suffering and resilience in medical journals, public forums, and advocacy campaigns.
- Collaborating with journalists, artists, and child rights organizations to *ethically* highlight children's experiences.
- Encouraging child participation in shaping postconflict health and education recovery programs.

Témoignage

Through the acts of *Témoignage*,[14] statistics can be transformed into lived realities, and empathy and political will mobilized. Clinical encounters can be transformed into testimony by documenting and ethically sharing children's stories of injury, loss, and resilience. By elevating children's voices through journals, media, and policy forums, data can be humanized and society compelled to confront the realities of the impact of humanitarian crises on children.

Systemic justice can be advanced by bearing witness to the structural causes of children's suffering—displacement, inequality, war crimes, crimes against humanity, genocide—by the following:

- Using clinical data to expose systemic patterns of harm (eg, targeting hospitals, malnutrition due to blockades).

- Partnering with human rights and humanitarian law experts to testify before commissions, courts, and national and international bodies.
- Promoting policies that protect children's rights to health, safety, and development.

Advocacy can be shifted from symptom relief to addressing the root cause determinants of the violation of children's rights to life and optimal survival and development.

Medical Care

The provision of medical care to children by professionals prepared and available to do so is a necessary component of humanitarian pediatrics. For example, care givers should understand child development and how this impacts the experience and expression of trauma. It is also imperative to have access to specialized medical care and resources capable of responding to the needs of children across the age continuum from infancy through adolescence. It is important to engage local providers who are familiar with the tools and resources necessary to deliver optimal care in the settings in which they work. In addition to care, indigenous providers can provide the most credible and legitimate form of *Temoignage*.

Education and Research

Evidence and expertise that improves care and advocacy can be established by the following:

- Conducting and supporting research documenting the health impacts of armed conflict.
- Including humanitarian pediatrics and child rights in child health training curricula.
- Mentoring young clinicians and public health professionals in ethical witnessing and advocacy.

Scientifically grounded and ethically informed pediatric voices in humanitarian discourse can be expanded. Through rigorous research and education, child health professionals can document the health and developmental impacts of armed conflict, climate change, globalization and other humanitarian crises, develop evidence-based interventions, and train future health professionals to respond ethically and effectively. These actions transform witnessing into knowledge and action.

Policy Development

Existing and novel platforms can be used to ensure policies reflect children's realities, are informed by the principles of child rights and Humanitarian Pediatrics, and influence political decisions by the following:

- Presenting evidence to ministries, parliaments, and private and public sector international bodies.
- Contributing to policy briefs, child protection frameworks, and health reconstruction plans.
- Using professional associations as vehicles for advocacy statements and global appeals.

Insight and experience with recovery agendas can be embedded into policies. Pediatricians and child health professionals can use their credibility and access to data to shape the response to humanitarian crises.

Professional Associations and Networks

By engaging professional associations, media, and global health institutions, pediatricians and child health professionals can ensure children's experiences are central to reconstruction, justice, and peace efforts. The International Society for Social Pediatrics and Child Health (ISSOP) is an example of a global organization addressing humanitarian crises impacting children, including armed conflict, climate change, globalization and displacement.

Professional networks can be established to integrate our work, create solidarity, and strengthen moral courage and impact, by the following:

- Joining or forming national and international health professional coalitions.
- Collaborating with educators, social workers, and faith leaders to establish intersectoral coalitions.
- Engaging diaspora and local communities to amplify advocacy.

Individual witnessing can be converted into a global collective moral force by engaging and organizing the efforts of global organizations, for example, International Pediatric Association, ISSOP, nongovernment organizations, etc.

Child Rights

Pediatricians and child health professionals can translate the principles, standards, and norms of Child Rights into clinical care, systems development, policy generation, strategies, and tools to identify, articulate, and respond to rights violations. The CRC,[12] the CRC Optional Protocol on the Involvement of Children in Armed Conflict,[15] CRC General Comments, UN Convention on the Rights of People with Disabilities,[16] SDGs,[13] Geneva Conventions[2] and other global human rights conventions, resolutions, and treaties provide the foundation to integrate a child rights–based approach into humanitarian pediatrics.

Foundational child rights principles of universality, accountability, indivisibility and interdependence of rights, youth participation, transparency, and nondiscrimination[17] solidify and contribute to the relevance of a child rights–based approach to the roles, capacity, and responsibility of pediatricians and child health associations, and other stakeholders in children's health and wellbeing—to respond. A child rights–based approach[18] transforms children from passive victims and objects of rights into active subjects and holders of rights. It insists that the response to polycrises and oppression does not just restore services and infrastructure, but also advances justice, dignity, and agency for every child.

Though the United States remains the only country that has not ratified the CRC, its articles and the principles of child rights are as relevant to children in the United States as they are to children globally. As such, it is equally as important for US pediatric clinicians to apply a child rights–based approach to their efforts to advance the health and wellbeing of children as it is for colleagues globally. Our failure to do so as providers and health care systems is a source of the disparities in children's health in the United States in comparison to other high-income countries.

Advancing humanitarian pediatrics

Humanitarian pediatrics is the next step toward an aspirational era that coalesces current efforts and advances child rights. In this era the following are maintained,

- Life and optimal survival and development of children are recognized as the primary organizing principles and drivers for establishing social, economic, environmental, cultural, and political systems.

- Decisions impacting children and youth are rights, justice, and equity-based, particularly those related to humanitarian crises.
- Child wellbeing is a central measure of social justice, equity, and moral legitimacy.
- Conditions shaping children's health, development, and rights are understood as the defining lens for evaluating social, economic, environmental, and political systems.
- Institutions, policies, and systems protect and promote child wellbeing, as measured by population-level rights-based indicators.
- Moral and ethical imperatives exist to protect and maintain the material and legal conditions necessary for children's optimal survival and development.[19]

Advancing the practice of *Humanitarian Pediatrics* will require national and global pediatric and child health organizations, that is, International Pediatric Association, Union of Arab Pediatric Societies, Asia Pacific Pediatric Association, European Association of Paediatrics, Union of African Paediatric Societies and Associations, Latin American Pediatric Association, ISSOP, to integrate their work into an effective and sustained cooperative global network capable of participating in global responses to humanitarian crises affecting children. The generation and implementation of rights-respecting child health services, systems, and policies are components of this effort. Familiarity with definitions, meaning, and relevance of International Human Rights Law, including the terminology of genocide, war crimes, crimes against humanity, and the Geneva Conventions,[2] is essential. Genuine presence in national and global public and private sector organizations and agencies, committees and boards, academic institutions, and other venues where decisions are made about children will help to build the field of humanitarian pediatrics. Strategies for educating professionals about the principles and practice of child rights and implementing elements of advocacy and *Témoignage* will be necessary.[14] Contribution to and participation in national and international judicial systems is critical.

In this regard, it is critically important for pediatrics to adopt *humanitarian pediatrics* as its next stage of development (see **Fig. 1**) and recognize it as core to its mission, by the following:

- Explicitly engaging a focus on child rights and SDGs.[13]
- Redefining pediatric professionalism to include clinical care, systems development, policy generation, and defense of children's rights—especially in contexts of climate disruption, armed conflict, globalization, and democratic erosion.
- Shifting from a primary focus on disease treatment to addressing the social, political, economic, cultural, commercial and environmental conditions that determine child health outcomes.
- Bearing witness to violations of children's rights to optimal survival and development through the practice of *Témoignage*,[14] and speak with authority.
- Recognizing pediatricians and pediatric societies have unique moral and scientific legitimacy—silence in the face of preventable harm to children is not neutrality—it is complicity.
- Training and preparing the next generation of child health professionals to understand and intervene in systems that shape child health.

If pediatricians, child health professionals, and child health professional societies accept a future in which child suffering is normalized—in which climate change, armed conflict, displacement, authoritarianism, and violations of children's rights to optimal survival and development happen with impunity—preventable harm becomes inevitable. Climate instability, poverty, violence, discrimination, authoritarianism and oppression have emerged as existential challenges to children's health, wellbeing, and identity. *Humanitarian pediatrics*, with its focus on child rights,[12] equity, and social justice offers tools and a roadmap to prevent what medicine cannot repair.

INSIGHTS TO ACTION

- Child health and wellbeing–globally and in the US–is increasingly being defined by polycrises.
- Humanitarian Pediatrics is a child rights-based evolving discipline responding to the effects of polycrises on children.
- Pediatricians in the future need to be trained in child rights-based principles and practice of Humanitarian Pediatrics.

DECLARATION OF AI AND AI-ASSISTED TECHNOLOGIES IN THE WRITING PROCESS

During the preparation of this work, the authors used GenAI to edit the article. After using this tool/service, the authors reviewed and edited the content as needed and take full responsibility for the content of the publication.

DISCLOSURE

The authors have no financial disclosures or conflicts of interest to disclose.

REFERENCES

1. Children's Villages SOS. Impact of the polycrisis: how do we protect and care for children?. 2023. Available at: https://www.sos-childrensvillages.org/news/polycrisis#:~:text=The%20polycrisis%20is%20a%20set%20of%20multiple%2C,*%20**Physical%20health%20concerns**%20*%20**Extreme%20trauma**. Accessed January 15, 2026.
2. International Committee of the Red Cross. The Geneva conventions and their commentaries. Available at: https://www.icrc.org/en/law-and-policy/geneva-conventions-and-their-commentaries#:~:text=Treaty%20database:%20full%20texts%2C%20commentaries,conflicts:%20Applying%20international%20humanitarian%20law. Accessed January 21, 2026.
3. Feeding America. Child hunger keeps kids from reaching their full potential. 2026. Available at: https://www.feedingamerica.org/hunger-in-america/child-hunger-facts. Accessed January 21, 2026.
4. National Center for Education Statistics. Concentration of public school students eligible for free or reduced-price lunch. Condition of education. U.S. Department of Education, Institute of Education Sciences; 2024. Available at: https://nces.ed.gov/programs/coe/indicator/clb. Accessed January 21, 2026.
5. Lebrun-Harris LA, Sandel M, Sheward R, et al. Prevalence and correlates of unstable housing among US children. JAMA Pediatr 2024;178(7):707–17. PMID: 38767882; PMCID: PMC11106712. Available at: https://pmc.ncbi.nlm.nih.gov/articles/PMC11106712/#:~:text=In%202022%2C%2017.1%25%20(95,other%20types%20of%20hardships%20examined). Accessed January 21, 2026.
6. Johns Hopkins Center for Gun Violence Solutions. Gun violence in the United States 2022 examining the burden among children and teens. Available at: https://

publichealth.jhu.edu/sites/default/files/2024-09/2022-cgvs-gun-violence-in-the-united-states.pdf. Accessed January 21, 2026.
7. Nam-Sonenstein B, Sawyer W. Youth confinement: the whole pie 2025. Prison Policy Initiative; 2025. Available at: https://www.prisonpolicy.org/reports/youth2025.html. Accessed January 21, 2026.
8. Oberg C, Kivlahan C, Mishori R, et al. Treatment of migrant children on the US Southern border is consistent with torture. Pediatrics 2021;147(1):e2020012930. https://doi.org/10.1542/peds.2020-012930. Epub 2020 Oct 27. [Erratum in: Pediatrics. 2021 May;147(5):e2021050943. doi: 10.1542/peds.2021-050943]. PMID: 33109743. Available at: https://pubmed.ncbi.nlm.nih.gov/33109743/. Accessed January 21, 2026.
9. Hornor G, Chiocca EM. Trauma exposure in migrant children: implications for mental and physical health. J Pediatr Health Care 2025;39(5):836–47. PMID: 40897443. Available at: https://pubmed.ncbi.nlm.nih.gov/40897443/. Accessed January 21, 2026.
10. Economic Policy Institute. Child labor laws are under attack in states across the country. 2023. Available at: https://www.epi.org/publication/child-labor-laws-under-attack/. Accessed February 25, 2026.
11. Woolf SH. The youth mental health crisis in the United States: epidemiology, contributors, and potential solutions. Pediatrics 2025;156(5):e2025070849.
12. United Nations Human Rights Office of the High Commissioner. Convention on the rights of the child. 1989. Available at: https://www.ohchr.org/en/instruments-mechanisms/instruments/convention-rights-child. Accessed February 13, 2026.
13. United Nations Department of Economic and Social Affairs Sustainable Development. The 17 goals. 2015. Available at: https://sdgs.un.org/goals. Accessed February 13, 2026.
14. Patel A, Alayyan A, Haq HA, et al. Bearing witness: témoignage as a tool for child advocacy during armed conflict. PLOS Glob Public Health 2025;5(9):e0004947. PMID: 40929085; PMCID: PMC12422417. Available at: https://pubmed.ncbi.nlm.nih.gov/40929085/. Accessed January 21, 2026.
15. UN of the Special Representative of the Secretary-General for Children and Armed Conflict. Optional Protocol to the Convention on the Rights of the Child on the involvement of children in armed conflict. 2000. Available at: https://childrenandarmedconflict.un.org/tools-for-action/optional-protocol/. Accessed January 21, 2026.
16. UN Department of Economic and Social Affairs Social Inclusion. Convention on the rights of persons with disabilities (CRPD). Available at: https://social.desa.un.org/issues/disability/crpd/convention-on-the-rights-of-persons-with-disabilities-crpd#:~:text=The%20Convention%20follows%20decades%20of,fastest%20negotiated%20human%20rights%20treaty. Accessed January 21, 2026.
17. United Nations Population Fund. Human rights principles. 2005. Available at: https://www.unfpa.org/resources/human-rights-principles. Accessed January 21, 2026.
18. Unicef. United Kingdom. Child friendly cities and communities. A child rights-based approach. Available at: https://www.unicef.org.uk/child-friendly-cities/crba/. Accessed January 21, 2026.
19. Laraque D. A moral imperative for children. JAMA 2009;302(8):892–3.
20. Save the Children. Stop the war on children – security for whom?. 2025. Available at: https://resourcecentre.savethechildren.net/document/stop-the-war-on-children-security-for-whom-2025?_gl=1*17urotf*_gcl_au*MTcyMDY1ODM0NC4xNzY4MzE0NTQ4*_ga*MTEyNDM2MDIwNS4xNzY4MzE0NTQ4*_ga_GRKVSTV36C*czE3Njgz

MTQ1NDckbzEkZzAkdDE3NjgzMTQ1NDgkajYwJGwwJGgw. Accessed January 15, 2026.
21. ReliefWeb. Children affected by armed conflict (1990-2024). 2024. Available at: https://reliefweb.int/report/world/children-affected-armed-conflict-1990-2024. Accessed January 15, 2026.
22. UNICEF. Nearly 50 million children uprooted worldwide. 2025. Available at: https://www.unicef.org/press-releases/nearly-50-million-children-uprooted-worldwide. Accessed January 15, 2026.
23. UNICEF. Climate displacement report (English). 2025. Available at: https://www.unicef.org/media/145951/file/Climate%20displacement%20report%20(English).pdf. Accessed January 15, 2026.
24. ReliefWeb. About 8 million babies born from conflicts and climate disasters. 2025. Available at: https://reliefweb.int/report/world/about-8-million-babies-born-conflicts-and-climate-disasters-2025. Accessed January 15, 2026.
25. EPA. CLiME final report. 2023. Available at: https://www.epa.gov/system/files/documents/2023-04/CLiME_Final%20Report.pdf. Accessed January 15, 2026.
26. Arráiz de Fernández C, Fernández Soto G, Rojas Conde L, et al. Effects of malnutrition on child neurodevelopment and mental health. Salud, Ciencia y Tecnología 2024;4:742. *Article 868/200*. Revision 2025. Available at: https://sct.ageditor.ar/index.php/sct/article/view/868/200. Accessed January 15, 2026.
27. Thapa S, Giri S, Ross AG. Extreme weather and climate-related adverse childhood experiences are a humanitarian crisis during the 21st century. Commun Med 2025;5:357. Available at: https://www.nature.com/articles/s43856-025-01089-x. Accessed January 15, 2026.
28. IIED. Report 20441G. 2021. Available at: https://www.iied.org/sites/default/files/pdfs/2021-09/20441G.pdf. Accessed January 15, 2026.
29. Harvard Developing Child. ECSCEE heat paper. 2024. Available at: https://developingchild.harvard.edu/wp-content/uploads/2024/10/ECSCEE-Heat-Paper.pdf. Accessed January 15, 2026.
30. Poverty Child. Street children – everything about this global humanitarian crisis. 2025. Available at: https://povertychild.org/street-children-everything-about-this-global-humanitarian-crisis/. Accessed January 15, 2026.
31. UNICEF. Global estimates of child labour – executive summary (2025). 2025. Available at: https://data.unicef.org/wp-content/uploads/2025/06/2024-Global-Estimates-of-Child-Labour-Executive-Summary-ENGLISH.pdf. Accessed January 15, 2026.
32. Sage Publishers. Urban studies – street children. 2025. Available at: https://sk.sagepub.com/ency/edvol/urbanstudies/chpt/street-children#_. Accessed January 15, 2026.
33. Noncommunicable Diseases Alliance. Harmful marketing – selling a sick future to children and teens. 2025. Available at: https://ncdalliance.org/stories/media-hub/videos/harmful-marketing-selling-sick-future-children-and-teens#:~:text=Industries%20involved%20in%20tobacco%2C%20alcohol%2C%20junk%20food,consumers%2C%20exploiting%20their%20naivete%2C%20vulnerability%20and%20emotions. Accessed January 15, 2026.
34. Abdi YH, Abdi MS, Bashir SG, et al. Understanding global health inequality and inequity: causes, consequences, and the path toward justice in healthcare. Public Health Chall 2025;4(4):e70156. PMID: 41146749; PMCID: PMC12553980. Available at: https://pmc.ncbi.nlm.nih.gov/articles/PMC12553980/#:~:text=The%20findings%20highlight%20that%20structural%20determinants%2C%20such,and

%20increased%20mortality%20rates%20in%20disadvantaged%20populations. Accessed January 15, 2026.
35. Vaghri Z, Tessier Z, Whalen C. Refugee and asylum-seeking children: interrupted child development and unfulfilled child rights. Children (Basel) 2019;6(11):120. PMID: 31671545; PMCID: PMC6915556. Available at: https://pmc.ncbi.nlm.nih.gov/articles/PMC6915556/. Accessed January 15, 2026.
36. UNICEF. Children's well-being: the wealthiest countries took a sharp turn for the worse following COVID-19. 2025. Available at: https://www.unicef.org/press-releases/childrens-wellbeing-worlds-wealthiest-countries-took-sharp-turn-worse-wake-covid-19. Accessed January 15, 2026.

Sexual Violence Against Children in Humanitarian Settings

Eugene Kongnyuy, MD, PhD, Christine Apio, MSc, MA*

KEYWORDS

- Gender-based violence • Conflict-related sexual violence
- Sexual violence against children in humanitarian settings • Child sexual abuse

KEY POINTS

- Children in humanitarian settings face heighened risks of sexual violence, including rape, sexual slavery, and exploitation, driven by conflict, displacement, and collapsed protective systems.
- Reliable data are scarce, but UN reports indicate rising conflict-related sexual violence against children, with significant under-reporting driven by stigma, fear, and limited services.
- An effective response requires robust, intersectoral coordination between gender-based violence and child protection agencies, guided by international humanitarian standards to provide life-saving, child-sensitive care.
- Evidence gaps persist, particularly on sexual violence against boys and technology-facilitated abuse, limiting effective prevention, detection and response efforts in humanitarian emergencies.

INTRODUCTION

Article 1 of the Convention on the Rights of the Child defines a child as any person under 18, unless majority is reached earlier under national law. Sexual violence is any sexual act, attempt, unwanted advance, or exploitation involving coercion, threats, or force, regardless of the perpetrator's relationship to the victim (World Health Organization, 2002, as cited in Inter-Agency Standing Committee, 2015, p. 322).[1] Against children, it includes any deliberate or exploitative act of a sexual nature—completed or attempted—that causes or risks physical or psychological harm (UNICEF, 2024).[2]

During emergencies, there is a heightened risk of sexual violence, exploitation, and abuse of children due to large-scale displacement, presence of armed groups, weak

United Nations Population Fund, Humanitarian Response Division, Rue de Varembe 7, 1202, Geneva, Switzerland
* Corresponding author.
E-mail address: chapio@unfpa.org

Pediatr Clin N Am 73 (2026) 943–951
https://doi.org/10.1016/j.pcl.2026.04.005 **pediatric.theclinics.com**

Abbreviations	
CAAC	Children and Armed Conflicts
GBV	gender-based violence
IRC	International Rescue Committee
PoLR	provider of last resort
UNFPA	United Nations Population Fund

rule of law and social protection institutions, overcrowded camps, separation from caregivers, and food insecurity. At the same time, national systems, including health and legal systems, and community and social support networks, weaken. This breakdown of systems can reduce access to critical life-saving services, such as health, protection, and legal services, leading to an environment of impunity in which perpetrators go unaccounted. When systems and services are disrupted or destroyed, children face an even higher risk of human rights violations, such as sexual violence, including sexual exploitation and abuse.

According to the Inter-Agency Standing Committee Guidelines (2015), humanitarian settings require urgent attention to sexual violence due to its immediate, life-threatening health consequences and the critical role of timely medical care in prevention and response.[3]

DISCUSSION

Policy and Legal Frameworks

At the international level, the Convention on the Rights of the Child (and its Optional Protocols), United Nations Security Council resolutions on Conflict-Related Sexual Violence and Children and Armed Conflicts (CAAC) frameworks create obligations to prevent, punish, and remedy sexual violence against children.[4–6] Specifically, CAAC reports and monitors violations for advocacy and sanctions. At the national level, many crisis-affected states have weak legal frameworks and/or weak enforcement, and non–child-sensitive procedures where frameworks exist, as well as the near-collapse of justice systems in active conflict, which produces impunity. Humanitarian settings expose these enforcement gaps acutely.

Forms and Manifestations of Sexual Violence Among Children

Sexual violence takes many forms, including rape, sexual slavery and/or trafficking, forced pregnancy, sexual harassment, sexual exploitation and/or abuse, and forced abortion. In a UNICEF Evidence Review (2015),[7] child sexual abuse is the involvement of a child in sexual activity that they do not fully comprehend, are unable to give informed consent to, or for which the child is not developmentally prepared and cannot give permission, or that violates the laws or social taboos of society. This may include, but is not limited to, the inducement or coercion of a child to engage in any unlawful sexual activity, the exploitative use of a child in prostitution or other illegal sexual practices, including the exploitative use of children in pornographic performances and materials. Generally, children are unable to provide informed consent because they do not have the ability and/or experience to anticipate the implications of an action, and they may not understand or be empowered to exercise their right to refuse.

Children in humanitarian settings experience a wide range of sexual violence forms. These forms commonly overlap (polyvictimization) and are shaped by displacement, armed presence, and breakdown of the rule of law:

- Contact sexual violence (rape, gang rape, sexual slavery, and sexual exploitation).

- Noncontact sexual violence (harassment, grooming, and exposure to pornography).
- Use of child marriage and transactional sex as perceived protective or survival strategies. As documented in Syria, Chad, northern Cameroon, Nigeria, and Afghanistan, among other humanitarian contexts, families who have lost livelihoods, land, and homes due to crisis may perceive marrying off a daughter as a coping strategy to alleviate acute economic hardship and to reduce the number of dependents within a household. In some crisis-affected environments, families often anticipate heightened insecurity and violence and may view marriage as a means of *protecting* girls from perceived risks, despite the well-documented harms associated with child marriage (Girls Not Brides, 2018). Similarly, in Ethiopia and South Sudan, drought-induced food insecurity compounded by ongoing armed conflict has contributed to increases in early marriage, including instances in which girls are married in exchange for livestock to support household survival (Castañeda and colleagues, 2020).
- Abduction, detention-related sexual violence and use of sexual violence as a tactic of war.

In terms of perpetration, children are most likely to experience sexual abuse perpetrated by someone known to them, typically as an adult or older child who is a family member, relative, family friend, or an individual in a position of trust or authority.[8,9] Evidence consistently demonstrates that the predominant perpetrators of sexual violence against children are those within their immediate social environment, including family members, peers, and intimate partners.[7]

Data and Trends of Sexual Violence Against Children in Humanitarian Settings

Drawing on the Inter-Agency Standing Committee Guidelines for Integrating Gender-Based Violence Interventions in Humanitarian Action,[10] prevalence data on sexual violence in emergencies are notoriously difficult to obtain due to security risks, limited services, and ethical concerns. As a result, most information comes from qualitative research, anecdotal accounts, monitoring tools, and service statistics.

No reliable prevalence data exist for sexual violence against children in armed conflict, though evidence from specific contexts shows widespread abuse of women and girls. UNICEF global data indicate that in fragile and conflict-affected settings, childhood rape and sexual assault occur at twice the global average,[11] with actual cases vastly under-reported due to stigma, fear, harmful norms, lack of services, and impunity.

The United Nations Annual Report of the Secretary-General on Children and Armed Conflict (June 2025) found sexual violence against children rose 35% in 2024, with gang rape cases surging. Haiti reported the highest verified cases (566), followed by Nigeria (419), the Democratic Republic of Congo (358), and Somalia (267). The report underscores persistent under-reporting driven by stigma, reprisals, and systemic gaps.[12]

Save the Children's analysis of UN annual reports shows verified cases of sexual violence against children in conflict reached 1938 in 2024—the highest since records began—marking a 50% increase since 2020.[13]

Number of verified cases of conflict-related sexual violence perpetrated against children:[12–15]

- 2025 report for 2024 figures: 1938 cases;
- 2024 report for 2023 figures: 1470 cases;
- 2023 report for 2022 figures: 1165 cases;

- 2022 report for 2021 figures: 1326 cases;
- 2021 report for 2020 figures: 1268 cases

Data from International Rescue Committee (IRC)–supported gender-based violence (GBV) programs in conflict-affected settings reveal the high prevalence of sexual violence against children. In the Central African Republic, nearly half of GBV survivors receiving IRC support were girls under 18. In Sierra Leone, 73% of female survivors were under 18, including 23% under 11. Almost all reported cases involved sexual violence, predominantly rape—97% among children aged 0% to 11% and 96% among those aged 12 to 18.[a,16]

Impacts of Sexual Violence on Children

Sexual violence has profound and lasting impacts on children, their families, and communities. As emphasized in the Inter-Agency Standing Committee Guidelines and the Inter-Agency Minimum Standards for GBV programming in emergencies, GBV—including sexual violence—undermines survivors' immediate sexual, physical, and psychological health and heightens risks of future health problems. For children, the consequences can be devastating: increased infant mortality, low birth weight, malnutrition, disrupted schooling, physical impairments, developmental delays, and long-term mental health conditions. Impacts range from physical injury, sexually transmitted infections (STIs) (including HIV), and unwanted pregnancy to post traumatic stress disorders (PTSD), depression, suicidal ideation, stigma, and intergenerational harm. In emergencies, limited access to medical, psychosocial, and legal support exacerbates these outcomes.[17]

Save the Children underscores that sexual violence against children fundamentally destroys futures: survivors often suffer severe injuries due to their developing bodies, including reproductive damage leading to incontinence, infertility, chronic pain, and heightened risk of STIs.[18] Pregnant girls face life-threatening complications, forced school dropout, and social exclusion. UNICEF (2024) warns that childhood is a critical period to intervene, as survivors risk revictimization or becoming perpetrators later in life.[2]

Intersectional Needs of Children

Children's vulnerabilities and experiences of sexual violence are shaped by intersecting identities—including gender, race, religion, geography, and physical ability—which influence their exposure to risks, protective factors, service needs, and help-seeking behaviors.[19] Despite this, major data gaps remain, particularly concerning sexual violence against boys and noncontact forms of abuse.[11] Boys associated with armed actors or held in detention may be subjected to rape, sexual torture, genital mutilation, sexual humiliation, sexual enslavement, and forced incest.[19] Addressing the needs of male survivors requires an intersectional approach that recognizes how sexual violence affects them and ensures safe, appropriate, and responsive entry points for services tailored to their circumstances.

The United Nations Response to Child Survivors of Sexual Violence in Humanitarian Settings

As the global lead agency for gender-based violence (GBV) and the designated Provider of Last Resort for GBV services, the United Nations Population Fund (UNFPA) coordinates GBV prevention, risk mitigation and response efforts within the Protection

---

[a] These figures are derived from cases reported to IRC-supported GBV programmes and recorded in the GBVIMS; they do not represent population-level prevalence estimates.

Cluster led by the United Nations High Commissioner for Refugees (UNHCR). Through its technical leadership and coordination functions, UNFPA supports the establishment and strengthening of survivor-centered, multi-sectoral service delivery systems and referral pathways with the aim of improving access to quality care and protection services for GBV survivors, child survivors of sexual violence.[20] In 2025, a major reform was introduced to make humanitarian work more efficient and accountable. As a part of this change, the global coordination system was simplified, reducing the number of clusters from 11 to 8 broader, integrated clusters. One of these is the Global Protection Cluster. It covers several areas of protection, including GBV, child protection, mine action, and protection monitoring. Its main job is to help keep civilians safe during emergencies.

Like other clusters, the Protection Cluster has a lead agency and brings together local, national, and international organizations that work to protect people affected by crises. The cluster is led by the UN Refugee Agency (UNHCR). UNFPA and UNICEF act as *providers of last resort* (PoLRs) for GBV and child protection. This means that if no organization is available to deliver essential services in these areas, the PoLR must step in and make sure the support is provided.[21]

Recognizing the interconnected needs of child and adolescent survivors, GBV and child protection actors share overlapping responsibilities in the prevention, mitigation, and response to sexual violence against children in humanitarian settings. As crises become increasingly complex, collaboration across disciplines is essential to understand and address the evolving needs affecting children. Both the GBV and child protection minimum standards emphasize the importance of intersectoral coordination.[24,26]

COUNTRY CASE STUDIES

Sudan

In Sudan, UNICEF analysis of GBV data shared by service providers recorded 221 rape cases against children since early 2024, including survivors as young as 1 year old (**Fig. 1**).[22] While the dataset is limited, it highlights the grave risks facing women

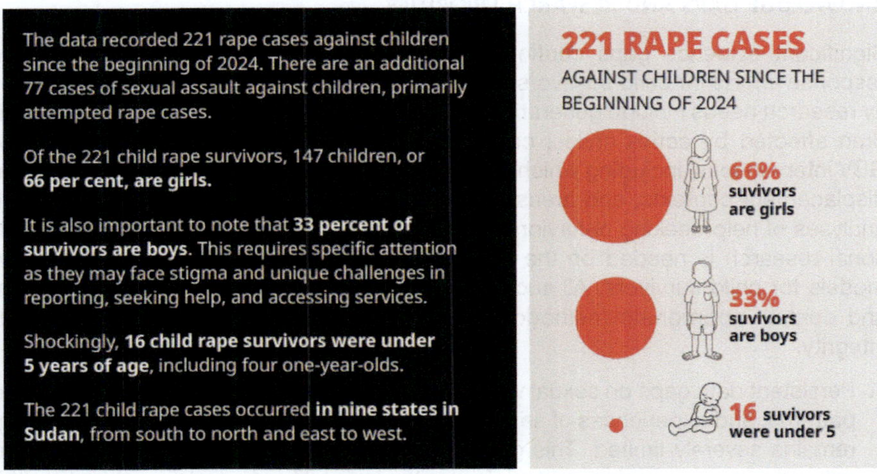

Fig. 1. Sudan's child rape and sexual violence crisis. (*Source* UNICEF. Over 370 Million Girls and Women Globally Subjected to Rape or Sexual Assault as Children - First-Ever Global Estimates on Sexual Violence in Childhood. New York, NY: UNICEF; 2024. Accessed November 21, 2025. Available at: https://www.unicef.org/eap/press-releases/over-370-million-girls-and-women-globally-subjected-rape-or-sexual-assault-children.)

and children and underscores the urgent need for survivor-centered services and safe, ethical data systems. According to the GBV Area of Responsibility led by UNFPA, now consolidated under the Protection Cluster, a coordination structure that brings together local, national, and international organizations delivering services to protect people affected by GBV in humanitarian crises in Sudan, many survivors remain unable to access life-saving services due to insecurity, restricted humanitarian access, and looting of medical supplies and facilities.[23]

Democratic Republic of the Congo

The 2024 *Children and Armed Conflict* report of the UN Secretary-General verified 662 cases of sexual violence against children (7 boys and 655 girls), aged 1 to 17.[14] These included rape (386), forced marriage (106), gang rape (100), sexual slavery (65), and attempted rape. Survivors included children as young as 3. Despite high prevalence, sexual violence remains under-reported due to fear of reprisals, stigma, and social exclusion.[14]

Haiti

In Haiti, sexual violence has been systematically used by armed gangs to instill fear, punish, subjugate, and control local populations. Gang members abduct, rape, and sexually assault girls during neighborhood attacks and during daily activities such as commuting to school.[24,25] Children engaged in commercial sex acts are victims of exploitation and collective rape by gangs requires specialized health care. This abuse remains substantially underreported, widespread impunity and fear of reprisals further impede survivors' access to justice and accountability mechanisms, and the GBV Area of Responsibility, now consolidated under the protection cluster, reported that sexual violence is used to instill fear and control populations, yet remains widely under-reported. Survivors often lack access to postrape treatment kits, heightening risks of HIV, STIs, and unwanted pregnancies, while impunity and fear of reprisals block access to justice.[25,26]

KNOWLEDGE GAPS AND RESEARCH PRIORITIES

Significant evidence gaps continue to limit the effectiveness of prevention and response efforts for child survivors of sexual violence in humanitarian settings. Priority research needs include generating reliable prevalence and incidence data for children affected by active crises; conducting rigorous evaluations of child-sensitive GBV interventions, including which models are most effective in camp settings, urban displacement contexts, and areas of ongoing conflict; and undertaking systematic analyses of help-seeking behaviors disaggregated by age, sex, and disability. Additional research is needed on the cost-effectiveness of integrated service delivery models for child survivors. All such research must be grounded in careful, ethical, and context-appropriate methodologies to avoid traumatization and ensure data integrity.

1. Persistent data gaps on sexual violence against boys. Evidence on the prevalence, patterns, and experiences of sexual violence among boys in humanitarian settings remains severely limited. This gap obscures the scale of the problem, hampers tailored service provision, and reinforces the invisibility of boys' experiences within GBV and child protection systems.
2. Insufficient evidence on technology-facilitated sexual abuse and exploitation. Although internet access and mobile connectivity have expanded rapidly, research on the nature, scale, and dynamics of these emerging harms—particularly in

humanitarian contexts—remains scarce. Better data are needed to understand risk pathways, perpetrator tactics, and effective prevention and response strategies for digitally mediated forms of sexual abuse against children.

SUMMARY

Sexual violence against children in humanitarian settings remains one of the most severe and underaddressed protection concerns in contemporary crises. Although global policy frameworks and humanitarian standards recognize children's heightened vulnerability, evidence across multiple contexts shows that existing systems often fail to prevent, identify, or adequately respond to these violations. The scarcity of reliable data, particularly on boys, adolescents, and technology-facilitated forms of abuse, continues to obscure the full scale and complexity of the problem, limiting the effectiveness of prevention and response efforts. At the same time, evolving patterns of conflict, displacement, and digital connectivity are generating new risks that outpace current research and programming models.

INSIGHTS TO ACTION

- Pediatric clinicians in all settings should be aware that children from humanitarian crisis backgrounds are at significantly heightened risk for sexual violence and its associated physical and mental health sequelae.
- A trauma-informed, survivor-centered approach is critical when dealing with any child suspected of being a survivor of sexual violence. This includes ensuring privacy, confidentiality, and informed consent (from the child, where possible and appropriate).
- Be familiar with and able to provide or refer for essential clinical services for child survivors of sexual violence, including postexposure prophylaxis for HIV, emergency contraception, STI prophylaxis, and medical-legal documentation.
- Recognize that boys are also survivors of sexual violence, though they may be even less likely to disclose. Avoid gendered assumptions about who can be a victim.
- Coordination with on-site or local GBV and child protection specialists is essential for ensuring a holistic response that addresses safety, psychosocial, and legal needs beyond the clinical setting.

DISCLOSURE

The authors have no financial disclosures or conflicts of interest to disclose.

REFERENCES

1. Inter-Agency Standing CommitteeGuidelines for integrating gender-based violence interventions in humanitarian action, 2015, Inter-Agency Standing Committee; Geneva, Switzerland, Available at: https://gbvguidelines.org/wp/wp-content/uploads/2015/09/2015-IASC-Gender-based-Violence-Guidelines_lo-res.pdf (Accessed 21 November 2025).
2. UNICEF, Over 370 million girls and women globally subjected to rape or sexual assault as children – First-Ever global estimates on sexual violence in childhood, 2024, UNICEF, New York; Available at: https://www.unicef.org/eap/press-releases/over-370-million-girls-and-women-globally-subjected-rape-or-sexual-assault-children (Accessed 21 November 2025).
3. Inter-Agency Standing CommitteeGuidelines for integrating gender-based violence interventions in humanitarian action, 2015, Inter-Agency Standing Committee;

Geneva, Switzerland, Available at: https://gbvguidelines.org/wp/wp-content/uploads/2015/09/2015-IASC-Gender-based-Violence-Guidelines_lo-res.pdf (Accessed 21 November 2025).

4. United Nations General Assembly, Convention on the rights of the child United Nations, *Treaty Series*, 1577, 1990, 3, Adopted November 20, 1989. Entered into force.
5. United Nations Security Council, Resolution 1820 (2008) on Sexual Violence in Conflict. S/RES/1820,2008.
6. United Nations Security Council, Resolution 1882 (2009) on Children and Armed Conflict. S/RES/1882, 2009. United Nations; New York.
7. UNICEF, Evidence review: sexual violence against children, 2015, UNICEF; New York, Available at: https://www.unicef.org/protection/files/UNICEF_Evidence_Review_Sexual_Violence_Children_2015.pdf (Accessed 21 November 2025).
8. Pinheiro PS. World report on violence against children. Geneva, Switzerland: United Nations; 2006.
9. UNICEF. Hidden in Plain sight: a statistical analysis of violence against children. New York: UNICEF; 2015.
10. Inter-Agency Standing Committee, Guidelines for integrating gender-based violence interventions in humanitarian action, 2015, Inter-Agency Standing Committee; Geneva, Switzerland, Available at: https://gbvguidelines.org/wp/wp-content/uploads/2015/09/2015-IASC-Gender-based-Violence-Guidelines_lo-res.pdf (Accessed 21 November 2025).
11. UNICEF, *When numbers demand action: Confronting the global scale of sexual violence against children*, UNICEF, 2024; New York, New York, Available at: https://data.unicef.org/resources/when-numbers-demand-action/ (Accessed 21 November 2025).
12. United Nations. Annual report of the secretary-general on children and armed conflict. New York: United Nations; 2025. Available at: https://childrenandarmedconflict.un.org/2025/06/annual-report-of-the-secretary-general-on-children-and-armed-conflict-2025. Accessed November 21, 2025.
13. Save the Children. Analysis of United Nations annual reports of the secretary-general on children and armed conflict: sexual violence against children in conflict. London, UK: Save the Children; 2025. Available at: https://www.savethechildren.net/news/sexual-violence-against-children-conflict-highest-records-began. Accessed November 21, 2025.
14. United Nations. Annual report of the secretary-general on children and armed conflict. New York: United Nations; 2024. Available at: https://childrenandarmedconflict.un.org/2024/06/annual-report-of-the-secretary-general-on-children-and-armed-conflict-2024. Accessed November 21, 2025.
15. United Nations. Annual report of the secretary-general on children and armed conflict. New York: United Nations; 2023. Available at: https://childrenandarmedconflict.un.org/2023/06/annual-report-of-the-secretary-general-on-children-and-armed-conflict-2023. Accessed November 21, 2025.
16. International Rescue Committee, Caring for Child Survivors of Sexual Abuse: Guidelines for health and psychosocial service providers in humanitarian settings, 2014, IRC; New York, Available at: https://www.gbvresponders.org/wp-content/uploads/2014/07/CCS-Guidelines-lowres.pdf (Accessed 21 November 2025).
17. World Health Organization. Violence against children: key facts. Geneva, Switzerland: World Health Organization; 2022. Available at: https://www.who.int/

news-room/fact-sheets/detail/violence-against-children. Accessed November 21, 2025.

18. Save the Children, Sexual Violence Against Children in Conflict Surges 50% in 5 Years to Worst Level Ever, 2025. Save the Children Press Release; London, Available at: https://www.savethechildren.org.uk/news/media-centre/press-releases/2025/sexual-violence-against-children-conflict-surges-50-5-years (Accessed 21 November 2025).
19. Family for Every Child. A systematic review of literature on the sexual abuse of boys. London, UK: Family for Every Child; 2018. Available at: https://familyforeverychild.org/report/a-systematic-review-of-literature-on-the-sexual-abuse-of-boys. Accessed November 21, 2025.
20. United Nations Population Fund (UNFPA). UNFPA's role as global lead agency for gender-based violence in emergencies. New York: UNFPA; 2020. Available at: https://www.unfpa.org/resources/gender-based-violence-emergencies. Accessed November 21, 2025.
21. Inter-Agency Standing Committee, *Guidance Note on Cluster Simplification and Adapting In-Country Coordination to Context*, 2026, Inter-Agency Standing Committee; Geneva, Switzerland, Available at: IASC Guidance Note on Cluster Simplification and Adapting In-Country Coordination to Context (Accessed 30 May 2026).
22. UNICEF. Sudan's child rape and sexual violence crisis. New York: UNICEF; 2024. Available at: https://www.unicef.org/press-releases/sudan-child-rape-sexual-violence-crisis. Accessed November 21, 2025.
23. GBV *Area of responsibility. Sudan GBV response services update*, 2024, UNFPA; Sudan, Available at: https://gbvaor.net (Accessed 21 November 2025).
24. Amnesty International. Haiti: sexual violence by armed gangs. London, UK: Amnesty International; 2024. Available at: https://www.amnesty.org/en/documents/amr36/2024/haiti-sexual-violence-report. Accessed November 21, 2025.
25. United Nations Integrated Office in Haiti and, Office of the United Nations High Commissioner for Human Rights, *Sexual Violence in Port-au-Prince: A Weapon Used by Gangs to Instill Fear*, United Nations. 2022. Port-au-Prince, Haiti and Geneva, Switzerland. Available at: https://haiti.un.org/en/203684-sexual-violence-port-au-prince-weapon-used-gangs-instill-fear?utm_source=chatgpt.com (Accessed 8 June 2026).
26. GBV *Area of responsibility. Haiti GBV response services update*, 2024, UNFPA; Port -au- Prince, Haiti, Available at: https://gbvaor.net (Accessed 21 November 2025).

Impact of Humanitarian Crises on Child Health

Pediatric Vaccination and Pandemic Preparedness in Humanitarian Settings

Annalicia Pickering, MD[a,*], Paul H. Wise, MD, MPH[b], Yvonne (Bonnie) Maldonado, MD[c]

KEYWORDS

• Pediatric immunization • Zero-dose children • Pandemic preparedness • One health • Vaccine equity • Infodemic management • Last mile • Health system resilience

KEY POINTS

- Humanitarian crises amplify pediatric vulnerability to infectious diseases due to disrupted systems and social determinants.
- Zero-dose children are concentrated in fragile and conflict-affected settings, necessitating targeted immunization strategies.
- Community engagement, trust, and infodemic management are central to vaccination success.
- Health system resilience depends on integrated services, adaptive logistics, and robust surveillance.
- Ethical, data-driven, and One Health approaches are essential for future pandemic preparedness.

INTRODUCTION

The magnitude and frequency of disease outbreaks have escalated in recent decades, highlighting the complex dynamics contributing to emerging and reemerging pediatric infectious diseases.[1] Many contributing factors are in and of themselves major challenges, ranging from climate change and geopolitical tensions to deeply entrenched systemic disparities restricting access to health care. Childhood immunization and

[a] Department of Pediatrics, Faculty Fellow, Center for Innovation in Global Health, Maternal Child Health Research Institute, Stanford University School of Medicine, Palo Alto, CA, USA; [b] Freeman Spogli Institute for International Studies, Stanford University, CA, USA; [c] Department of Pediatrics, Stanford University School of Medicine, Lucile Packard Children's Hospital at Stanford, CA, USA

* Corresponding author. Center for Academic Medicine General Pediatrics, Stanford University, 453 Quarry Road, MC 5660, Stanford, CA 94304.

E-mail address: annalicia.pickering@stanford.edu

Pediatr Clin N Am 73 (2026) 953–964
https://doi.org/10.1016/j.pcl.2026.04.006 **pediatric.theclinics.com**
0031-3955/26/

Abbreviation	
CDE	common data element

outbreak prevention hold enormous potential to reduce morbidity and mortality in crisis-affected populations. Despite their proven efficacy, vaccine coverage and outbreak response in many humanitarian settings remain suboptimal, presenting major challenges for child health protection.[2,3]

CONTEXT AND BURDEN IN HUMANITARIAN SETTINGS

In 2024, there were 14.3 million children globally who did not receive a single vaccine. Recent studies suggest a significant portion of the world's zero-dose children, or those who have not received a single dose of a routine vaccine, are located in conflict zones or humanitarian contexts. Among lower-income countries, nearly 30% (~2.9 million) of zero-dose children live in fragile and conflict-affected settings.[4–7] With approximately half a billion children exposed to armed conflict, natural disasters or humanitarian crises, recognition of the destabilizing impacts of these environments is critical to maintain effective infectious disease prevention and control.[8–10] In these fragile contexts, the vulnerability of children to communicable diseases is dramatically increased due to disrupted health systems, population displacement, and reduced access to essential services. Armed conflicts systematically destroy the social determinants of health that protect children from infectious diseases.[11,12] Children's immature immune systems, dependence on adult caregivers, and elevated metabolic needs place them at increased risk when facing conditions such as malnutrition, overcrowding, and poor sanitation, all of which contribute to increased transmission risk and disease severity.

In an era of escalating armed conflicts and increasingly protracted humanitarian crises, safeguarding children from infectious disease threats requires an understanding of the complex intersection between environmental, socioeconomic, and health determinants in these settings. Prioritizing immunization and pandemic preparedness is not only a public health necessity but an ethical imperative to upholding the fundamental right to health for all children, regardless of where they live.[13] This article examines the critical components necessary to advance these goals and highlights strategies to strengthen vaccination systems and pandemic preparedness in humanitarian contexts.

DISEASE THREAT LANDSCAPE

Several emerging and reemerging viral threats demand attention in humanitarian pediatric settings. These include: measles, which has seen concerning resurgence globally since 2016 due to declining vaccination coverage; polio, which continues to defy eradication efforts in conflict-affected regions; and various arboviral diseases like Zika, dengue, and chikungunya, whose vector ecology is predicted to expand with climate shifts. Each presents unique challenges for public health programs in humanitarian settings, requiring tailored approaches for prevention and control. The role that children play in disease transmission is often underestimated, and identification of illness in children can be challenging in regions lacking pediatric-trained health care workers. Additionally, the ever-present specter of *Disease X*, a hypothetical pathogen with pandemic potential, underscores the need for preparedness measures that anticipate the emergence of new or unknown diseases.[1]

COMMUNITY ENGAGEMENT

Equitable community engagement has proven to be a foundational unifying mechanism for improving vaccination outcomes across nearly all intervention types in humanitarian settings. The most effective strategies involve engagement across multiple levels and sectors. Engaging local leaders, recruiting community mobilizers, and addressing context-specific concerns about vaccines have demonstrated success in building trust and increasing demand. This is particularly important in settings where distrust of authorities may be high due to ongoing conflict or historical grievances. Effective community engagement goes beyond simple information dissemination to include meaningful participation of affected populations in program planning and implementation.[14] Acknowledgment of local priorities is paramount: many communities will be dismissive of vaccination efforts alone if they perceive that their more immediate suffering is being disregarded. However, while addressing upstream social determinants of health is crucial, this must be balanced with the moral imperative to provide highly effective technical interventions, including immunizations and life-saving medications.[12]

As with any public health campaign, vaccination and pandemic prevention efforts must be built atop a bedrock of trust and respect between local leaders, community members and public health officials. Trust-building can become complicated in situations of political instability, and international public health teams are encouraged to recognize the legitimacy and authority of adversarial factions when possible, since the denial of their authority will often cease all cooperation.

INFODEMIC MANAGEMENT

An additional component of trust involves agreement upon a shared set of facts. Misinformation encompasses both incorrect information that is spread inadvertently as well as disinformation or false information that is intentionally distributed. When applied to an infectious disease outbreak, the World Health Organization refers to this phenomenon as an infodemic. Efforts to combat this have centered on 2 areas: communication training for public health officials and health care workers (**Table 1**) and media literacy training for laypeople (**Table 2**), which can be incorporated into formal educational curricula or shared on an individual level. Arming communities with correct information and critical thinking skills before they are introduced to misinformation, also known as *prebunking*, is generally accepted to be most effective.[15] Medical communities are encouraged to proactively prioritize messaging when constructing disease mitigation strategies.

HEALTH SYSTEM RESILIENCE

Vaccination delivery in humanitarian contexts requires adaptive approaches that can function despite compromised security, damaged infrastructure, and mobile populations. Evidence suggests that vaccination campaigns remain a foundation of adaptive crisis response. Among these campaigns, the most successful initiatives employing multifaceted approaches leveraging a range of service delivery pathways alongside targeted recruitment and training of health care personnel.[14] Periodic Intensification of Routine Immunization (PIRI) has shown promise in boosting vaccination coverage in fragile contexts. This strategy typically involves scheduled, short-term vaccination campaigns through outreach or mobile teams. Though often short-term interventions, they can build on existing health system capacities to enhance resilience over time. For example, polio eradication infrastructure has been successfully leveraged in

Table 1
Health professionals' communication strategies[15–23]

Topic	Description
Risk communication basics	Use plain, audience-centered language and empathy to acknowledge concerns. Explain what is known/unknown and how guidance may change. Develop message maps so every spokesperson delivers the same 2–3 key points.
MI & presumptive recommendation	Open the conversation with a confident, routine recommendation (*you're due today*). Use ask–tell–ask and reflective listening to surface specific barriers. Affirm values, address risk perceptions with simple visuals, and close with a clear next step or follow-up.
Evidence-based debunking	Lead with the fact, briefly note the myth *without* repetition, and immediately explain why it's false using a simple causal story. Pair text with a single reinforcing graphic and a concrete action (where/when to vaccinate).
Infodemic management function	Stand up a small, multidisciplinary team linked to the clinical environment that continuously listens, analyzes, coordinates responses, and evaluates impact. Define roles, escalation paths, and decision rights so rumors are triaged and acted on quickly.
Ethical social listening & rumor logs	Follow circulating questions and rumors in addition to health behaviors and downstream health effects. Log items with date/source/harm potential and produce weekly insight briefs that inform messaging.
Diagnose barriers with BeSD analysis	Use standardized tools to measure drivers of vaccine uptake: opinions about vaccines, social processes, motivation to seek vaccination, and practical barriers. Tailor interventions (eg, clinic hours, messengers, frame) to the specific BeSD profile of each community.
Trusted 2-way channels	Deploy low-bandwidth, high-trust options such as WhatsApp or IVR chatbots, call centers, and clinic desk scripts that give consistent answers, capture new questions, and route complex cases.
Media/platform partnerships	Prenegotiate *fast lanes* with local media and platform reps for rumor escalation and corrective PSAs. Publish transparent situation updates (what changed and why) to sustain trust during evolving evidence.
Measurement & rapid learning	Track a small KPI set (ie, detection-to-response time, resolution rate, reach/recall, sentiment, BeSD shifts, and vaccine uptake) and run A/B tests on frames and messengers. Feed results into weekly ops huddles to adapt tactics.
Preparedness assets	Prebuild FAQ banks and message maps for priority pathogens and vaccines. Cocreate messages with faith/youth leaders, midwives and other community members. Ensure materials reflect local languages, norms and practical barriers (travel time, childcare, and so on).

Abbreviations: BeSD, behavioral and social drivers; FAQ, frequently asked question; IVR, interactive voice response; KPI, key performance indicator; MI, motivational interviewing; PSA, public service announcement.

Table 2
Community member education strategies[15,24–27]

Topic	Description
Media & health literacy microlessons	Learn quick checks like lateral reading (open a new tab, check *About* pages), verify sources and dates, and look for scientific consensus rather than single influencers. Practice using local examples and short role-plays
Prebunking: spotting manipulation	Share brief *inoculation* lessons that reveal common misinformation tactics such as scapegoating, false dichotomies, or fake experts, so people recognize them when you see them. Reinforce via short videos or social stories before major campaign pushes
Pause-before-share accuracy prompts	Encourage the use of simple reminders to think about accuracy before reposting. Take 30 s to check the headline against the article and see if other reputable sources confirm the claim
Where to find verified info	Bookmark official MOH/WHO channels and local hotlines/ WhatsApp services. When in doubt, call or message to confirm rather than relying on forwarded posts or screenshots
How to report rumors	Establish a simple *see-something, say-something* workflow: have them send a voice note or hotline message with the claim, where they heard it, and their question, thereby allowing responders to verify and get back to the community with accurate info
Protect yourself from online harms	Educate how to spot bots/trolls, set privacy controls, avoid sharing personal health data in public groups, and mute or report accounts that target or harass community members discussing vaccination

several contexts to support delivery of other antigens, demonstrating how disease-specific initiatives can strengthen broader immunization systems. While this has proven efficacious as a stopgap measure, further research is required to evaluate long-term efficacy and effectiveness in conflict-affected populations.[28]

Novel financing mechanisms such as community-based health insurance, *cash transfers* consisting of payment by formal or informal institutions directly to populations in need, and performance-based financing have potential to address some of the funding challenges inherent to protracted crises. However, their impact on health and well-being are often most successful when part of a wider set of health system reforms.[14,29] Decentralization of government decision-making and basic infrastructure to preserve transportation, communication and disease surveillance could empower more accurate and immediate monitoring of and response to outbreaks, especially in fragile settings and regions of evolving conflict.[11,28] However, evidence for these transformative interventions remains limited, underscoring the need for continued research and documentation of innovative approaches.

SERVICE INTEGRATION

Service integration can effectively improve vaccination coverage and overall health system resilience to disease outbreaks in crisis settings. Studies from South Sudan and other conflict-affected regions show that integrating immunization with nutrition services can substantially increase the number of children reached with vaccines through localized service delivery and the strategic use of existing community trust.[14] Similarly, integration with complementary sectors such as water-sanitation-hygiene can directly impact a community's ability to manage outbreaks through simultaneous reduction in vector transmission.[30] Importantly, these multifaceted campaigns can not only leverage existing trust within communities but also inspire new confidence when their immediate quality of life is improved.

LAST MILE LOGISTICS

Because many vaccines require refrigeration from creation to injection, vaccine supply chain logistics, often referred to as cold chain, are highly sensitive to disruptions.[31] The Last Mile denotes the final, often most challenging segment of vaccination delivery due to a myriad of destabilizing effects. Recent synthesis reviews confirm that Last Mile efforts are increasingly shaped around the realities of conflict, displacement and fragility.[32] Efforts like the Global Alliance for Vaccines and Immunization's Zero-Dose Immunization Program explicitly target complex emergencies.[33]

Mobile health teams and drone delivery of vaccinations have shown effectiveness in improving access, particularly among marginalized communities where security concerns limit fixed-site service delivery.[14,34] These approaches create important collateral channels, bringing vaccines and potentially other resources to populations that might otherwise remain unreached. Looking forward, current and future research efforts devoted to heat-stable vaccinations could reduce many of the present-day barriers posed by cold chain logistics. Needle-free formulations have been promoted by the Coalition for Epidemic Preparedness Interventions due to offering a thermostable solution that simultaneously overcomes the barrier of needle-aversion.[35,36]

SURVEILLANCE, DATA, AND CROSS-BORDER COORDINATION

Building truly resilient vaccination and disease monitoring systems in humanitarian contexts requires moving beyond adaptive responses toward actively strengthening underlying health system capacities.[14] Timely monitoring that is consistent across countries and regions is imperative for early recognition, rapid epidemiologic analysis, targeted response and mitigation of spread. Health information systems that facilitate real-time monitoring and decision-making are especially valuable in unstable environments, allowing for rapid adjustment of strategies as conditions change.[37] Additionally, cross-border coordination has shown promise in improving vaccination coverage among mobile populations.[38]

To standardize clinical research metrics as well as operational frameworks, various members of the international community have developed common data elements (CDEs) and communities of practice on vaccination and disaster response. CDEs, or a set of variables where standardized questions are met with specified responses, can enhance multicountry coordination, thereby improving outcomes.[37]

The World Health Organization (WHO) and United Nations Children's Fund (UNICEF) have established one of the most comprehensive global systems for immunization data collection through the electronic joint reporting form. This online data collection portal tracks annual vaccination data from all WHO Member States, Reporting Entities and Associate Members and covers a wide range of domains including standard performance indicators, financial data and quality metrics. These comprehensive data allow for monitoring of global and regional implementation strategies, informing vaccine-preventable disease burden estimates, and contributing to national immunization coverage estimates.[39]

The Immunization Agenda 2030 Data Action Framework, a similarly broad data set, reflects the international community's shift toward data-driven vaccination strategies, while also emphasizing flexibility to respond effectively to emerging challenges.[40]

The ISARIC-WHO Clinical Characterization Protocol monitors emerging pathogens and is used in conflict zones.[41] The WHO Early Warning, Alert and Response System Minimum Dataset includes case definitions and minimal variables to expedite outbreak detection. Designed for conflict and other humanitarian emergencies, these field kits allow teams to begin surveillance within 48 hours, regardless of access to internet.[42]

While current models have vastly improved the international community's capacity for coordination and access to high-quality data, challenges persist in achieving harmonization across crises. More attention must be paid to the rising prevalence of violence and other disruptive factors directly influencing vaccine access and disease outcomes.

PREPAREDNESS AND RESPONSE

The disaster cycle of preparedness, response, recovery, and mitigation becomes severely compromised in settings where governance structures have collapsed or become actively hostile to civilian populations. Inappropriate diagnosis and drug regimens can contribute to pathogen resistance, and international spread of diseases can be accelerated by movement of refugees, international aid workers and animals.[37,38,43] Building capacity for pediatric pandemic preparedness requires strategic investment in key areas. Health care workers require pediatric-specific training, and strong infrastructure capable of supporting pediatric care during pandemics must be sustained, even during active conflicts.[37] This includes maintaining reserves of pediatric-specific supplies and developing protocols for the safe evacuation of critically ill children when local capacity is exceeded.

LESSONS FROM COVID-19

The COVID-19 pandemic introduced additional layers of complexity to vaccination delivery in humanitarian settings. While the pandemic disrupted routine immunization services worldwide, it also catalyzed innovations in service delivery and highlighted the critical importance of building system resilience. The rapid development and deployment of SARS-CoV-2 vaccines demonstrated both the potential of modern vaccine technology and the persistent inequities in global vaccine access as well as personal protective equipment and life-saving medical interventions. Children in humanitarian settings have been particularly affected by these disparities, with many crisis-affected countries struggling to return to prepandemic routine vaccination levels.[7,39,44]

ONE HEALTH/PLANETARY HEALTH

The adoption of a One Health/Planetary Health approach is an integrated framework for addressing the interconnected challenges of emerging infectious diseases in humanitarian contexts. By acknowledging the linkages between human, animal, and ecosystem health, attention can be focused on preventing zoonotic spillover events that can lead to new outbreaks.[45] Crisis-affected communities are often disproportionately exposed to environmental risks, and this framework can enhance both equity and resilience by addressing root causes of disease emergence rather than simply responding to outbreaks after they occur.[1]

GLOBAL GUIDANCE & GOVERNANCE QUALITY

While there has been a proliferation of guidance documents by multilateral organizations and national governments, critical appraisal suggests many of these resources would benefit from improved scientific rigor both in their creation and postimplementation assessment. Both transparency in their evidence selection and accountability in the development process are essential to reinforcing the credibility of these resources, a major driver of adherence by target groups.[3] Moreover, embedding mechanisms for continuous revision based on emerging evidence is vital to maintaining their relevance and effectiveness in rapidly evolving humanitarian and public health contexts.

ETHICAL CONSIDERATIONS

Ethical considerations must guide all aspects of pediatric vaccination and pandemic preparedness in humanitarian settings. The key ethical principles guiding clinical medicine and public health establish the framework informing decisions made in times of crisis, namely: beneficence, nonmaleficence, distributive justice, and autonomy in the form of consent. Tension between individual good and the common good can manifest in many ways: the prioritization of limited resources during acute crises, prevention of unactualized harm versus the consequences of inaction, and considerations of autonomy and consent each present nuanced ethical challenges.[46] A robust understanding of the risk of contagion of various diseases and local vaccination coverage is necessary for strategic vaccination selection. This requires not only adequate funding and political will but also calls for vaccine formulations and delivery strategies appropriate to crisis settings, such as simplified dosing schedules.

FUTURE RESEARCH PRIORITIES

Looking ahead, preparation for future pandemics in humanitarian settings will require sustained investment in vaccination delivery systems capable of absorbing, adapting to, and transforming in response to acute and protracted shocks. Strengthening the evidence base through targeted research remains critical, with particular emphasis on pediatric vaccination strategies, the integration of immunization with other essential health services, and approaches to reaching mobile and displaced populations. Additional research is needed on the application of digital tools for vaccine tracking and surveillance, the design of cross-sectoral coordination mechanisms that align health, humanitarian, and development efforts, and the education and capacity-building of health care workers to recognize pediatric presentations of disease and sustain immunization activities under crisis conditions. Innovation in vaccine technologies will be pivotal to advancing equitable access in challenging environments. This research agenda is essential to improving the sustainability, effectiveness, and equity of future preparedness and response efforts.

SUMMARY

In conclusion, safeguarding children from infectious diseases in humanitarian settings demands agile, multifaceted strategies capable of addressing both immediate needs and fostering long-term system resilience. In the face of dynamic challenges inherent to complex humanitarian crises, integration of evidence-based delivery approaches, robust community engagement, comprehensive service models, and adaptive governance structures is essential. As global threats from emerging and reemerging infectious diseases continue to intensify, strengthening these systems is not only a humanitarian imperative but also a cornerstone of global health security. Sustained investment and coordinated global action are required to ensure that the world's most vulnerable children are afforded the protection they rightfully deserve against preventable diseases.

INSIGHTS TO ACTION

- Trust and recognition of a community's priorities are integral to any successful vaccination campaign.
- There are proven strategies to combat misinformation, but these tactics often require coordination among team members and proactive outreach.
- Integrating vaccination and pandemic preparedness with other public health efforts such as nutrition services can dramatically increase effectiveness.

DECLARATION OF AI AND AI-ASSISTED TECHNOLOGIES IN THE WRITING PROCESS

During the preparation of this work the authors used ChatGPT to assist with synopsis preparation, collation of strategies to address misinformation, and preliminary scoping of gray literature, publicly available toolkits and data sources. After using this tool/service, the authors reviewed and edited the content as needed and take full responsibility for the content of the publication.

DISCLOSURE

The authors have no financial disclosures or conflicts of interest to disclose.

REFERENCES

1. Hoffman SA, Maldonado YA. Emerging and re-emerging pediatric viral diseases: a continuing global challenge. Pediatr Res 2024;95(2):480–7.
2. Warsame A, Murray J, Gimma A, et al. The practice of evaluating epidemic response in humanitarian and low-income settings: a systematic review. BMC Med 2020;18(1):315.
3. Allison LE, Alhaffar M, Checchi F, et al. A systematic review of vaccination guidance for humanitarian responses. Vaccines 2023;11(12):1743.
4. Bile AS, Ali-Salad MA, Mahmoud AJ, et al. Assessing vaccination delivery strategies for zero-dose and under-immunized children in the fragile context of Somalia. Vaccines 2024;12(2):154.
5. International Vaccine Access Center (IVAC), Gavi, the Vaccine Alliance. Equity in crisis: zero-dose children in humanitarian settings: an advocacy brief. International vaccine access center. Johns Hopkins Bloomberg School of Public Health; 2022. Available at: https://publichealth.jhu.edu/sites/default/files/2024-02/zero-doseadvocacy-brief-maintaining-equity-in-crisisax.pdf. Accessed May 27, 2025.
6. Shearer F, Sodha S, Danovaro C, et al. Progress toward achieving immunization agenda 2030 (IA2030) targets — worldwide, 2023. Morb Mortal Wkly Rep 2024; 73(43):1053–9.
7. World Health Organization. Immunization coverage. World Health Organization; 2025. Available at: https://www.who.int/news-room/fact-sheets/detail/immunization-coverage. Accessed May 27, 2025.
8. United Nations. Children and armed conflict: report of the secretary-general. United Nations; 2024. Available at: https://childrenandarmedconflict.un.org/

wp-content/uploads/2024/08/2410784_CAAC_AnnualReport_Summary_2023_WEB-23Jul24.pdf. Accessed October 17, 2025.
9. Humanitarian Outcomes. Aid worker security report 2024: balancing advocacy and security in humanitarian action — summary of key findings. Humanitarian Outcomes; 2024. Available at: https://humanitarianoutcomes.org/sites/default/files/publications/awsr_2024.pdf. Accessed October 17, 2025.
10. Humanitarian Outcomes. Major attacks on aid workers: summary statistics. 2025. Available at: https://www.aidworkersecurity.org/incidents/report. Accessed October 17, 2025.
11. Singh NS, Ataullahjan A, Ndiaye K, et al. Delivering health interventions to women, children, and adolescents in conflict settings: what have we learned from ten country case studies? Lancet 2021;397(10273):533–42.
12. Wise PH, Shiel A, Southard N, et al. The political and security dimensions of the humanitarian health response to violent conflict. Lancet 2021;397(10273):511–21.
13. United Nations General Assembly. Convention on the rights of the child 1989. Available at: https://www.ohchr.org/en/instruments-mechanisms/instruments/convention-rights-child. Accessed May 30, 2025.
14. Ismail SA, Lam ST, Bell S, et al. Strengthening vaccination delivery system resilience in the context of protracted humanitarian crisis: a realist-informed systematic review. BMC Health Serv Res 2022;22(1):1277.
15. Lewandowsky S, Cook J, Lombardi D. Debunking handbook 2020 2020. https://doi.org/10.17910/B7.1182.
16. World Health Organization. WHO strategic communications framework for effective communications. World Health Organization; 2020. Available at: https://iris.who.int/handle/10665/259807. Accessed May 25, 2025.
17. World Health Organization. Health worker module - conversations: talking about vaccination. Presented at: January 2025; Geneva. Available at: https://cdn.who.int/media/docs/default-source/immunization/demand/health-worker-module—conversations_jan2025_en.pptx?sfvrsn=9377f79d_4. Accessed May 25, 2025.
18. World Health Organization. WHO competency framework: building a response workforce to manage infodemics. World Health Organization; 2021. p. 120. Available at: https://www.who.int/publications/i/item/9789240035287. Accessed May 25, 2025.
19. World Health Organization. Social listening in infodemic management for public health emergencies: guidance on ethical considerations. World Health Organization; 2025. Available at: https://www.who.int/publications/i/item/9789240108202. Accessed October 20, 2025.
20. World Health Organization. Behavioural and social drivers of vaccination: tools and practical guidance for achieving high uptake. World Health Organization; 2022. Available at: https://www.who.int/publications/i/item/9789240049680. Accessed October 20, 2025.
21. International Telecommunication Union, World Health Organization. Digital tools and strategies in COVID-19 infodemic response: case studies and discussion. International Telecommunication Union; 2021. Available at: https://www.itu.int/pub/D-STR-ICT_APP-2021-01. Accessed October 20, 2025.
22. World Health Organization. EPI-WIN: WHO information network for epidemics. Available at: https://www.who.int/teams/epi-win. Accessed October 20, 2025.
23. UNICEF, The Public Good Projects. Vaccine misinformation management guide: guidance for addressing a global infodemic and building demand for immunization. UNICEF; 2021. Available at: https://vaccinemisinformation.guide/. Accessed October 20, 2025.

24. European Centre for Disease Prevention and Control. *Countering online vaccine misinformation in the EU/EEA*. European centre for disease prevention and control. ECDC); 2021. Available at: https://www.ecdc.europa.eu/en/publications-data/countering-online-vaccine-misinformation-eu-eea. Accessed October 20, 2025.
25. United Nations Department of Global Communications. Pledge to pause: take a moment to stop the spread of misinformation. Available at: https://shareverified.com/pledge-to-pause/. Accessed October 20, 2025.
26. World Health Organization. Be careful what you share: things aren't always what they seem online. Available at: https://www.who.int/news/item/22-09-2021-be-careful-what-you-share.-things-aren-t-always-what-they-seem-online. Accessed October 20, 2025.
27. UNICEF Office of Research - Innocenti. Digital misinformation/disinformation and children. UNICEF; 2021. Available at: https://www.unicef.org/innocenti/reports/digital-misinformation-disinformation-and-children. Accessed October 20, 2025.
28. World Health Organization. IMMUNIZATIONbasics project. Periodic intensification of routine immunization: lessons learned and implications for action 2009. Available at: https://www.technet-21.org/en/resources/presentation/periodic-intensification-of-routine-immunisation-piri-lessons-learned-and-implications-for-action. Accessed May 29, 2025.
29. Bogale B, Scambler S, Khairuddin ANM, et al. Health system strengthening in fragile and conflict-affected states: a review of systematic reviews. PLoS One 2024;19(6):e0305234. https://doi.org/10.1371/journal.pone.0305234.
30. World Health Organization. Aiming for zero cholera in South Sudan. 2022. Available at: https://www.who.int/about/accountability/results/who-results-report-2020-mtr/country-story/2022/aiming-for-zero-cholera-in-south-sudan. Accessed May 27, 2025.
31. Intelsius. COVID-19 vaccine transport: last mile delivery. Intelsius news. Available at: https://intelsius.com/news/covid-19-vaccine-transport-last-mile-delivery/. Accessed February 9, 2025.
32. Ingle EA, Shrestha P, Seth A, et al. Interventions to vaccinate zero-dose children: a narrative review and synthesis. Viruses 2023;15(10):2092.
33. Zero-dose children and missed communities. Available at: https://www.gavi.org/our-alliance/strategy/phase-5-2021-2025/equity-goal/zero-dose-children-missed-communities. Accessed May 28, 2025.
34. Ospina-Fadul MJ, Kremer P, Stevens SE, et al. Cost-effectiveness of aerial logistics for immunization: a model-based evaluation of centralized storage and drone delivery of vaccines in Ghana using empirical data. Soc Sci Res Netw 2024;21. https://doi.org/10.2139/ssrn.4775458.
35. Adigweme I, Yisa M, Ooko M, et al. A measles and rubella vaccine microneedle patch in the Gambia: a phase 1/2, double-blind, double-dummy, randomised, active-controlled, age de-escalation trial. Lancet 2024;403(10439):1879–92.
36. Coalition for Epidemic Preparedness Innovations. CEPI and micron biomedical accelerate needle-free vaccines against disease X. 2025. Available at: https://cepi.net//cepi-and-micron-biomedical-accelerate-needle-free-vaccines-against-disease-x. Accessed May 30, 2025.
37. Pediatric Disaster Science. Understanding needs, highlighting imperatives, and leveraging opportunities - NAM. Available at: https://nam.edu/perspectives/pediatric-disaster-science-understanding-needs-highlighting-imperatives-and-leveraging-opportunities/. Accessed May 29, 2025.

38. Buback L, Martin S, Pardo E, et al. Using the WHO building blocks to examine cross-border public health surveillance in MENA. Int J Equity Health 2025; 24(1):38.
39. World Health Organization. WHO/UNICEF joint reporting process. Available at: https://www.who.int/teams/immunization-vaccines-and-biologicals/immunization-analysis-and-insights/global-monitoring/who-unicef-joint-reporting-process. Accessed May 26, 2025.
40. Immunization Agenda 2030 Data Strategy Working Group. A data action framework: data to support the immunisation agenda 2030 - a global strategy to leave no one behind. Immunization agenda 2030. 2021. Available at: https://www.immunizationagenda2030.org/resources/34-ia2030-data-action-framework.
41. International Severe Acute Respiratory and emerging Infection Consortium. ISARIC CCP toolkit. ISARIC. Available at: https://isaric.org/resources/clinical-characterisation-protocol/. Accessed May 29, 2025.
42. Sheel M, Collins J, Kama M, et al. Evaluation of the early warning, alert and response system after Cyclone Winston, Fiji, 2016. Bull World Health Organ 2019;97(3):178–189C.
43. Gayer M, Legros D, Formenty P, et al. Conflict and emerging infectious diseases 2007;13(11):1625–31. https://doi.org/10.3201/eid1311.061093.
44. Aiken D. Vaccination barriers in complex settings. MSF OCBA Centre for Applied Reflection on Humanitarian Practice (ARHP); 2024. Available at: https://arhp.msf.es/wp-content/uploads/2024/12/Vaccination-Barriers-in-Complex-Settings_FV.pdf. Accessed May 29, 2025.
45. Whitmee S, Haines A, Beyrer C, et al. Safeguarding human health in the anthropocene epoch: report of the Rockefeller Foundation–Lancet Commission on planetary health. Lancet 2015;386(10007):1973–2028.
46. Moodley K, Hardie K, Selgelid MJ, et al. Ethical considerations for vaccination programmes in acute humanitarian emergencies. Bull World Health Organ 2013;91(4):290–7.

When Care Coordination Meets Crisis

Tameir Holder, MPH[a,*], Jonathan Sury, MPH, CPH[b,c]

KEYWORDS

• Noncommunicable diseases • Children • Humanitarian crises • Emergencies
• Care coordination • Health systems readiness

KEY POINTS

- Inequities in noncommunicable disease (NCD) burden are evident, given that high prevalence in low- and middle-income countries (LMICs) renders children in humanitarian settings exceptionally susceptible to poor health outcomes.
- Weaknesses in LMIC health system infrastructure, such as insufficient funding, inadequate access to medical supplies, and workforce attrition, hinder proper care coordination which enhances NCD burden after a crisis.
- The contextual setting of a humanitarian response requires comprehensive multisector planning. It is necessary to maintain a pediatric-inclusive lens while continually investing in health systems strengthening and health systems readiness.
- Collectively, operational guidelines, frameworks pertaining to child well-being and survival, and select care models offer valuable insights to manage pediatric NCDs in humanitarian settings.
- Three domains emerged from the reviewed literature: (1) pediatric clinical care, (2) NCD management, and (3) humanitarian crises. More work is needed to develop literature that addresses the intersection of these domains.

INTRODUCTION

The Role of Care Coordination

Meeting the health care needs of a given population is a complicated endeavor that requires adoption of systematic strategies and care plans. Care coordination meets this requirement and refers to the organization of health care processes across a variety of facilities, settings, and providers in an effort to facilitate procurement of efficient, high-quality, and timely patient health care services.[1–4] Evidence suggests

[a] Department of Epidemiology, Mailman School of Public Health, Columbia University, New York, NY, USA; [b] National Center for Disaster Preparedness, Columbia Climate School, Columbia University, New York, NY, USA; [c] Heilbrunn Department of Population and Family Health, Mailman School of Public Health, Columbia University, New York, NY, USA
* Corresponding author. Department of Epidemiology, Columbia University, Mailman School of Public Health, 722 West 168th Street, New York, NY 10032.
E-mail address: tah2129@columbia.edu

Pediatr Clin N Am 73 (2026) 965–984
https://doi.org/10.1016/j.pcl.2026.04.007 **pediatric.theclinics.com**
0031-3955/26/

Abbreviations	
AKI	acute kidney injury
LMIC	low- and middle-income country
NCD	noncommunicable disease
T1D	type 1 diabetes mellitus
UNHCR	United Nations High Commissioner for Refugees
WHO	World Health Organization

that implementation of coordinated tasks and care planning have the potential to successfully improve patient outcomes, while reducing morbidity, adverse outcomes, rehospitalization, and mortality.[5–7] In this fashion, globally, establishing care coordination in primary care settings is often hailed as an effective tool for facilitating disease prevention and management.[1,3,4,8] Key functions of care coordination include improving patient safety, developing patient health care plans or activities, streamlining communication across providers, bridging gaps in service delivery, and reducing fragmentation, among others.[1,2,4,9,10] As expected, coordination efforts and strategies may vary by (1) geographic region, (2) characteristics of the health system's infrastructure, readiness, and financing, (3) demographics of the target population, and (4) diseases or conditions of interest. In low- and middle-income countries (LMICs), implementation of care coordination activities is met by many barriers such as financial constraints, weak health system infrastructure, poor health record data quality, and lack of quality resources.[3,11–13] Furthermore, the durability of care coordination tasks may falter in the midst of a humanitarian crisis or emergency, which often occur in LMICs, thus exposing the potential vulnerabilities and weaknesses of the given health system.[14] Over the past several decades, bodies such as the World Health Organization (WHO), World Bank, Médicines Sans Frontières, International Rescue Committee, The International Federation of Red Cross and Red Crescent Societies, the United States Agency for International Development, a variety of United Nations organizations such as the United Nation's Children Fund and the United Nations High Commissioner for Refugees (UNHCR), as well as nongovernmental organizations including the NCD Alliance and Sphere, among others, have played an instrumental role in addressing these systemic weaknesses. These global health actors have generally addressed these weaknesses by supplying humanitarian aid, facilitating direct service delivery, advocating for policy reform, setting standards of care, and establishing multisector coordination in humanitarian settings.[15–17] Multinational commitments such as WHO's *Global Action Plan for the Prevention and Control of Noncommunicable Diseases 2013* to *2020* (now extended through 2030), have placed NCDs on the global agenda.[18,19]

This piece is designed to address noncommunicable disease (NCD) burden within the context of the resources and best practices that have been used to systematically manage NCDs in children during humanitarian crises that take place in LMICs. A visual tool for understanding relevant literature that has informed this narrative is presented herein and is to serve as a resource for humanitarian actors and pediatric clinicians who practice in LMICs and respond to emergencies. Throughout this piece, the term *LMIC* is defined by World Bank classifications which range from low income to upper-middle income. A list of key terms can be found in Appendix 1.

Global Mission and Priorities: Addressing Noncommunicable Diseases

Defined as chronic conditions that are often characterized by multiple risk factors and generally require long-term care, NCDs serve as a substantial source of disability, functional impairment, and death globally.[20–23] Generally influenced by environmental, behavioral, and genetic risk factors, NCDs are typically prevented and managed via a combination of approaches including screening, lifestyle modifications, and medical intervention.[22,24–31] Key NCDs include cardiovascular diseases, cancer, diabetes mellitus, stroke, chronic obstructive pulmonary disease, dementia, injury, and mental illnesses such as anxiety and depression.[20–22,25,27,29] Globally, life expectancy at birth increased from 65.4 in 1990 to 73.5 in 2019, which contributed to an aging population before the COVID-19 pandemic.[32,33] While life expectancy at birth drastically declined during the COVID-19 pandemic, sources indicate that it has been partially restored to prepandemic levels in certain regions as of 2023.[32,34,35] This rapidly aging population represents a demographic shift that increases the prevalence of NCDs, fueling the urgent need to promote effective NCD prevention and management strategies.[36] The increase in NCD prevalence is partially attributable to the childhood diabetes and obesity epidemics as well as medical advancements that have enhanced survival rates among children who have various cancers or congenital and rheumatic heart diseases, although survival rates vary by region.[23,37–40] Accordingly, developing coordinated efforts to address the rising NCD burden has been recognized as one of many global priorities.[41,42] The *2030 Agenda for Sustainable Development* serves as a collective commitment to promote human rights and well-being, while addressing essential drivers of poor global health such as poverty, violence, and climate change, among others.[43] Curated by all members of the United Nations, this agenda offers a blueprint for addressing 17 key objectives and "*Reduce pre-mature NCD mortality by one-third through prevention and treatment and promote mental health and well-being*" serves as Sustainable Development Goal Target 3.4.[43–45]

NONCOMMUNICABLE DISEASE BURDEN

Pediatric Noncommunicable Disease Morbidity and Mortality: Inequities in Low- and Middle-Income Countries

NCDs are responsible for 74% of deaths globally, with stroke, diabetes, and ischemic heart disease serving as the most prevalent conditions.[29] The global burden of NCDs in children is well-documented. Worldwide, among children and adolescents less than the age of 20, NCDs account for one-third of dsability life-adjusted years,[46] with more than 2.1 billion people being affected in this age group.[27] Each year, among children in this age group, mortality due to treatable NCDs is more than 15.9%, which amounts to 1 million deaths.[27] Moreover, the percent of global deaths due to NCDs in children increased from 10.5% in 1990 to 17.2% in 2023 (**Fig. 1**), illustrating the rising mortality due to NCDs in the pediatric population.[47]

The extreme disparity in NCD mortality is evident, given that 82% of all global premature NCD deaths (death before the age of 70) occur in LMICs.[29,48,49]

Given this disproportionately high mortality burden in LMICs, children in these countries are exceptionally vulnerable and susceptible to poor health outcomes. NCD prevalence among children less than the age of 20 in LMICs ranges from 85.5% to 87.8%.[50] This high prevalence is partially due to an epidemiologic shift in the pattern of disease burden in LMICs.[20,51] Explicitly, while communicable and neonatal diseases were traditionally responsible for high child mortality in these regions, medical advancements in the early 1900s progressively decreased deaths due to infectious disease, while increases in urbanization, aging, and certain behavioral risk factors have contributed to the rise of chronic disease prevalence.[51,52] This phenomenon is widely recognized as a *double burden* whereby LMICs must contend with the coexistence of communicable and NCDs as a result of lower child mortality and the aforementioned changes in population, environmental, and behavioral factors.[52–55]

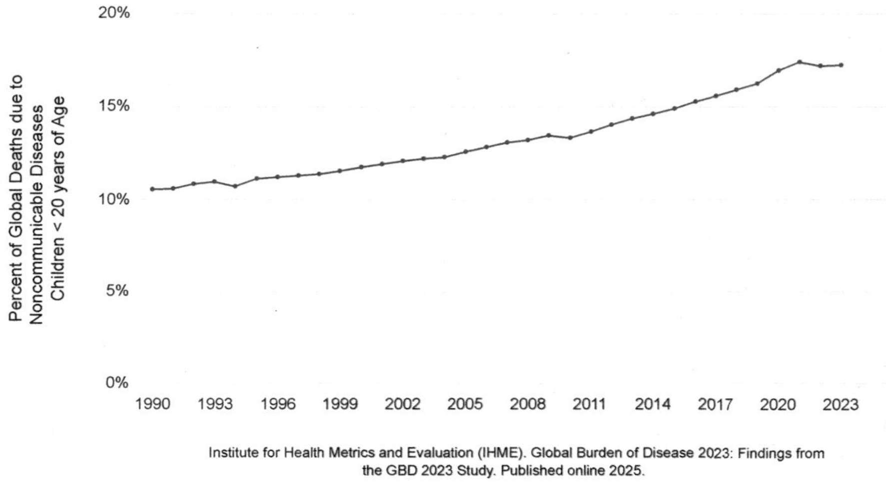

Fig. 1. Global deaths due to NCDs in children less than 20 years. (*Source* Institute for Health Metrics and Evaluation. Used with permission. All rights reserved.)

Within LMICs, key chronic conditions that are prevalent in this age group include cancers, chronic respiratory disorders, injuries, nutritional deficiencies, obesity, and mental illness, while severe onset diseases include type 1 diabetes (T1D), heart diseases (congenital and acquired), and sickle cell diseases.[28,38,56–58] Factors such as malnutrition, poverty, food insecurity and poor diet, physical inactivity, and tobacco exposure increase the risk for developing certain of the aforementioned conditions.[28,51,56–58] From a lifecourse perspective, particular risk factors are most salient during certain age ranges, and accordingly, these distinct windows of vulnerability illustrate that burden of disease patterns vary by age subgroup.[31,59] For example, poor sanitation, lack of access to quality foods, and exposure to poverty, render children in LMICs at risk for nutritional deficiencies. The prevalence of nutritional deficiencies including protein-energy malnutrition, as well as deficiencies in vitamin A, iron, and dietary iron, ranges from 25.6% to 64.1% among children less than the age of 5 years and ranges from 16.2% to 47.3% among children ages 5 to 14. Similarly, behavioral and psychosocial changes peak during adolescence and accordingly in LMICs, the prevalence of mental disorders ranges from 17% to 20%, among adolescents ages 15 to 19.[50] These distinct windows of vulnerability offer insight into the key risk factors that contribute to disease burden throughout the child and adolescent lifecourse.

Humanitarian Crises and Disruptive Events: Exacerbation of Noncommunicable Disease Burden

As compared to the general population, the risk of NCD burden is enhanced in crisis-affected populations following humanitarian crises, and this exacerbation is primarily due to weaknesses in LMIC health system infrastructure, such as lack of access to key medical resources and medicines, insufficient food supply, health care worker attrition, and disrupted health system operations.[11,49,60] Management of NCDs requires long-term care and crisis-affected populations are often unable to present to health care facilities in a timely fashion which leads to discontinuity of essential care. This cascade substantially precludes effective follow-up and health care action planning, thus increasing the likelihood that these crisis-affected populations will experience long-term NCD complications.[60,61]

Emergence of other past and ongoing disruptive events also influence NCD burden. Globally, the COVID-19 pandemic exposed the fault lines and systemic vulnerabilities that had a substantial impact on those with NCDs. In 2021, COVID-19 accounted for 8.7 million deaths globally and accordingly surfaced as a leading cause of death worldwide.[62] Notably, NCDs such as cardiovascular disease, diabetes, and stroke, among others, increased the risk of severe infection from SARS-CoV2,[20,63] rendering certain individuals, such as young children, exceptionally vulnerable to disability and potential death.[64] Natural disasters serve as another source of disruption. In a systematic review of chronic NCDs in disaster settings, Ngariuiya and colleagues found multiple risk factors for NCDs both directly and independent of disaster exposure.[65] Specifically, their review noted that the mental and physical stressors serve as risk factors for NCDs and increase NCD-related morbidity. The loss of family members, displacement, and proximity to the disasters were also found to increase morbidity, as was refugee status as an independent predictor. Notably, malnutrition and food insecurity were identified as drivers of diabetes, while reduced access to monitoring supplies was a factor that hindered the ability to manage the disease. The compounding effects of climate change, which drive global and local weather extremes, place children at a great risk for direct and indirect health effects.[66] Planning humanitarian responses to these events requires multisectoral preparedness. This form of preparation supports both endogenous health systems and response organizations in effectively meeting the special health care needs of children who are in humanitarian settings and are exposed to this changing environment.

NATURE OF THE PROBLEM

Health System Infrastructure in Low- and Middle-Income Countries: Contextualizing the Provision of Noncommunicable Disease Care in Crises

In a given disaster or humanitarian emergency setting, there is a confluence of actors who aim to provide a wide variety of services, including (1) medical, social, psychological, or supportive resources such as supplies, logistics, and supply chain management or (2) donation management: in-kind, cash, or otherwise. A strong situational understanding is necessary to appropriately plan for and coordinate with the local context of the affected areas, to facilitate appropriate staffing, resources, and coordination with local and national actors.[67] These contextual factors may include health system baseline and readiness capabilities, as well as geopolitical, cultural, religious, demographic, topographic, historical, and security considerations.[28,68] Adequate understanding of these forces may help improve outcomes in child health throughout the response and recovery phases of the given disaster.

There are 4 types of local organizational responses to disasters where local actors will interact with external response organizations. There is (1) the *established* organized response: local organizations with a bureaucratic structure who provide disaster response services, (2) the *expanding* organized response: local organizations, often composed of volunteers who organize to provide direct services, (3) the *extending* organized response: local organizations who add new mission areas in response to the disaster or emergency, and (4) the *emergent* organized response: local organizations which nascently appear to fulfill a hyperlocal need.[69,70] Responding organizations standing up clinics or providing staff to support various local efforts should be aware of these types of organizations, their capacities to provide pediatric-specific care, and the connections they may have to procure and deliver the necessary supplies to support the unique needs of children. The health cluster model of humanitarian coordination, led by the WHO, provides a framework and structure to manage assistance from the global to local level, with the intention of collaboratively reducing morbidity and mortality in humanitarian crises.[71]

Responding pediatric clinicians, and their organizations with whom they work, must be cognizant of the medical service delivery context in which they are entering. **Fig. 2**, developed by Bausch and colleagues, illustrates the 2x2 matrix of pre-event NCD burden and pre-event health system capabilities.[67] These pre-event health system capabilities are likely positively correlated with the level of national development and economic status. This context should be incorporated into operational planning considerations to facilitate coordination with local pediatric clinicians, clinics, community health workers, pediatric-specific medical and pharmaceutical supply chains, transportation and logistics infrastructure, and access to other supportive services such as mental health and psychosocial support. Relatedly, health systems readiness is closely tied to health security. Improved preparedness and planning for health systems and its actors is paramount to reducing loss of life from future natural disasters, anthropogenic climate change, and pandemics - as was experienced during COVID-19.

Disrupted Care Coordination: Impact on Children

Children are not little adults as they differ anatomically and developmentally. As such, they are exceptionally vulnerable to (1) NCD care disruption during emergencies and crises, (2) the psychological trauma of both direct and indirect exposure to the causal event, and (3) clinical care that is not age, physiologically, or size-appropriate.[72] Clinical guidelines that are age and setting-appropriate must be prepositioned and meet consensus within the pediatric clinician community through improved multisector preparedness, a call to action that has been made within the practice community.[67,73–75] There is “no health without mental health”,[76] and the exposure to trauma, both at the individual and community level, may increase the incidence of mental disorders.[74] Continuity of care for previously diagnosed NCDs for children with special health care needs requires multisectoral planning and preparedness, which may be more challenging in low-resource regions with less-developed child-specific health systems.[28,77,78]

The 2023 Türkiye–Syria Earthquake

On February 6, 2023, 2 major earthquakes, magnitude 7.8 and 7.5, struck the Karamanmaraş region of Türkiye and Northern Syria, leading to extensive death, injuries, and damage to homes and infrastructure.[79,80] In Türkiye, the official death toll exceeded 50,000, and in Syria, estimates range between 5,000 and 8,000.[80] Damage

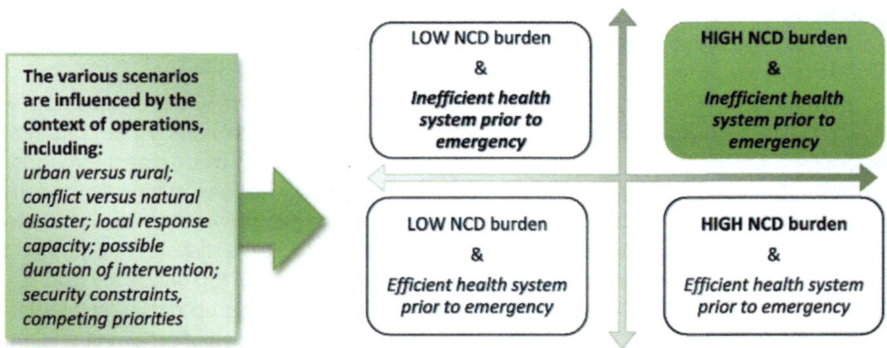

Fig. 2. Relationship between pre-event and post-event health system status and NCD burden (Bausch and colleagues, 2021). (*Source* Bausch FJ, Beran D, Hering H, et al. Operational considerations for the management of noncommunicable diseases in humanitarian emergencies. Confl Health. 2021 Feb 25;15(1):9. https://doi.org/10.1186/s13031-021-00345-w. PMID: 33632275; PMCID: PMC7905755.)

severity and remoteness in the affected areas slowed the initial response and influx of humanitarian assistance. More than 518,000 buildings were deemed uninhabitable due to collapse or severe damage.[80] The building collapse resulted in a high rate of crush injuries, internal organ damage, and amputations.

Several studies highlighted challenges in post-disaster pediatric NCD management for T1D,[81] celiac disease,[82] and the therapeutic care of crush syndrome–related acute kidney injury (crush-related AKI).[83,84] Trabzon and colleagues found in their T1D study that in the aftermath of the earthquake, 36.7% of patients had disrupted insulin therapy and 77.2% experienced glycemic control issues, which were associated with child and parental mental health.[81] Dağ and colleagues found poor access to appropriate food for celiac patients, citing infrastructure and logistical challenges, low diet compliance, exacerbation of symptoms due to psychological distress, and poor access to clinical services.[82] Crush-related AKI, due to the severe muscle tissue damage, can lead to kidney failure if untreated. Bakkaloğlu and colleagues studied cases seen by pediatric nephrologists across 40 sites in Türkiye.[83] Of these patients (n = 903), 74.8% had crush injury, 34.8 developed crush-related AKI, 20.9% required dialysis, 21.7% required fasciotomy, and 10.6% required amputation. The authors note that, with appropriate care coordination and resources, including pediatric nephrology specialists, crush-AKI is treatable.

Shortly after the earthquakes, the editors of The Turkish Journal of Pediatrics stated, "*The central organization of the medical response, which initially requested surgeons but not pediatricians or internists to the affected area, highlights a well-known flaw in the approach to trauma: the misconception that trauma is exclusively in the domain of surgery.*"[85] Pediatric care in low-resource humanitarian settings is beyond communicable disease management, and in this case, beyond pre-existing NCD management. It requires integrating pediatric clinician expertise in postacute, recovery, rehabilitative, and continuity of care for new-onset and pre-existing conditions. These challenges point to the need for comprehensive disaster plans that address the unique needs of children with NCDs locally, regionally, and nationally.

DISCUSSION

Promoting Noncommunicable Disease Care and Child Health in the Wake of an Emergency: Frameworks and Care Models

Historically, NCD care management in primary care has been underprioritized and underdeveloped in humanitarian settings, given that communicable diseases such as malaria and tuberculosis have garnered the vast majority of government resources and fiscal support.[11,61] However, within the past 2 to 3 decades, humanitarian actors have been making an effort to conceptualize strategies and models of care for addressing the rising burden of NCDs in crisis-affected settings.[67] Much of the work done to date has involved leveraging the lessons learned from communicable disease care approaches and other care models to adapt those measures to build strategies that are effective for NCD management.[11,49] In the midst of this shift, a series of evidence-based frameworks and guidelines have been adopted to enhance NCD management and child health in the wake of a crisis or emergency.

Child Well-Being and Survival: Lifecourse Perspective

Grounded in the notion that humanitarian crises serve as a source of toxic stress for children, the *Nurturing Care Framework* is designed to support response during the acute phase of a disaster.[86] The framework promotes early childhood development by offering a toolkit that actors can use to develop and implement policies and interventions that support nurturing care. Key components of the framework include good health, opportunities for early learning, security and safety, responsive caregiving, and adequate nutrition.[86] Relatedly, Reif and colleagues conducted a scoping review of lifelong care models for adolescents and children in LMICs to identify commonalities throughout the literature and to support ongoing program development. They identified emerging themes including (1) common care model components, such as social and community services, mental health and psychosocial well-being, as well as family education to facilitate self-management, (2) service delivery approaches which included provision of care that was either decentralized or accessible and patient-centered, and (3) resources such as chronic care training for health workers.[46] Other resources address how families, educational systems, and communities play a critical role in self-management among pediatric patients.[23]

Operational Guidance and Standards

Certain resources articulate the fundamental building blocks of NCD programming as well as the operational processes that should be followed when providing emergency services. Produced by the WHO, the *Manual for the Health Care of Children in Humanitarian Emergencies* offers guidance on priorities pertaining to triage and emergency response and likewise addresses integrated management strategies for common childhood illnesses.[87] In 2024, the WHO released a report that addressed the notion of strengthening NCD management during a humanitarian emergency response.[88] The following domains were identified as essential components that enhance NCD programming.

1. Collaborative Surveillance and Health Intelligence
2. Community Protection and Engagement
3. Safe and Scalable Care
4. Access to countermeasures to Prevent Service Disruption
5. Awareness of NCDs throughout coordination of Emergency Response
6. Strengthening NCD Governance and Financing during Emergencies

The domains of lifesaving care, community engagement, and health information systems were deemed valuable by the *UNHCR Operational Guide,* which contextualizes the ongoing efforts to integrate NCD prevention care and management into primary care facilities within humanitarian settings.[89] Notably, the guide offers a framework that addresses actions that should be addressed during both the acute phase (0–6 months post-disaster) and the ongoing phase (>6 months post-disaster). Actions are contextualized into key domains such as (1) *Needs Assessment and Planning*, which addresses response activities and mobilizing resources, and (2) *Implementation*, which addresses coordination and partnerships, service delivery, human resources, supplies, health information, monitoring and evaluation, transition to national health services, as well as advocacy and research. Methods for operationalizing essential components of NCD management are offered within the context of the *Humanitarian Program Cycle*, a framework that illustrates the cyclic relationship between these aforementioned domains.[89] To further assist in preparedness and planning, Perone and colleagues have compiled a list of 10 essential questions to guide the intervention design for medical response in humanitarian settings.[73] These clear and concise questions (**Fig. 3**), can help improve contextually appropriate response to the service delivery setting.

Care Model Selection and Integration

The aforementioned resources addressed certain fundamental components of NCD programming as well as operational processes that should be followed when providing emergency services and nurturing pediatric care. In tandem, much work

1. What are the existing capacities of the local health system?
2. Which NCDs to address?
3. Who is the target population?
4. What kind of interventions needed to ensure continuum and continuity of care?
5. Which algorithms or guidelines to use?
6. What medications to be integrated in the basic essential drug list?
7. What are the ethical implications?
8. How to ensure accountability to patients?
9. How to monitor interventions?
10. What to do beyond provision of health services for "classical" NCDs?

Fig. 3. Ten essential questions for developing a humanitarian response to NCDs (Perone and colleagues,2027). (*Source* Aebischer Perone S, Martinez E, du Mortier S, Rossi R, Pahud M, Urbaniak V, Chappuis F, Hagon O, Jacquérioz Bausch F, Beran D. Non-communicable diseases in humanitarian settings: ten essential questions. Confl Health. 2017 Sep 17;11:17. https://doi.org/10.1186/s13031-017-0119-8. PMID: 28932259; PMCID: PMC5602789.)

has been done to identify NCD care models while designating key barriers and facilitators that impact the ability to execute effective health planning and coordination in humanitarian settings. A systematic review conducted by Nguyen and colleagues addressed the factors that impact implementation of pediatric NCD programs and policies in LMICs and noted that key barriers and facilitators span the following 6 WHO health system building blocks: (1) health service delivery, (2) health workforce, (3) leadership and governance, (4) financing, (5) health information systems, and (6) access to essential medicines.[28,90] Their review revealed that, within *leadership and governance*, competing public health priorities hinder successful pediatric program and policy implementation, while multisectoral coordination and ministry support serve as facilitators. System fragmentation was identified as a barrier within *health service delivery*, while integrating new programs into pre-existing programs serves as a strategy that facilitates effective implementation within this domain. Notably, within *health information systems*, limited pediatric surveillance data is a bottleneck that precludes effective monitoring, while strong research capacity facilitates program and policy implementation.[28]

These aforementioned themes have been observed in the general population as well. Obstacles such as care fragmentation, lack of prioritizing NCDs during emergencies, understaffing, delivering NCD care in hospitals which lack fortified referral systems, and minimal government commitment have generally hindered the ability to provide effective, continuous, and comprehensive NCD care.[11,60,61] Many of these barriers were identified by a qualitative study that ascertained health actors' perspectives around continuity of hypertension and diabetes care for Syrian refugees and vulnerable Lebanese based in Lebanon.[91]

Overcoming these service constraints and resource limitations remains an essential objective. Integrated NCD care models have largely been recognized as an ideal approach for preventing and managing other diseases and as such, work has been done to conceptualize how care integration can be used to best standardize NCD clinical and system-level decisions for refugees and internally displaced people in crisis-affected settings.[60] In this context, integration refers to the notion of embedding health service coordination and delivery at the primary care level. This includes provision of comprehensive, patient-centered care that operates via multidisciplinary teams. In humanitarian settings, NCD care delivery is often fragmented with distinct teams overseeing individual functional tasks. Accordingly, adaptation of an integrated model of care would promote cross-functional communication, collaboration, and ultimately, improved patient outcomes. To this end, key facilitators to NCD care model integration include communication among multidisciplinary stakeholders, colocation of key services to facilitate easy access for patients, and well-defined process improvement plans.[60] Enhancing disaster preparedness for patients with NCDs has also been accomplished by articulating key recommendations that health care providers should follow, and advocating for interagency collaboration postdisaster. Other strategies include fostering patient education, ensuring continuity of medication management, and promoting use of digital health modalities that either support widespread communication (system-wide text alerts) or facilitate self-management (such as home blood pressure monitoring).[92,93]

Findings illustrate that model selection and integration are context-dependent and may still be met with challenges. Ansbro and colleagues conducted semistructured qualitative interviews with global experts to synthesize opinions regarding models of care that should be used to manage hypertension and diabetes in humanitarian settings.[94] Their findings demonstrated that many gaps in hypertension and diabetes care management persisted, primarily with regard to coordinating actions with other humanitarian actors, care standardization, and care integration. Selection of the ideal care model relied on certain factors such as the organization implementing the care model, the type of humanitarian crisis, the characteristics of the target population, the health system's level of readiness to manage hypertension and diabetes crises, and overall resilience in the midst of an emergency.[94] Relatedly, work conducted by Asgary and colleagues affirms that the feasibility of care model implementation varies by setting.[61]

Contextualizing Key Domains

As demonstrated, within the context of leveraging resources to effectively manage NCDs in humanitarian settings, it is evident that there is a wealth of reviewed literature that addresses organizational strategies, frameworks pertaining to child health and survival, operational standards, and NCD care models. Herein, we present a visual tool (**Fig. 4**) that illustrates the 3 key domains that emerged from the literature. These domains include (1) pediatric clinical care, (2) NCD management, and (3) humanitarian crises. This tool is designed to support pediatric clinicians who plan to engage with the literature and resources that inform this narrative.

In **Fig. 4**, an intersection corresponds to an overlap in 2 domains. Accordingly, each identified piece of literature was assigned to a specific intersection (A, B, C, or D) based on the content that it addressed and examined (Appendix 2). For example, publications that were assigned to intersection "A" intentionally addressed both pediatric clinical care and NCD management within the LMIC setting, while a publication assigned to intersection "B" intentionally addressed both NCD management and humanitarian crises within this respective setting. Examining this compendium illustrates that very few publications, which were reviewed for this particular piece, were assigned to intersection "A" and intersection "D", respectively. This uneven distribution may imply that more work is needed to develop studies and resources that intentionally address (1) both pediatric clinical care and NCD management in LMICs (intersection A) and (2) clinical management of pediatric NCDs in the wake of a humanitarian crisis in LMICs (intersection D - which represents all 3 domains). Nonetheless, a key limitation is that this piece is not a structured literature review, and as such, a more comprehensive review may be warranted. Furthermore, there is a wealth of other cited publications that contribute to

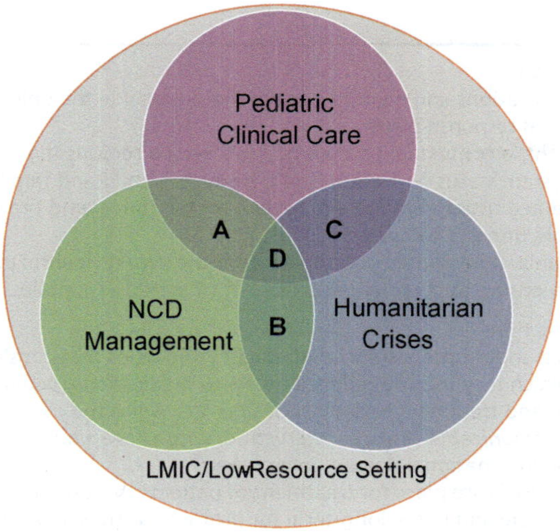

Fig. 4. Venn Diagram which represents key domains that emerged from the literature. Pieces of literature were categorized into overlapping domains according to the content addressed. Overlapping Domains include **A**: Pediatric Clinical Care and NCD Management; **B**: NCD Management and Humanitarian Crises; **C**: Pediatric Clinical Care and Humanitarian Crises; **D**: Pediatric Clinical Care, NCD Management, and Humanitarian Crises.

this narrative, yet were not included in the final compendium as they addressed fewer than 2 domains or did not address the LMIC setting.

SUMMARY

A substantial amount of work has been done to articulate the value of adapting a life-course approach when caring for children in humanitarian settings and similarly, operational standards for emergency response serve as a continued resource for humanitarian actors and pediatric clinicians. Furthermore, while context may present challenges and determine implementation feasibility, integrated care models serve as an evidence-based approach for addressing the systemic bottlenecks that exist within humanitarian settings. Findings from the presented visual tool may imply that advancing efforts to support humanitarian pediatric care should involve further development of literature and resources that are intentionally designed to address all 3 critical domains that inform this narrative.

Promoting this work must also operate within the context of the organizational environment and certain sociocultural factors that will impact the provision of pediatric NCD care and health service delivery in LMICs. Explicitly, pediatric clinicians must remain aware of the medical service delivery context they are engaging with, as well as the 4 distinct organizational responses that are adopted, postdisaster. Moreover, changes to international aid and funding will impact LMIC health system infrastructure and will influence sustainability of care model integration. Humanitarian actors and pediatric clinicians will be charged with the task of developing strategies to promote this agenda despite the changing policy landscape. The rising NCD burden in children is the driving force behind this task, and the field must work collaboratively and strategically to overcome and address the systemic weaknesses and contextual nuances. The expectation is that such efforts will promote improved health outcomes among children in crisis-affected settings.

INSIGHTS TO ACTION

Organizational Actions

- Responding organizations and health agencies should include the unique needs of children in their operational response plans.
- Before deployment, a contextual analysis of the affected regions should be conducted to include health system status (pre-event and post-event), child and family demographics, sociocultural characteristics, refugee and asylum seeker status, and prevalence of noncommunicable diseases by age.
- Responding organizations should coordinate with the World Health Organization Global Health Cluster to ensure appropriate deployment of staff and supplies.[71,87]

Pediatric Clinician Actions

- Pediatric clinicians should preposition clinical care guidelines that consider low-resource environments, which may include reduced access to medications, pediatric-appropriate medical supplies, and treatment settings. Consider exploring the use of the *Package of Essential Non-Communicable Diseases Interventions for Humanitarian Settings (PEN-H)* developed by the International Rescue Committee.[95]
- Consider continuity of care plans for treatment of patients throughout the disaster response and recovery life cycle and in the long-term for protracted crises and complex humanitarian emergencies.
- Integrate and coordinate mental health and psychosocial support services for children and family members.

DISCLOSURE

The authors have no financial disclosures or conflicts of interest to disclose.

REFERENCES

1. Khatri R, Endalamaw A, Erku D, et al. Continuity and care coordination of primary health care: a scoping review. BMC Heal Serv Res 2023;23(1):750.
2. Council On Children With Disabilities And Medical Home Implementation Project Advisory Committee. Patient- and family-centered care coordination: a framework for integrating care for children and youth across multiple systems. Pediatrics 2014;133(5):e1451–60.
3. Foo CD, Logan K, Eu E, et al. Starfield's 4Cs of NCD management in primary healthcare: a conceptual framework development from a case study of 19 countries. BMJ Glob Heal 2025;10(1):e017578.
4. Ju HH. Improving care coordination of patients with chronic diseases. J Nurse Pr 2022;18(8):833–6.
5. Chang GM, Tung YC. Impact of care coordination on 30-Day readmission, mortality, and costs for heart failure. Am J Manag Care 2024;30(4):e116–23.
6. Misra V, Sedig K, Dixon DR, et al. Prioritizing coordination of primary health care. Can Fam physician Med Fam Can 2020;66(6):399–403.
7. Elliott MN, Adams JL, Klein DJ, et al. Patient-reported care coordination is associated with better performance on clinical care measures. J Gen Intern Med 2021;36(12):3665–71.
8. Karam M, Chouinard MC, Poitras ME, et al. Nursing care coordination for patients with complex needs in primary healthcare: a scoping review. Int J Integr Care 2021;21(1):16.
9. Looman WS, Presler E, Erickson MM, et al. Care coordination for children with complex special health care needs: the value of the advanced practice nurse's enhanced scope of knowledge and practice. J Pediatr Heal Care 2013;27(4):293–303.

10. World Health Organization (WHO). Continuity and coordination of care: a practice brief to support implementation of the WHO framework on integrated people-centred health services. 2018. Available at: https://www.who.int/publications/i/item/9789241514033.
11. Tesema AG, Abimbola S, Mulugeta A, et al. Health system capacity and readiness for delivery of integrated non-communicable disease services in primary health care: a qualitative analysis of the Ethiopian experience. PLOS Glob Public Heal 2021;1(10):e0000026.
12. Odhus CO, Kapanga RR, Oele E. Barriers to and enablers of quality improvement in primary health care in low- and middle-income countries: a systematic review. PLOS Glob Public Heal 2024;4(1):e0002756.
13. Langlois EV, McKenzie A, Schneider H, et al. Measures to strengthen primary health-care systems in low- and middle-income countries. Bull World Heal Organ 2020;98(11):781–91.
14. Kohrt BA, Mistry AS, Anand N, et al. Health research in humanitarian crises: an urgent global imperative. BMJ Glob Heal 2019;4(6):e001870.
15. United Nations Children's Fund (UNICEF). *UNICEF Annual Report 2024*. UNICEF; 2025. https://www.unicef.org/reports/unicef-annual-report/2024.
16. Cavalcanti DM, de Oliveira Ferreira S, da Silva AF, et al. Evaluating the impact of two decades of USAID interventions and projecting the effects of defunding on mortality up to 2030: a retrospective impact evaluation and forecasting analysis. Lancet 2025;406(10500):283–94.
17. Besançon S, Sidibé A, Sow DS, et al. The role of non-governmental organizations in strengthening healthcare systems in low- and middle-income countries: lessons from Santé Diabète in Mali. Glob Heal Action 2022;15(1):2061239.
18. World Health Organization (WHO). Global action plan for the prevention and control of noncommunicable diseases 2013-2020. World Health Organization; 2013. Available at: https://www.who.int/publications/i/item/9789241506236.
19. World Health Organization (WHO). Implementation roadmap 2023-2030 for the Global action plan. Available at: https://www.who.int/teams/noncommunicable-diseases/governance/roadmap. Accessed October 31, 2025.
20. Hacker K. The burden of chronic disease. Mayo Clin Proc: Innov, Qual Outcomes 2024;8(1):112–9.
21. Piovani D, Nikolopoulos GK, Bonovas S. Non-communicable diseases: the invisible epidemic. J Clin Med 2022;11(19):5939.
22. Anderson E, Durstine JL. Physical activity, exercise, and chronic diseases: a brief review. Sports Med Heal Sci 2019;1(1):3–10.
23. Mastorci F, Lazzeri MFL, Ait-Ali L, et al. Chronic disease in pediatric population—A narrative review of psychosocial dimensions and strategies for management. Children 2025;12(8):967.
24. Basu S. Chronic disease accumulation: aetiological basis, the unexplained remainder, and the way ahead. Lancet Heal Longev 2025;6(5):100716.
25. Watson KB, Wiltz JL, Nhim K, et al. Trends in multiple chronic conditions among US adults, by life stage, behavioral risk factor surveillance system, 2013–2023. Prev Chronic Dis 2025;22:E15.
26. Rappaport SM, Smith MT. Environment and disease risks. Science 2010;330(6003):460–1.
27. UNICEF. Non-communicable diseases. 2021. Available at: https://www.unicef.org/health/non-communicable-diseases.
28. Nguyen GT, Gauvreau C, Mansuri N, et al. Implementation factors of non-communicable disease policies and programmes for children and youth in low-

income and middle-income countries: a systematic review. BMJ Paediatr Open 2024;8(1):e002556.
29. World Health Organization (WHO). Noncommunicable diseases. 2025. Available at: https://www.who.int/news-room/fact-sheets/detail/noncommunicable-diseases. Accessed January 21, 2026.
30. Geng X, Liang F, Wang P. The global burden of non-communicable diseases attributable to behavioral risk factors and its trends from 1990 to 2021. J Adv Res 2025. https://doi.org/10.1016/j.jare.2025.09.022.
31. Budreviciute A, Damiati S, Sabir DK, et al. Management and prevention strategies for non-communicable diseases (NCDs) and their risk factors. Front Public Heal 2020;8:574111.
32. World Health Organization (WHO). Global health estimates: life expectancy and healthy life expectancy. Available at: https://www.who.int/data/gho/data/themes/mortality-and-global-health-estimates/ghe-life-expectancy-and-healthy-life-expectancy.
33. Xi JY, Liang BH, Zhang WJ, et al. Effects of population aging on quality of life and disease burden: a population-based study. Glob Heal Res Polic 2025;10(1):2.
34. World Health Organization (WHO). COVID-19 eliminated a decade of progress in global level of life expectancy. 2024. Available at: https://www.who.int/news/item/24-05-2024-covid-19-eliminated-a-decade-of-progress-in-global-level-of-life-expectancy. Accessed January 19, 2026.
35. Institute for Health Metrics and Evaluation (IHME). Global burden of disease (GBD) key findings. Available at: https://www.healthdata.org/research-analysis/gbd-key-findings. Accessed January 21, 2026.
36. Sun X, Li X. Editorial: aging and chronic disease: public health challenge and education reform. Front Public Heal 2023;11:1175898.
37. Hu Y, He T, Zhang Y, et al. Analysis of the global burden of diabetes and attributable risk factor in children and adolescents across 204 countries and regions from 1990 to 2021. Front Endocrinol 2025;16:1587055.
38. Di Cesare M, Sorić M, Bovet P, et al. The epidemiological burden of obesity in childhood: a worldwide epidemic requiring urgent action. BMC Med 2019;17(1):212.
39. Fahmi A, Safa F, Mariya S, et al. Long-term cardiovascular outcomes in childhood cancer survivors: a systematic review. Cureus 2025;17(6):e85670.
40. Deng Y, Tian R, Zhao J, et al. Global survival trends in congenital heart disease: temporal, regional, and sex disparities from global burden of disease analyses. Int J Cardiol 2026;443:133925.
41. Ngowi JE, Munishi C, Ndumwa HP, et al. Efforts to address the burden of non-communicable diseases need local evidence and shared lessons from high-burden countries. Ann Glob Heal 2023;89(1):78.
42. Horton R. Chronic diseases: the case for urgent global action. Lancet 2007;370-(9603):1881–2.
43. World Health Organization (WHO). Sustainable development goals: target 3. Available at: https://www.who.int/europe/about-us/our-work/sustainable-development-goals/targets-of-sustainable-development-goal-3.
44. Thakur JS, Nangia R, Singh S. Progress and challenges in achieving noncommunicable diseases targets for the sustainable development goals. FASEB Bioadv 2021;3(8):563–8.
45. World Health Organization (WHO). SDG target 3.4 non-communicable diseases and mental health. Available at: https://www.who.int/data/gho/data/themes/topics/sdg-target-3_4-noncommunicable-diseases-and-mental-health. Accessed January 21, 2026.

46. Reif LK, Olmen J van, McNairy ML, et al. Models of lifelong care for children and adolescents with chronic conditions in low-income and middle-income countries: a scoping review. BMJ Glob Heal 2022;7(7):e007863.
47. Institute for Health Metrics and Evaluation (IHME). GBD compare data visualization. IHME, University of Washington; 2025. Available at: https://vizhub.healthdata.org/gbd-compare. Accessed October 31, 2025.
48. Heine M, Hanekom S. Chronic disease in low-resource settings: prevention and management throughout the continuum of care—A call for papers. Int J Environ Res Public Heal 2023;20(4):3580.
49. Jaung MS, Willis R, Sharma P, et al. Models of care for patients with hypertension and diabetes in humanitarian crises: a systematic review. Heal Polic Plan 2021;36(4):509–32.
50. Institute for Health Metrics and Evaluation (IHME). GBD results. 2025. Available at: https://vizhub.healthdata.org/gbd-results/. Accessed November 1, 2025.
51. Bollyky TJ, Templin T, Cohen M, et al. Lower-income countries that face the Most rapid shift in noncommunicable disease burden are also the least prepared. Heal Aff (Proj Hope) 2017;36(11):1866–75.
52. Gulis G, Zidkova R, Meier Z. Changes in disease burden and epidemiological transitions. Sci Rep 2025;15(1):8961.
53. Li Z, Shi J, Li N, et al. Temporal trends in the burden of non-communicable diseases in countries with the highest malaria burden, 1990–2019: evaluating the double burden of non-communicable and communicable diseases in epidemiological transition. Glob Heal 2022;18(1):90.
54. Marshall SJ. Developing countries face double burden of disease. Bull World Heal Organ 2004;82(7):556. Available at: https://pubmed.ncbi.nlm.nih.gov/15500291/.
55. Basto-Abreu A, Barrientos-Gutierrez T, Wade AN, et al. Multimorbidity matters in low and middle-income countries. J Multimorb Comorbidity 2022;12:26335565221106074.
56. Liu J, Qi X, Wang X, et al. Evolving patterns of nutritional deficiencies burden in Low- and middle-income countries: findings from the 2019 global burden of disease study. Nutrients 2022;14(5):931.
57. Yue T, Zhang Q, Li G, et al. Global burden of nutritional deficiencies among children under 5 years of age from 2010 to 2019. Nutrients 2022;14(13):2685.
58. UNICEF. Placing children at the heart of the non-communicable disease and mental health agenda. 2025. Available at: https://www.unicef.org/documents/advocacy-ncd-mental-health. Accessed October 31, 2025.
59. Jones NL, Gilman SE, Cheng TL, et al. Life course approaches to the causes of health disparities. Am J Public Heal 2019;109(S1):S48–55.
60. Vijayasingham L, Ansbro É, Zmeter C, et al. Implementing and evaluating integrated care models for non-communicable diseases in fragile and humanitarian settings. J Migr Heal 2024;9:100228.
61. Asgary R, Garland V, Ro V, et al. A systematic review of effective strategies for chronic disease management in humanitarian settings; opportunities and challenges. Prev Med 2022;161:107154.
62. World Health Organization (WHO). Global health estimates: leading causes of death - cause specific mortality, 2000-2021. Available at: https://www.who.int/data/gho/data/themes/mortality-and-global-health-estimates/ghe-leading-causes-of-death.
63. Jung HS, Choi JW. Association between COVID-19 and incidence of cardiovascular disease and all-cause mortality among patients with diabetes. Front Endocrinol 2023;14:1230176.

64. Tsankov BK, Allaire JM, Irvine MA, et al. Severe COVID-19 infection and pediatric comorbidities: a systematic review and meta-analysis. Int J Infect Dis 2021;103: 246–56.
65. Ngaruiya C, Bernstein R, Leff R, et al. Systematic review on chronic non-communicable disease in disaster settings. BMC Public Heal 2022;22(1):1234.
66. Garcia DM, Sheehan MC. Extreme weather-driven disasters and children's health. Int J Heal Serv 2016;46(1):79–105.
67. Bausch FJ, Beran D, Hering H, et al. Operational considerations for the management of non-communicable diseases in humanitarian emergencies. Confl Heal 2021;15(1):9.
68. Yapa CM. Primary health care service delivery by international actors in humanitarian emergencies. Australia: The Australian National University; 2019.
69. Quarantelli EL, Dynes RR. *Different types of organizations in disaster responses and their operational problems.* Disaster research center. University of Delaware; 1977. Available at: http://udspace.udel.edu/handle/19716/414. Accessed October 30, 2025.
70. Schlegelmilch J, Sury J, Brooks J, et al. A philanthropic approach to supporting emergent disaster response and recovery. Disaster Med Public 2020;14(1): 158–60.
71. World Health Organization (WHO). Health cluster guide: a practical handbook. 2020. Available at: https://wkc.who.int/resources/publications/i/item/9789240004726.
72. Burton A. Caring for children amidst chaos: guidelines to maintain health. Environ Heal Perspect 2006;114(10):A584–91.
73. Perone SA, Martinez E, du Mortier S, et al. Non-communicable diseases in humanitarian settings: ten essential questions. Confl Heal 2017;11(1):17.
74. Garcia DM, Amsalu R, Harkensee C, et al. Humanitarian paediatrics: a statement of purpose. PLOS Glob Public Heal 2022;2(12):e0001431.
75. Johnson HL, Gaskins SW, Seibert DC. Clinical skill and knowledge requirements of health care providers caring for children in disaster, humanitarian and civic assistance operations: an integrative review of the literature. Prehospital Disaster Med 2013;28(1):61–8.
76. Prince M, Patel V, Saxena S, et al. No health without mental health. Lancet 2007; 370(9590):859–77.
77. Maliqi B, Hinton R, Chowdury M, et al. Prepared health systems provide quality care at all times. BMJ 2023;380:e072698.
78. Ansbro É, Cooper K, Tharwat M, et al. Non-communicable diseases in emergencies: time for action on converging crises. Lancet 2025;406(10509): 1197–200.
79. Schmitt R, Herman M, Barnhart W, et al. The 2023 Kahramanmaras, Turkey earthquake sequence. U.S. Geological Survey StoryMap; 2024. Available at: https://earthquake.usgs.gov/storymap/index-turkey2023.html. Accessed January 20, 2026.
80. T.C. Cumhurbaşkanlığı Strateji ve Bütçe Başkanlığı. Kahramanmaraş and Hatay earthquakes report, 2023. 2023. Available at: https://www.sbb.gov.tr/wp-content/uploads/2023/03/2023-Kahramanmaras-and-Hatay-Earthquakes-Report.pdf.
81. Trabzon G, Sarı SA, Yüce S, et al. The impact of the 2023 Türkiye earthquakes on glycemic control and stress levels in children with type 1 diabetes: single-center experience. J Clin Res Pediatr Endocrinol 2025;17(3):288–96.
82. Dağ YS, Zengin M, Yayan EH, et al. The difficulties experienced by children with celiac disease in the Kahramanmaras centered earthquake in Turkey: a qualitative research. J Pediatr Heal Care 2025;39(3):387–95.

83. Bakkaloğlu SA, Delibaş A, Döven SS, et al. Pediatric kidney care experience after the 2023 Türkiye earthquake. Nephrol Dial Transplant 2024;39(9): 1514–22.
84. Taner S, Tabel Y, Bakkaloğlu SA. The devastating Turkey-Syria earthquake from the perspective of pediatric nephrology. J Pediatr Res 2023;10(4):244–8.
85. Düzova A, Akgül S, Utine GE, et al. The Türkiye-Syria earthquake: a response from the editors of the Turkish Journal of Pediatrics. Turk J Pediatr 2023;65(1):1–2.
86. Kadir A, Doull L, Patterson JM, et al. Improving humanitarian health responses for children through nurturing care. Child Prot Pr 2024;2:100035.
87. World Health Organization (WHO). Manual for the Health Care of Children in Humanitarian Emergencies. https://www.who.int/publications/i/item/9789241596879.
88. World Health Organization (WHO). Strengthening services for NCDs in all-hazards emergency preparedness, resilience and response: a WHO report (Draft). 2024. Available at: https://www.who.int/publications/m/item/strengthening-services-for-ncds-in-all-hazards-emergency-preparedness–resilience-and-response.
89. UNHCR IRC. Informal Inter-Agency Group on NCDs in humanitarian settings. Integrating non-communicable disease care in humanitarian settings: an operational guide. 2020. Available at: https://www.unhcr.org/us/media/integrating-non-communicable-disease-care-humanitarian-settings-2020-pdf.
90. World Health Organization (WHO). Monitoring the building blocks of health systems: a handbook of indicators and their measurement strategies. World Health Organization; 2010. Available at: https://iris.who.int/handle/10665/258734.
91. Akik C, Dirani ZE, Willis R, et al. Providing continuity of care for people living with noncommunicable diseases in humanitarian settings: a qualitative study of health actors' experiences in Lebanon. J Migr Heal 2024;10:100269.
92. Tomio J, Sato H. Emergency and disaster preparedness for chronically ill patients: a review of recommendations. Open Access Emerg Med 2014;6(0):69–79.
93. Arrieta MI, Foreman RD, Crook ED, et al. Insuring continuity of care for chronic disease patients after a disaster: key preparedness elements. Am J Med Sci 2008;336(2):128–33.
94. Ansbro É, Issa R, Willis R, et al. Chronic NCD care in crises: a qualitative study of global experts' perspectives on models of care for hypertension and diabetes in humanitarian settings. J Migr Heal 2022;5:100094.
95. International Rescue Committee. Package of essential non-communicable diseases interventions for humanitarian settings (PEN-H). International Rescue Committee; 2020. Available at: https://www.rescue.org/report/package-essential-non-communicable-diseases-interventions-humanitarian-settings-pen-h.

APPENDIX 1: GLOSSARY

- *Care Model:* A framework that addresses the organization of health care services and is applied in clinical or community settings to facilitate the systematic well-being of a specific patient population, via the application of certain theories and evidence-based practices.
- *Crisis-affected Population:* Vulnerable people who are critically affected by humanitarian crises or emergencies such as refugees, internally displaced people, and other community-dwellers.
- *Humanitarian Crisis:* A disruptive event such as famine, war, emergency, or a natural disaster, that threatens the lives, safety, and well-being of the target population such that corrective action is needed to enforce protection and survival.

Substantial external aid and resources are required to meet the needs of the target population.

- *LMIC:* A term that encompasses countries that are designated by the World Bank as either low-income, lower-middle income, or upper-middle income.
- *NCDs:* A group of chronic conditions that are often characterized by multiple risk factors, generally require long-term care, and serve as a substantial source of disability, functional impairment, and death.

APPENDIX 2: COMPENDIUM OF MULTIDOMAIN REFERENCES (SEE FIG. 4)

The display below provides references categorized into key overlapping domains that emerged from the literature as depicted in **Fig. 4**. All pieces addressed LMIC settings.

A	**Pediatric Clinical Care + NCD Management**
	Di Cesare, M., Sorić, M., Bovet, P., Miranda, J. J., Bhutta, Z., Stevens, G. A., Laxmaiah, A., Kengne, A.-P., & Bentham, J. (2019). The epidemiologic burden of obesity in childhood: a worldwide epidemic requiring urgent action. *BMC Medicine, 17*(1), 212. https://doi.org/10.1186/s12916-019-1449-8 Reif, L. K., Olmen, J. van, McNairy, M. L., Ahmed, S., Putta, N., Bermejo, R., Nugent, R., Paintsil, E., Daelmans, B., Varghese, C., Sugandhi, N., & Abrams, E. J. (2022). Models of lifelong care for children and adolescents with chronic conditions in low-income and middle-income countries: a scoping review. *BMJ Global Health, 7*(7), e007863. https://doi.org/10.1136/bmjgh-2021-007863
B	**NCD Management + Humanitarian Crises**
	Akik, C., Dirani, Z. E., Willis, R., Truppa, C., Zmeter, C., Perone, S. A., Roswall, J., Hamadeh, R., Blanchet, K., Roberts, B., Fouad, M. F., Perel, P., & Ansbro, É. (2024). Providing continuity of care for people living with noncommunicable diseases in humanitarian settings: A qualitative study of health actors' experiences in Lebanon. *Journal of Migration and Health, 10*, 100269. https://doi.org/10.1016/j.jmh.2024.100269 Ansbro, É., Cooper, K., Tharwat, M., Kehlenbrink, S., Pratap, B., Hag, E., Perel, P., & Laarsen, L. B. (2025). Non-communicable diseases in emergencies: time for action on converging crises. *The Lancet, 406*(10509), 1197–1200. https://doi.org/10.1016/s0140-6736(25)01852-5 Arrieta, M. I., Foreman, R. D., Crook, E. D., & Icenogle, M. L. (2008). Insuring Continuity of Care for Chronic Disease Patients After a Disaster; Key Preparedness Elements. *The American Journal of the Medical Sciences, 336*(2), 128–133. https://doi.org/10.1097/maj.0b013e318180f209 Asgary, R., Garland, V., Ro, V., Stribling, J. C., & Waldman, R. (2022). A systematic review of effective strategies for chronic disease management in humanitarian settings; opportunities and challenges. *Preventive Medicine, 161*, 107154. https://doi.org/10.1016/j.ypmed.2022.107154 Bausch, F. J., Beran, D., Hering, H., Boulle, P., Chappuis, F., Dromer, C., Saaristo, P., & Perone, S. A. (2021). Operational considerations for the management of non-communicable diseases in humanitarian emergencies. *Conflict and Health, 15*(1), 9. https://doi.org/10.1186/s13031-021-00345-w Iyer, A., Bookstein, A., Kim, G., & Po, J. (2025). Community-based solutions for chronic disease management during natural disasters: A systematic review. *PLOS Global Public Health, 5*(8), e0004997. https://doi.org/10.1371/journal.pgph.0004997 Jaung, M. S., Willis, R., Sharma, P., Perone, S. A., Frederiksen, S., Truppa, C., Roberts, B., Perel, P., Blanchet, K., & Ansbro, É. (2021). Models of care for patients with hypertension and diabetes in humanitarian crises: a

systematic review. *Health Policy and Planning, 36*(4), 509–532. https://doi.org/10.1093/heapol/czab007

MD, R. L., DTM&H, A. S., MD, MSc, MPH, R. B., MD, L. W., MPH, A. H., MD, MPH, P. A., MD, MLS, D. H., & DTM&H, C. N., MD, MSc,. (2021). A review of interventions for noncommunicable diseases in humanitarian emergencies in low- and middle-income countries. *American Journal of Disaster Medicine, 16*(4), 297–311. https://doi.org/10.5055/ajdm.2021.0412

NCD Alliance. (2024). *Neglected and in Crisis: NCDs as a priority in humanitarian settings*. NCD Alliance. https://ncdalliance.org/resources/neglected-and-crisis-ncds-priority-humanitarian

Ngaruiya, C., Bernstein, R., Leff, R., Wallace, L., Agrawal, P., Selvam, A., Hersey, D., & Hayward, A. (2022). Systematic review on chronic non-communicable disease in disaster settings. *BMC Public Health, 22*(1), 1234. https://doi.org/10.1186/s12889-022-13399-z

Perone, S. A., Martinez, E., Mortier, S. du, Rossi, R., Pahud, M., Urbaniak, V., Chappuis, F., Hagon, O., Bausch, F. J., & Beran, D. (2017). Non-communicable diseases in humanitarian settings: ten essential questions. *Conflict and Health, 11*(1), 17. https://doi.org/10.1186/s13031-017-0119-8

SPHERE Alliance. (2018). *The Sphere Handbook: Humanitarian Charter and Minimum Standards in Humanitarian Response* (fourth edition). Sphere Association. https://spherestandards.org/handbook/

UNHCR, IRC, & Informal Inter-Agency Group on NCDs in Humanitarian Settings. (2020). *Integrating Non-communicable Disease Care in Humanitarian Settings: An Operational Guide*. https://www.unhcr.org/us/media/integrating-non-communicable-disease-care-humanitarian-settings-2020-pdf

Vijayasingham, L., Ansbro, É., Zmeter, C., Abbas, L. A., Schmid, B., Sanga, L., Larsen, L. B., Perone, S. A., & Perel, P. (2024). Implementing and evaluating integrated care models for non-communicable diseases in fragile and humanitarian settings. *Journal of Migration and Health, 9*, 100228. https://doi.org/10.1016/j.jmh.2024.100228

WHO. (2024). *Strengthening services for NCDs in all-hazards emergency preparedness, resilience and response: A WHO report (draft)*. https://www.who.int/publications/m/item/strengthening-services-for-ncds-in-all-hazards-emergency-preparedness–resilience-and-response

Yapa, C. M. (2019). *Primary Health Care Service Delivery by International Actors in Humanitarian Emergencies*. The Australian National University (Australia).

C Pediatric Clinical Care + Humanitarian Crises

Johnson, H. L., Gaskins, S. W., & Seibert, D. C. (2013). Clinical Skill and Knowledge Requirements of Health Care Providers Caring for Children in Disaster, Humanitarian and Civic Assistance Operations: An Integrative Review of the Literature. *Prehospital and Disaster Medicine, 28*(1), 61–68. https://doi.org/10.1017/s1049023x12001550

Kadir, A., Doull, L., Patterson, J. M., Khan, M., Cummings, R., Noble, D. J., & Banerjee, A. (2024). Improving humanitarian health responses for children through nurturing care. *Child Protection and Practice, 2*, 100035. https://doi.org/10.1016/j.chipro.2024.100035

Kocik, V. I., Borgman, M. A., April, M. D., & Schauer, S. G. (2023). A scoping review of 2 decades of pediatric humanitarian care during wartime. *Journal of Trauma and Acute Care Surgery, 95*(2S), S170–S179. https://doi.org/10.1097/ta.0000000000004005

Lai, B. S., & Greca, A. L. (2020). *Understanding the Impacts of Natural Disasters on Children* (Child Evidence Brief). Society for Research in Child Development.

World Health Organization. (2008). *Manual for the health care of children in humanitarian emergencies.*

D	Pediatric Clinical Care + NCD Management + Humanitarian Crises
	International Rescue Committee. (2020). *Package Of Essential Non-Communicable Diseases Interventions For Humanitarian Settings (PEN-H).* https://www.rescue.org/report/package-essential-non-communicable-diseases-interventions-humanitarian-settings-pen-h Nguyen, G. T., Gauvreau, C., Mansuri, N., Wight, L., Wong, B., Neposlan, J., Petricca, K., & Denburg, A. (2024). Implementation factors of non-communicable disease policies and programmes for children and youth in low-income and middle-income countries: a systematic review. *BMJ Paediatrics Open*, *8*(1), e002556. https://doi.org/10.1136/bmjpo-2024-002556 World Health Organization (WHO). (2013). *Global action plan for the prevention and control of noncommunicable diseases 2013–2020.* World Health Organization. https://www.who.int/publications/i/item/9789241506236

Mental Health and Wellness Following Large-Scale Catastrophic Events

The Role of the Pediatric Clinician

Bruce D. Perry, MD, PhD[a,b,*]

KEYWORDS

- Trauma • Post-traumatic stress • Mass casualty • Catastrophic event
- Natural disaster

KEY POINTS

- Humanitarian crises are often created by catastrophic traumatic events.
- The scope and scale of the mental health needs following catastrophic trauma overwhelm even the most resourced mental health systems.
- Pediatric clinicians play key leadership roles in the individual, community and systemic responses to catastrophic trauma.
- Many symptoms of an acute stress response and posttraumatic stress disorders present primarily as *physical health* issues (eg, syncope, chest, and gastrointestinal pain, headaches, lethargy and mental status changes mimicking absence seizures).
- Education about the known and predictable physical and mental health impacts of traumatic stress should be incorporated into graduate and postgraduate training for pediatric health care providers.

INTRODUCTION

Each year millions of children, youth and their families are impacted by natural disasters (eg, flood, earthquake, hurricane, tsunami, tornado, wildfire, and famine) and human-induced large scale traumatic events (war, school or public shootings, forced displacement, cultural, and active genocide). This overview is based upon lessons learned from over 30 years of direct clinical care, community consultation and program development in a wide range of major traumatic events and humanitarian crises.[1–5] These include high profile incidents (eg, Branch Davidian Siege and fire),

[a] School of Allied Health, Human Services and Sport, La Trobe University, Melbourne, Victoria, Australia; [b] Neurosequential Network, Houston, TX, USA
* The Neurosequential Network, 3733-1 Westheimer Road, #1039, Houston, TX 77027.
E-mail address: bdp@neurosequential.com

Pediatr Clin N Am 73 (2026) 985–996
https://doi.org/10.1016/j.pcl.2026.04.008 pediatric.theclinics.com

Abbreviation	
PTSD	posttraumatic stress disorder

dozens of school shootings (eg, Columbine and Sandy Hook), terrorist actions (eg, Oklahoma City bombing, 9/11), natural disasters (eg, Hurricane Katrina, Tohoku tsunami, earthquakes in New Zealand, Turkey and Syria; wildfires and floods in the United States and Australia), mass migration humanitarian crises (eg, separation of child and parent at US border) and hundreds of other individual and family traumatic events (eg, suicide, murder, kidnapping, motor vehicle accidents, rape, and almost every version of human and natural traumatic). In each of these situations, pediatric clinicians had the opportunity to provide leadership to disorganized, overwhelmed and dysfunctional public systems struggling with the scope, scale and complexity of the physical and mental health challenges faced by children, youth and parents. In many of these major traumatic events, there were lost opportunities to optimize the healing process for children, families and the community. Thirty years ago, a major reason for this was simply a lack of awareness regarding the effects of stress, distress and trauma on the developing child (and everyone else involved in the catastrophic event). While the general knowledge about adversity and development[1,6] and posttraumatic stress disorder (PTSD), in general, has increased, challenges remain. This overview will highlight some areas of particular relevance for pediatric health care professionals.

Posttraumatic Impacts of Catastrophic Trauma

The pattern of stress caused by large-scale catastrophic events—uncontrollable, unpredictable, often extreme and prolonged—will predictably lead to alterations in the sensitivity and reactivity of stress response systems throughout the body.[2,3] This sensitization across the body's multiple stress response systems results in a pervasive impact on the immune, endocrine, autonomic and central nervous systems.[1,6] A cascade of alterations in these systems will influence cardiorespiratory, gastrointestinal, reproductive, musculoskeletal and brain-mediated functions. The result is a wide range of physical and mental health symptoms and signs.[7,8] Common posttraumatic symptoms include syncope, gastrointestinal issues (eg, pain and constipation), r/o seizure disorder, headaches, exhaustion, as well as sleep, anxiety, attention and mood problems along with the more commonly *known* posttraumatic stress symptoms of intrusive ideations, *reenactment* behaviors and pervasive physiologic reactivity (ie, the sensitization across multiple systems). The full range of these symptoms is beyond the scope of this overview, but the emerging field of disaster mental health has provided multiple excellent resources for the pediatric clinician.[9–13]

In many cases a pediatric health care provider is the first and most *logical* resource for families seeking help for a symptomatic child. Often the parents (and the clinical team) do not connect the symptoms to the traumatic experience. In the case of acute mental health symptoms such as anxiety with event-specific elements (eg, reenactment play, nightmares or evocative cues clearly reminiscent of the event) it is more apparent. The further away from the event and the less *mental health* related the symptoms or signs, the less likely a clinician will make the connection. This is most apparent in clinicians who have had minimal exposure to the emerging concepts related to stress, trauma and the multisystemic impacts of traumatic stress. The range and complexity of these clinical presentations often lead to diagnostic challenges and, most important, treatment inefficiencies. Posttraumatic physical and mental health symptoms act as *Great Imposters*—mimicking a myriad of syndromes or disease processes (eg, cardiac insufficiency and absence seizures) and complicating the presentation and control of other existing conditions (eg, diabetes, autoimmune disorders and irritable bowel syndrome [IBS]). This is where a full developmental history that includes nature, pattern and timing of adversity and, the counter-balancing, *protective* relational health is very helpful. Understanding the effects of developmental trauma can bring additional, often essential, insights to the diagnostic, and treatment planning process.

Understanding the Risk for the Development of Posttraumatic Problems

The risk of developing posttraumatic problems varies depending upon various factors (**Table 1**). A key factor in risk is the proximity to the event's *ground zero* or primary area of threat, destruction, and life-threatening impact (**Fig. 1**). Each event creates an event-specific trauma 'footprint' resulting from the pattern of immediate impact, chronic secondary effects and potential for ongoing evocative cues (eg, high profile events with Western media coverage that includes social media blasting creates an almost unavoidable flood of evocative cues). Displacement of a community following the death and destruction of an earthquake or tsunami will pose multiple year recovery issues impacting the capacity of a family and community to restore stability of housing and economic health all while grieving at multiple levels across many families. Personal grief is compounded by community or even cultural grief; loss of life, home, community, and collective identity often occurs during humanitarian crises created by war and major natural disasters. While each event is unique, there is emerging evidence to suggest that a key factor in risk following major catastrophic trauma is preevent mental health and attachment status.[14] Early life experiences create the filters through, which all future events are experienced—including major catastrophic trauma. The individuals with greatest risk for posttraumatic problems following any traumatic experience are those who go into that event with preexisting vulnerability.[1,5,14]

Whether the clinician is playing a leadership role in system-wide, family or individual responses, a major challenge is the way stress-related shifts in functioning create a *state-dependent* inefficiency in the capacity to process complex cognitive content.[2,3] Threat, stress, fear—all activate CNS responses intended to help the individual survive the perceived threat.[2] In the face of inescapable distress and pain, the mental (and physical) mechanism of dissociation is the dominant adaptive response.[1,3] A primary feature of dissociation is a graded disengagement from the external *world* with an increasing focus on the *internal* world; emotional numbness, a sense of *unreality*, a robotic mirroring quality to communication, which leads to a misunderstanding on the part of the pediatric clinician that the child/parent has actually attended to and internalized what you have been trying to communicate. When individuals are in this dissociative *state* traditional forms of communication and therapeutic work are often less efficient. This challenge in communication leads to misunderstandings and miscommunication, which only adds to the frustration, anger, disappointment and disengagement that is so often seen in crisis intervention efforts that are well-intended but trauma-unaware. Dissociation—numbness in the face of the unavoidable, uncontrollable pain of the traumatic event—dominates the acute posttraumatic period. Unfortunately, this means that when supports are most likely to be available and energized, the traumatized population is least capable of engaging and benefiting from the supports that are offered.

As mentioned earlier, there is a wide range of symptoms that are interrelated and trauma-induced; further when dealing with the acute traumatic situation, the nature of the primary symptoms will shift (**Fig. 2**). In the first few weeks during and after

Table 1
Factors influencing risk for developing posttraumatic mental health issues

	Event	Individual	Family and Social
Increase risk (prolong the intensity or duration of the acute stress response)	• Multiple or repeated events (eg, domestic violence, sexual abuse, and physical abuse) • Physical injury to child • Involves physical injury or death to loved one, particularly mother • Dismembered or disfigured bodies seen • Destroys home, school, or community • Disrupts community infrastructure (eg, earthquake) • Perpetrator is family member • Long duration (eg, flood)	• Female • Age (Younger more vulnerable) • Subjective perception of physical harm • History of previous exposure to trauma • No cultural or religious anchors • No shared experience with peers (experiential isolation) • Low intelligence quotient (IQ) • Preexisting neuropsychiatric disorder (especially anxiety related)	• Trauma directly impacts caregivers • Anxiety in primary caregivers • Continuing threats and disruption to family • Chaotic, overwhelmed family • Physical isolation • Distant caregiving • Absent caregivers
Decrease risk (decrease intensity or duration of the acute stress response)	• Single event • Perpetrator is stranger • No disruption of family or community structure • Short duration (eg, tornado)	• Cognitively capable of understanding abstract concepts • Healthy coping skills • Educated about normative posttraumatic responses • Immediate posttraumatic interventions • Strong ties to cultural or religious belief system	• Intact, nurturing family supports • Nontraumatized caregivers • Caregivers educated about normative posttraumatic responses • Strong family beliefs • Mature and attuned parenting skills

The development of significant posttraumatic mental health issues will vary depending upon a host of factors. Any factors that can decrease the intensity, duration and unpredictability of the individual's stress response (eg, strong relational supports) following the trauma will decrease the probability of lingering mental health effects. In large scale humanitarian events, the adults in the child's life have also been profoundly impacted. This can interfere with these important *stress-buffering* relationships and result in an increased risk for MH challenges in the entire family. For more detail see.[4,5]

Adapted with permission from Perry BD. *Stress, trauma, and posttraumatic stress disorders in children: an introduction*. Houston, TX: CTA press; 2007. https://www.childtrauma.org/_files/ugd/aa51c7_60c617d2160b417d9ee0f80e5ca8eaac.pdf.[4]

the primary traumatic event, anxiety and dissociation are the most common primary presentations as the 2 major *wings* of the stress response systems are recruited—the arousal continuum (ie, the *fight, flight* components of our stress response capabilities) and the dissociative continuum (ie, *preserve and prepare for injury* components).

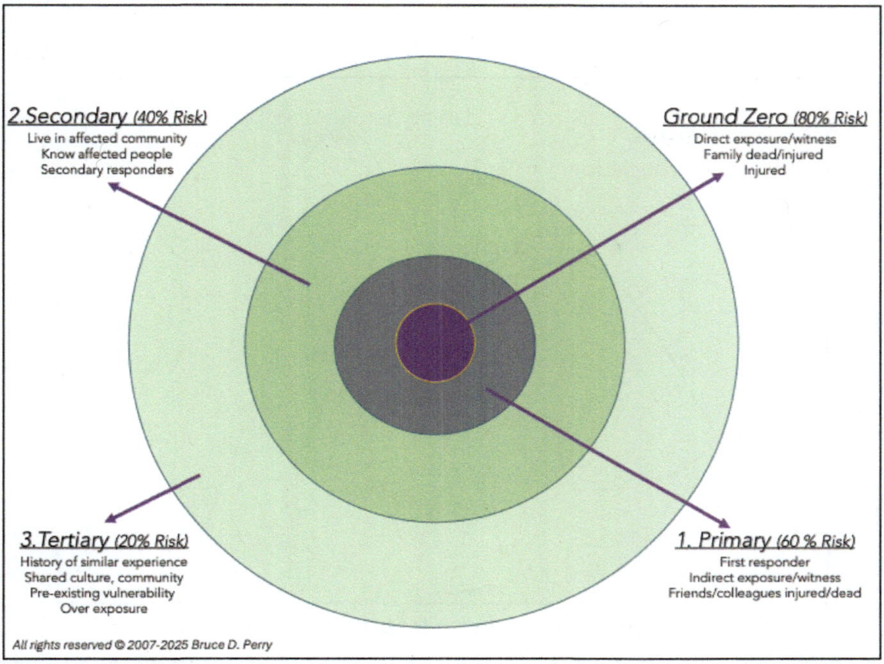

Fig. 1. Differential risk following traumatic event. Proximity to the traumatic event will influence nature and severity of the acute trauma response which, in turn, influences the risk for development of long-term or chronic health issues. Understanding this graded risk profile is helpful when pediatric health care providers are developing their differential diagnoses in children and youth who may have been impacted by a community-wide catastrophic event. Estimates of risk are based upon 30 + years of clinical experience and a variety of reports on the development of PTSD, post-traumatic stress symptoms (PTSS), and MH symptoms following various *types* of trauma.[14] (*Figure courtesy* Bruce D. Perry.)

These 2 major response patterns work together to help the individual, but they both are energy consuming[1,3]; the result is ultimately an exhaustion—both mental and physical. Over time, then, the primary symptoms shift and exhaustion and depression dominate—although both dissociative and anxiety continue. Lethargy, deep sadness, anhedonia, relational collapse and *robotic* engagement in everyday life characterize this heartbreaking grief. This is a time when mental health supports are most needed, and, ironically, it is a time when volunteer and affordable (or free) mental health supports are not usually available (**Fig. 3**). This is one of the most powerful and pervasive observations of our 30 years of work in this area—the mismatch between need and available supports. Many people and systems mobilize and rush in during the first weeks of a catastrophic trauma but 6 months later that attention, effort and concern have moved on—back to their preevent baselines.

This leaves the existing mental health and health care systems to deal with the morbidity from the traumatic event. Over the last 30 years, the disaster mental health field has grown. Research and clinical expertise have emerged and documented various challenges of catastrophic trauma.[10–16] A major challenge is a lack of capacity—the mental health (MH) needs following a traumatic event are greater than the available, well-trained MH supports. At baseline, almost all public mental health systems are already resource challenged, near or overcapacity and dealing with high

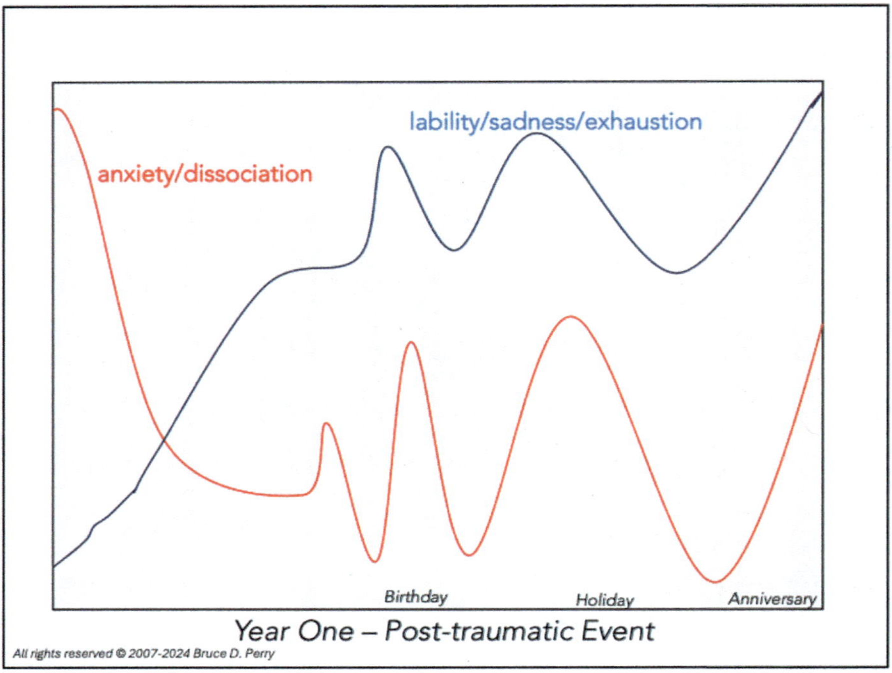

Fig. 2. Evolution of posttraumatic symptoms: Year 1. The nature of posttraumatic mental health symptoms evolve with time. While each person has a unique adaptive pattern that is influenced by many factors (see **Table 1**), a general trend of the waxing and waning of the type and intensity of symptoms is illustrated earlier. Anniversaries, holidays, family events all can be evocative cues in the months and years following catastrophic trauma. (*Figure courtesy* Bruce D. Perry.)

rates of burn out, turn over and nonstop systemic flux with constant leadership, policy and practice changes. Adding more MH needs in a community only magnifies these vulnerabilities. While there are excellent resources available to pediatric clinicians to help build *trauma-sensitive* capacity for their own clinical team, even a well-resourced, *trauma-sensitive* health care community is unable to meet the needs of even small-scale traumatic events (see further).

The Challenge of the Scope and Scale in Humanitarian Crises

Humanitarian crises pose major challenges due to the pervasive traumatic impact throughout a community. Major factors in providing support and therapeutic presence for the traumatized child are the adult relationships in the child's life—the parent, grandparent, neighbor, teacher, coach, and even the pediatric health care professional. But if all of these adults are also traumatized and overwhelmed by the same catastrophic event, their capacity to provide the safe, stable and regulating presence for the child is compromised. The scope of these events will often destabilize and impair the very systems intended to provide education, mental health and health care supports for the child. In short, catastrophic trauma and humanitarian crises overwhelm the capacity of the existing systems, including the mental health system. An additional confound in cases of armed conflict is the political climate, which is often permeated with blaming and *othering* that can influence the allocation of limited resources intended to meet the physical and mental health needs of children from all

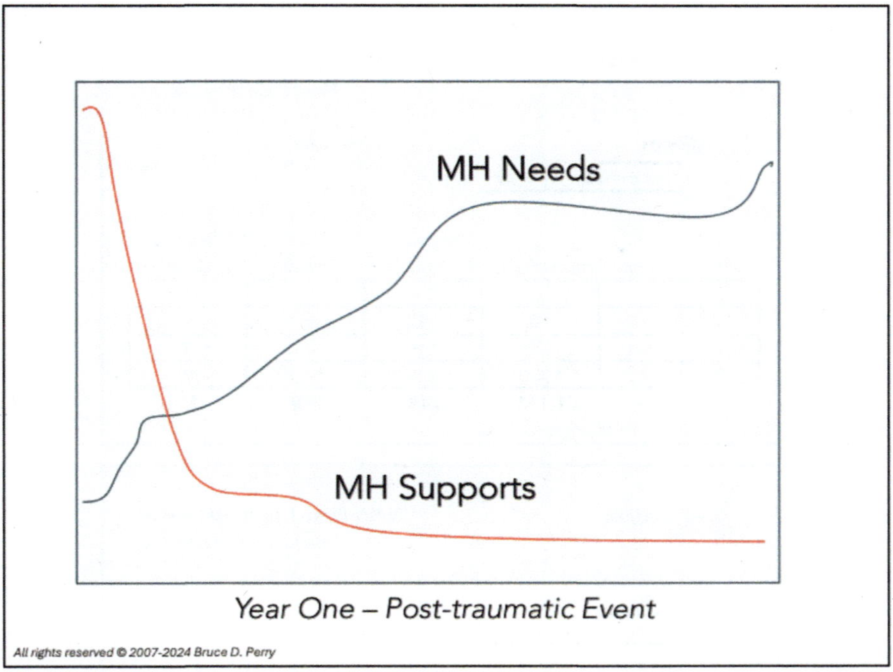

Fig. 3. Mismatch of MH needs and supports in Year 1. In high profile traumatic events it is very common for family, community and systemic supports to mobilize in the immediate aftermath. These supportive efforts are well-intended but often out of sync with the actual needs of those most impacted by the trauma. Mental health professionals often volunteer time and attention in these initial few weeks; yet traditional *therapeutic* assessment and treatment options may not be effective due to the overwhelming circumstances (ie, stress-related inefficiencies in concentration, reasoning, and reflection are common). Over time, the availability of easily accessed and affordable mental health supports shrinks. Ironically, when the most serious and enduring MH symptoms emerge and persist, the availability of MH supports has diminished. (*Figure courtesy* Bruce D. Perry.)

sides of the conflict. The traumatic effects of these conflicts impact children, youth and families independent of political, ethnic, religious or cultural status and should not influence the pediatric clinician's efforts to address the needs of all children.

A first step in planning clinical supports following a traumatic event is to better understand the scope (who has been impacted) and scale (how many people will require intervention) of the traumatic event. In our experience this is one of the major gaps in addressing the mental health needs during a humanitarian crisis, a fundamental misunderstanding of the enduring impact on individuals, families and communities. To estimate the potential mental health morbidity, we developed the Mental Health Risk Tool (**Fig. 4**). Using our experiences from thousands of traumatic events (from catastrophic, impacting hundreds of thousands—to community, impacting thousands—to individual, impacting hundreds) and the published literature about risk for development of Mental ea problems (eg, PTSD, major depressive disorder [MDD]) we have been able to use this tool to illustrate the capacity needs assuming the *1 hour, once a week* dosing of a traditional mental health intervention. In **Fig. 4** the top panel illustrates how a traumatic experience can have a ripple effect within a family, school and community. In this instance, 2 children witnessed the murder of their

NEUROSEQUENTIAL NETWORK™

NMN Post-Traumatic Event
Mental Health Risk Tool

Date: 2021
Event: *home invasion/murder*

Impact Ring	*Risk*	*Individuals*	*Highest Risk*	*"TAU" 1 hr/wk*	*Clinicians (20 hr/wk)*
0	0.8	2	1.6	1.6	0.08
1	0.6	10	6	6	0.3
2	0.4	100	40	40	2
3	0.2	1000	200	200	10
		1,112	***248***	***248***	***12***

NEUROSEQUENTIAL NETWORK™

NMN Post-Traumatic Event
Mental Health Risk Tool

Date: 2023
Event: *Türkiye Earthquake*

Impact Ring	*Risk*	*Individuals*	*Highest Risk*	*"TAU" 1 hr/wk*	*Clinicians (20 hr/wk)*
0	0.8	400,000	320000	320000	16000
1	0.6	800,000	480000	480000	24000
2	0.4	1,500,000	600000	600000	30000
3	0.2	2,000,000	400000	400000	20000
		4,700,000	***1,800,000***	***1,800,000***	***70,000***

Fig. 4. Top and down. MH Risk following catastrophic traumatic events. Risk for experiencing significant mental health symptoms following traumatic events has been estimated from our 40 years of experience studying traumatic events. We developed an MH Risk Tool to help systems and communities understand the *carrying capacity* of their existing mental health systems and the predictable increased demand following these events. We have used this tool for multiple school shootings, natural disasters, and higher profile traumatic events (eg, armed conflict, Branch Davidian siege and fire, September 11). Two examples are included (see text). *Ring* refers to the *distance* from the epicenter of the most destructive traumatic impact of the event (see **Fig. 1**). *Differential Risk* image, with 0 being *ground zero* where the individual is directly impacted by the traumatic event (see **Fig. 1**), and 2 and 3 refer to different populations that were less proximal to the direct traumatic experience. *TAU* refers to treatment as usual (1 hour a week of psychotherapeutic intervention). (*Figure courtesy* Bruce D. Perry.)

parents during a home invasion. Ten people were directly involved and impacted by the murder, 100 were family, church, school connected and close to the parents. The MH 'ripple' of that single traumatic event resulted in over 250 people who had significant MH symptoms that would benefit from, at a minimum, an assessment, psychoeducation and ongoing MH supports. To adequately respond to this, a mental health system would have to dedicate 12 clinicians who would have to clear their calendar so they could provide 20 hours of standard MH intervention to address the new MH morbidity from these murders.

All of this is complicated by major differences in how traditional mental health *help* from a stranger is viewed. At these most vulnerable times, a major challenge is finding and supporting a culturally-sensitive team that has existing connections in the community that will endure beyond the transient influx of mental health supports. The tendency for traditional mental health interventions to push *talking* about the trauma with debriefings or immediate implementation of *evidence-based* protocols with urgency can actually feel intrusive. This is one of the most universal comments our team has heard from thousands of people impacted by traumatic events over the last 40 years. In the immediate posttraumatic period quiet, respectful presence with attunement to the basic needs of the person—shelter, food, information—is what is needed. This stance will make the individual much more willing to consider more formal MH services later in the healing process; if the initial interactions feel disruptive and intrusive, future formal MH services are less attractive to the person—even if needed.

In the lower panel of **Fig. 4**, the initial calculations for the catastrophic earthquake on February 6, 2023, in Turkey and Syria are illustrated.[17] Over 55,000 people died, 40,000 buildings collapsed, 200,000 more were heavily damaged—it is estimated that more than 3 million people were displaced. The MH Risk Tool estimates, at a minimum, 1.8 million people were significantly impacted and would benefit from MH intervention. Yet, if a traditional MH 'dose' and intervention (1 hr/wk) was used, it would take 70,000 clinicians dedicating 50% of their time for this single catastrophic event. That is, of course, impossible. Turkey has roughly 25,000 psychiatrists, psychologists, and social workers combined[17]; even if each of them spent 100% of their time serving people impacted by this single catastrophic event, it would not meet the need.

Supporting Relational Health: the Healing Power of Connectedness

The best buffer for current stress is connectedness—to family, friends, classmates, neighbors. Relationships that are safe, stable and nurturing provide the optimal, and necessary, elements for healing from traumatic stress.[1,17] The major role that a pediatric clinician can play in the posttraumatic healing process is to help identify, support and enrich the relational milieu of the child. Through this relational *orchestration* the pediatric clinician plays the role of the conductor of the relational symphony that will provide the moments of therapeutic support that are regulating, rewarding and healing. There is no need to be the only one *playing an instrument*—providing the therapeutic input. Use the natural strengths and resources of the child's relational network—something we call the *therapeutic web*. In our work, and in others, the best predictor of positive outcomes is relational health—connection to family, community and culture.[1,17] In the face of an overwhelmed mental health system, the most effective and therapeutic interventions are through this therapeutic web in the child's life. Relational poverty creates ongoing risk while relational health—connectednessprovides opportunities for healing. The pediatric clinician, as the conductor of this relational orchestra – can educate, engage, direct and coordinate how others in the child's life understand and interact in ways that will be supportive, developmentally-sensitive and, ultimately, healing.

Systemic and Practice Recommendations

1. Improve pregraduate and postgraduate training about stress, distress, impact of developmental adversity, and relational health on global health wellness
2. Improve pregraduate and postgraduate training about key concepts essential to effective engagement and communication with stressed, distressed or traumatized children and families

3. Proactively create cross-sector work groups to *game* potential catastrophic events in community and begin to build leadership and communication structures with template agreements clarifying leadership roles and establishing funding flexibility
4. Have social and wellness *impact* mapping templates prepared in advance—to identify highest risk individuals for engagement and follow-up health surveillance and support
5. Screening for developmental risk should be a standard component in any comprehensive pediatric health assessment. This risk estimate can be derived from knowing the nature, timing and pattern of developmental adversities *and* counterbalancing relational anchors to family, community and culture (ie, relational health or *connectedness*).
6. Most therapeutic experiences occur outside of *therapy*. Sport, performing arts—drama and dance, creative arts—music, painting, sculpture, writing, and a host of culturally-specific community and group activities are all know to provide the regulation, reward and healing necessary to survive and thrive during and after catastrophic trauma.

Considerations for Clinical Care

The physical signs and symptoms related to a traumatic experience will vary depending upon a host of factors including proximity to the direct threat of the event, the age of the individual and preexisting mental health status (see **Table 1**). Further, these symptoms will wax, wane and evolve over time.

In the acute posttraumatic period, a primary adaptation is dissociation. In the face of inescapable and uncontrollable pain or distress, there is a cognitive and emotional disengagement from the external world and a *retreat* to the inner world. This graded emotional *flight* response can result in a robotic, unemotional presentation to others and a *numb* sense of unreality to the person. A primary clinical complication of this response is the impact this has on communication. The capacity to clearly process and act on advice, recommendations, prescribed treatment etc. will be significantly impaired. The resulting miscommunications will cause missed appointments, difficulty following through with prescribed treatments and misunderstandings between the clients and the health care professional.

Catastrophic traumatic stress is exhausting emotionally and physically. This will impact the capacity to function at the preexperience level. Students have a harder time learning and performing, parents have a harder time being as productive and engaged at work and home. This trauma-related impact on efficiency, effectiveness, mood and social functioning contributes to the MH morbidity of the catastrophic trauma. Psychoeducation and support are key to helping children and families through the long posttraumatic period.

Posttraumatic symptoms often mimic pediatric health conditions and should always be considered as potential factors during diagnostic process.

Relational health and connectedness to family, community and culture are the optimal developmental and therapeutic milieu.

INSIGHTS TO ACTION

- Expect overwhelming needs: Many children and families will need help, and existing systems may not be able to meet all needs.
- Physical symptoms are common: Trauma can cause headaches, stomach pains, abdominal cramping, light-headedness, fatigue and other physical complaints that may look like medical problems.

- Emotional and behavioral symptoms are common: Children, youth and adults may show anxiety, sadness, trouble sleeping, or act out; these may be present in the immediate post-event phase or appear later.
- Dissociation is frequent: Adults, youth and children may seem numb, disconnected, or robotic, making communication and treatment harder.
- Relational support is vital: Strong connections to family, friends, and community help recovery. Keep communication simple: Traumatized children and families may struggle to understand complex information; use clear, supportive language – and expect to repeat the same information multiple times.
- Prepare and educate: Clinicians should understand and be capable of teaching others, including children and youth, about the predictable effects of traumatic experience.
- Don't rush or overwhelm: Avoid pushing individuals to talk about trauma right away; focus on basic needs and gentle support. Give individuals the 'space' to control the timing and manner of 'revisiting' their traumatic experiences.

DECLARATION OF AI AND AI-ASSISTED TECHNOLOGIES IN THE WRITING PROCESS

During the preparation of this work the authors used MS Copilot in order to format the reference section. After using this tool/service, the author reviewed and edited the content as needed and takes full responsibility for the content of the publication.

DISCLOSURES

The author has no commercial interests to declare.

REFERENCES

1. Perry BD, Szalavitz M. The boy who was raised as a dog. 2nd edition. New York: Basic Books; 2017.
2. Perry BD, Pollard R, Blakely T, et al. Childhood trauma, the neurobiology of adaptation and "use-dependent" development of the brain: how "states" become "traits.". Infant Ment Health J 1995;16(4):271–91.
3. Perry BD, Pollard R. Homeostasis, stress, trauma, and adaptation: a neurodevelopmental view of childhood trauma. Child Adolesc Psychiatr Clin N Am 1998; 7(1):33–51.
4. Perry BD. Stress, trauma and post-traumatic stress disorders in children: an introduction. Houston (TX): CTA Press; 2007. Available at: https://www.childtrauma.org/_files/ugd/aa51c7_60c617d2160b417d9ee0f80e5ca8eaac.pdf.
5. Ungar M, Collin-Vezina D, Perry BD. Violence, trauma and resilience. In: Alaggia R, Vine C, editors. Cruel but not unusual: violence in families in Canada. 3rd ed. Waterloo (ON): Wilfrid Laurier University Press; 2022. p. 13–41. https://doi.org/10.51644/9781771125376-003.
6. Anda RF, Felitti VJ, Walker J, et al. The enduring effects of childhood abuse and related experiences: a convergence of evidence from neurobiology and epidemiology. Eur Arch Psychiatr Clin Neurosci 2006;256(3):174–86.
7. Ursano RJ, Fullerton CS, Weisaeth L, et al, editors. Textbook of disaster psychiatry. 2nd ed. Cambridge, England: Cambridge University Press; 2017.
8. Flynn BW, Vance MC, Morganstein JC. Curriculum recommendations for disaster health professionals: disaster behavioral health. 2nd ed. Center for the Study of Traumatic Stress. 2020. Available at: https://www.cstsonline.org/assets/media/documents/CSTS_Curriculum_Recommendations_2nd_ed.pdf.

9. Rahmani M, Muzwagi A, Pumariega AJ. Cultural factors in disaster response among diverse children and youth around the world. Curr Psychiatry Rep 2022;24(10):481–91.
10. Schauss E, Hawes K, Roberts S, et al, BRAIN Center at the University of Memphis. Examining the incidence of acute stress in pediatric trauma patients. Trauma Surg Acute Care Open 2022;7:e000946.
11. Medical traumatic Stress Working Group of National Child Traumatic Stress Network (NCTSN). Pediatric medical traumatic stress: a comprehensive guide. Available at: https://www.nctsn.org/sites/default/files/resources/pediatric_toolkit_for_health_care_providers.pdf.
12. Powell T, Cohen F, Ramchal M. Children's coping in disasters: developments, challenges, and future directions. Curr Psychiatry Rep 2026;28(3). https://doi.org/10.1007/s11920-025-01654-0.
13. Dixon KE, Layne CM, Ho Misiaszek KS, et al. Interpersonal, not existential, adversities predict postwar deterioration in youth social support. Academia Medicine 2024;1. https://doi.org/10.20935/AcadMed6252.
14. Powell T, Wegmann KM, Backode E. Coping and post-traumatic stress in children and adolescents after an acute onset disaster: a systematic review. Int J Environ Res Publ Health 2021;18:4865.
15. Heanoy EZ, Brown NR. Impact of natural disasters on mental health: evidence and implications. Healthcare 2024;12:1812.
16. Wood LCN. Impact of punitive immigration policies, parent-child separation and child detention on the mental health and development of children. BMJ Paediatrics Open 2018;2:e000338.
17. Perry BD. Understanding the challenge of catastrophic traumatic events 1: Turkey & Syria. Neurosequential Model YouTube Channel; 2023. Available at: https://youtu.be/oPmG-tPG4fc?si=xAik0yHcb5Ge9hLu. Accessed January 16, 2026.

Child Abuse and Neglect Risk in Times of Crisis

Melissa T. Merrick, PhD*, J. Bart Klika, MSW, PhD

KEYWORDS

• Child abuse • Child neglect • COVID-19 • Great recession • Public health

KEY POINTS

- Violence against children is a preventable public health problem.
- Humanitarian crises such as economic downturns (eg, Great Recession) and health emergencies (eg, coronavirus disease 2019) increase the risk for violence against children.
- Violence prevention is possible when proactive systems and strategies are in place to meet child and family needs before crisis occurs.

INTRODUCTION

More than half of the children in the world—1.6 billion children—experience regular violent punishment in the home.[1] Direct exposure to physical, sexual, or psychological violence in childhood and indirect exposure to potentially traumatic experiences in the home (eg, intimate partner violence, parental separation, untreated mental illness, or substance misuse), collectively referred to as adverse childhood experiences, can have lasting negative effects on health and life outcomes throughout the life course and often intergenerationally.[2–4] Importantly, for the youngest of children, child abuse and neglect are the most prevalent and impactful of such victimization experiences given the trajectory it sets in motion for children across their lifetimes.[5]

Experiencing child abuse and neglect impairs brain architecture and development, affects the nervous and immune systems, and even changes the way our genes express themselves, in part because of excessive, prolonged doses of toxic stress.[6] Childhood maltreatment makes it more likely for children to experience other types of violence, like peer violence and intimate partner violence, in adolescence and into adulthood, as well as to perpetrate violence throughout development. Experiencing child abuse and neglect is also associated with a host of health-risk behaviors, chronic diseases, mental health problems, and decreased productivity and life opportunities.[2,4,7]

Prevent Child Abuse America, 33 N. Dearborn Street, Suite 2300, Chicago, IL 60602, USA
* Corresponding author.
E-mail address: mmerrick@preventchildabuse.org

Pediatr Clin N Am 73 (2026) 997–1006
https://doi.org/10.1016/j.pcl.2026.04.009 **pediatric.theclinics.com**

Abbreviations	
COVID-19	coronavirus disease 2019
SNAP	supplemental nutrition assistance program

While the causes and sequelae of child abuse and neglect perpetration and victimization are complex, the many detrimental impacts on the individual child, family, community, and society are well-established.[8] Researchers have estimated the lifetime economic burden associated with addressing the consequences of abuse and neglect. Across their lifetime, each victim of child abuse or neglect is estimated to incur costs of nearly US$830,928 for services like child welfare, special education, medical care, and juvenile justice.[9] Further, this estimate includes projected losses in productivity as the child progresses through adulthood. While the individual does not necessarily pay out-of-pocket for these expenses, taxpayer dollars are used to pay for services and programs used by these individuals.

There is no single cause of child abuse and neglect.[10–12] The social-ecological model is a helpful one when examining the complex interplay of risk and protective factors for child abuse and neglect perpetration and victimization.[13] Indeed, there are risk and protective factors along each of the individual, interpersonal/relationship, community, and societal levels.[14] Further, the cumulative risk model helps to explain why not all individuals with the same risk factors go on to experience violence.[15,16] For purposes of this article, we focus on both the societal and community risk factors that set the context for violence to occur, and those risk factors that are exacerbated during humanitarian crises. We end with a call to action for boosting protective factors at every level to ultimately prevent child abuse and neglect from happening in the first place (primary prevention) and those required to mitigate harm, help families and communities recover from crises quicker, and promote resilience (secondary and tertiary prevention).

Societal and Community Risk Factors

The conditions in which individuals live, parents raise their children, and children develop are critical to their lifelong health, well-being, prosperity, and ability to be resilient.[17] The connection between structural and societal conditions and exposure to childhood adversity has been well-established.[18] In any society, there are sociopolitical and cultural factors that can support and even enhance health, well-being, and prosperity, and those that can marginalize, penalize, and disadvantage people from experiencing their full health and life potential.[19] The laws in any country, state, even locality, along with the accompanying narratives, can promote the conditions in which child abuse and neglect can occur. For example, if the societal norm is to society is to engage in harsh discipline and these behaviors are promoted on television and in media, it is more likely that child maltreatment occurs as a matter of course, even absent acute crises. Similarly, when gender norms make it such that mothers and female caregivers take on the majority of childcare responsibilities, absent social and concrete supports, vulnerability to child abuse and neglect is magnified.

Economic pressures also significantly impact family functioning and child safety, even in precrisis times. High rates of poverty and unemployment create additional stressors, like housing instability, food insecurity, and reduced access to health care and educational opportunities, all of which can add additional strain to parenting capacity and increase child maltreatment risk.[14] Resource constraints, too, like limited access to high-quality affordable childcare, transportation, mental health and substance use services, and other essential family supports create additional stressors on parents. Communities lacking social cohesion and support systems, and neighborhoods with high crime and violence rates, with easy access to drugs, alcohol, and firearms can place a heavier toll on families.[14,20]

Other Risk Factors

Factors at the individual and relational level can also confer risk for child abuse and neglect. While children are never responsible for their victimization, children aged younger than 4 years[21] and those with intellectual and physical disabilities[22–24] have been associated with increased incidence of child abuse and neglect victimization. Caregivers with mental health problems like depression and substance use disorders, those with unrealistic expectations of childhood development, and those experiencing high levels of stress or with low education and income have also been found to engage in child maltreatment perpetration.[8,11,12,14] Another key risk factor is one's experience of their own childhood victimization, perhaps because they develop attitudes that support, justify, or normalize violence and aggression. In a similar vein, families that have high conflict in the home or experience other types of violence in the home have an increased likelihood of experiencing child maltreatment. Families with household members who are incarcerated or have little social support are also likely to struggle with child abuse and neglect.[14]

Humanitarian Crises and Risk for Child Maltreatment

Writing this article from Chicago, Illinois in 2025, we would be remiss not to describe the many ways in which children, families, and communities are actively experiencing preventable crises. Currently, there is palpable fear and tension in communities as visible threats of helicopters and armed vehicles target minoritized communities. There is a lack of childcare availability and affordability in the United States, forcing hard-working families to decide between employment or caring for their children. The legal rights of Lesbian, Gay, Bisexual, Transgender, Queer/Questioning, Intersex, and Asexual/Aromantic/Agender (LGBTQIA)+ communities are being challenged, leaving many fearful for their safety and prosperity. To make matters worse, the public health infrastructure put into place as a safety net for families is eroding through the intentional actions of key decision-makers. The stress and pressures on families are immense and opportunities for support are dwindling. Families, especially those with minoritized identities, are left to fend for themselves, creating greater isolation for those most in need. This article is framed with the backdrop of ongoing crisis that is the "normal" for so many communities in the United States. As the Great Recession and coronavirus disease 2019 (COVID-19) are discussed later in this article, we recognize that these 2 crises occurred amid a series of intersectional crises disproportionately experienced by minoritized communities, including racial and civil unrest. The need for robust public health infrastructure—what we term a "primary prevention ecosystem"—is more needed than ever to ensure families have what they need before they find themselves in crisis, or they have support once a crisis exponentiates their challenges.

Rubenstein and Stark[25] provide a conceptual framework for understanding the ecological factors associated with an increased risk for child maltreatment during times of humanitarian crisis. The authors note that risk for child abuse and neglect varies based on the type of crisis experienced, the stage of the crisis (eg, ongoing, after-the-fact), the socio-political context where the crisis occurs, as well as the presence of risk and protective factors—at each level of the social ecology—that exacerbate or mitigate crisis.

In this article, we review 2 acute crises that occurred in the United States since the turn of the century—The Great Recession and COVID-19—and how these crises elevated the risk for child abuse and neglect. There are many forms of humanitarian crises that we do not cover, including war, famine, and forced migration and we acknowledge this as a limitation. Further, we have limited our discussion of humanitarian crises to the United States as this is where we work and where our implications will be most relevant. There is an intentional focus on child abuse and neglect *risk* during times of crisis, not on official rates of child abuse and neglect. Public health surveillance and methodological challenges can influence the actual rates of child abuse and neglect, so we focus instead on risk factors. For a discussion of the surveillance issues, see Klika and colleagues[26] and Klika and colleagues.[27]

Great Recession

Major downturns in the economy have been linked to increases in child abuse and neglect.[28] The groundbreaking work of Elder[29] studying children of the Great Depression and, later, Conger and colleagues[30] studying children in rural Iowa who endured a major farming crisis, provide a strong foundation for understanding how economic hardship can lead to increased violence in the home. The Family Stress Model[31–33] is one framework that helps explain the complex relationship between stress, particularly economic stress, and later violence. As caregivers experience economic hardship, through factors like job loss, they begin to experience financial pressure to make ends meet. Mounting economic pressures can lead to immense psychological distress, including anxiety, excessive worry, and depression. These factors can interfere with a caregiver's ability to respond appropriately to the physical and emotional needs of children (or partners), leading to child neglect, physical abuse, or intimate partner violence.[33]

The Great Recession is a recent economic downturn, beginning in 2007 and ending in 2009, which created disruption for families across the United States and beyond.[34] Employment losses, housing precarity, and ensuing stress and mental health challenges brought about by the Great Recession created an environment of increased risk for child abuse and neglect.[35] It is estimated that nearly 2.3 million children were living in families who lost their home to foreclosure at some point during the Great Recession.[36] One-third of children were living in homes that were spending more than 30% of their income on housing expenses (ie, cost-burdened).[36] Approximately 1 in 9 children (8.1 million) were living with at least one parent experiencing unemployment.[37] Increases in food assistance programs like the supplemental nutrition assistance program (SNAP) and the Special Supplemental Nutrition Program for Women, Infants, and Children and health insurance coverage (ie, Children's Health Insurance Program [CHIP]) helped buffer and mitigate the effects of the Great Recession.[36]

These findings all point to an increased risk for child abuse and neglect during the Great Recession. However, the research findings on rates of child abuse and neglect during the Great Recession are mixed. For example, Berger and colleagues[38] observed increases in rates of abusive head trauma (AHT) in hospital settings during the Great Recession compared to years prior. Home foreclosures were linked to increased probability of child welfare involvement, a concerning finding in light of the growing number of children experiencing home foreclosure during the Great Recession.[39] Schneider and colleagues[35] documented significant increases in parental self-reported physical and psychological aggression linked to higher rates of unemployment associated with the Great Recession; however, rates of physical and supervisory neglect decreased. While findings on rates of child abuse and neglect during the Great Recession are mixed, the evidence is clear that the risk for child abuse and neglect was significantly elevated during this period.

Coronavirus disease 2019

In March of 2020, the World Health Organization declared the coronavirus as a pandemic in the United States. The White House followed quickly with guidance on how to slow its spread.[40] At that time, professionals began to worry about the overall well-being of children and their families. As COVID-19 progressed, families experienced significant interruptions to daily living.[41] In-person schooling ceased, hospitals provided directives to only come to the hospital for extreme emergencies, and care arrangements such as daycares and after-school programs closed.[42–45] Over 140,000 US children lost a caregiver at some point during COVID-19.[46] Caregivers were left to balance work, remote learning, and the growing restrictions on social spaces, including grocery stores, parks, and places of worship.[47] Put another way, the stress and pressure on caregivers increased significantly, while the opportunity for physical and social connection was largely removed, leading to conditions of increased risk for maltreatment.[40]

Attuned to the mounting risk factors that families were experiencing, Lee and colleagues[40,47] conducted a survey to understand how families were coping with the chaos and uncertainty of COVID-19. Their results highlighted what many expected. Parental self-reports of mental health challenges such as anxiety and depression, conflict in the home, stress regarding financial stability, and increasing use of harsh parenting were but a few of the risk factors for child maltreatment highlighted in the survey.

A recent literature review examined child maltreatment during COVID-19.[27] The authors conclude that while studies using child welfare and hospital/emergency department data largely show decreases in child maltreatment during COVID-19, these declines should be understood in light of policies and protocols that may have affected these data. For example, child welfare practices and protocols changed during COVID-19 to accommodate health and safety measures for families and workers.[48] As a result, there were fewer child welfare investigations during COVID-19. Russel and colleagues[43] speculate that decreases in emergency department visits could be, in part, due to the fear of contracting COVID-19. Importantly, Sanford and colleagues[44] document reductions in emergency department visits for motor vehicle-related crashes, all-terrain vehicle (ATV), bicycle, and other sports-related injuries during COVID-19, highlighting a decreasing trend in all-cause emergency department visits, not just for child abuse and neglect. As was true during the Great Recession, risk for child abuse and neglect was elevated during COVID-19 even if official rates of abuse and neglect do not reflect that reality. This trend could be due to obvious limitations in our violence surveillance systems; however, it could also signal that sources of protection are buffering risk exposure.[49]

DISCUSSION AND PREVENTION

Humanitarian crises hold up a magnifying glass to expose the extreme gaps, cracks, and absence of a robust social safety net for families here in the United States.[50] The magnitude and gravity of widespread poverty (and near-poverty) is brought to the fore during these times. All too many families live paycheck-to-paycheck, without adequate medical insurance, and with no financial savings to manage an acute crisis. Humanitarian crises exacerbate and exponentiate financial, physical, and social stress, leading to the conditions in which the risk for child maltreatment is elevated.[25]

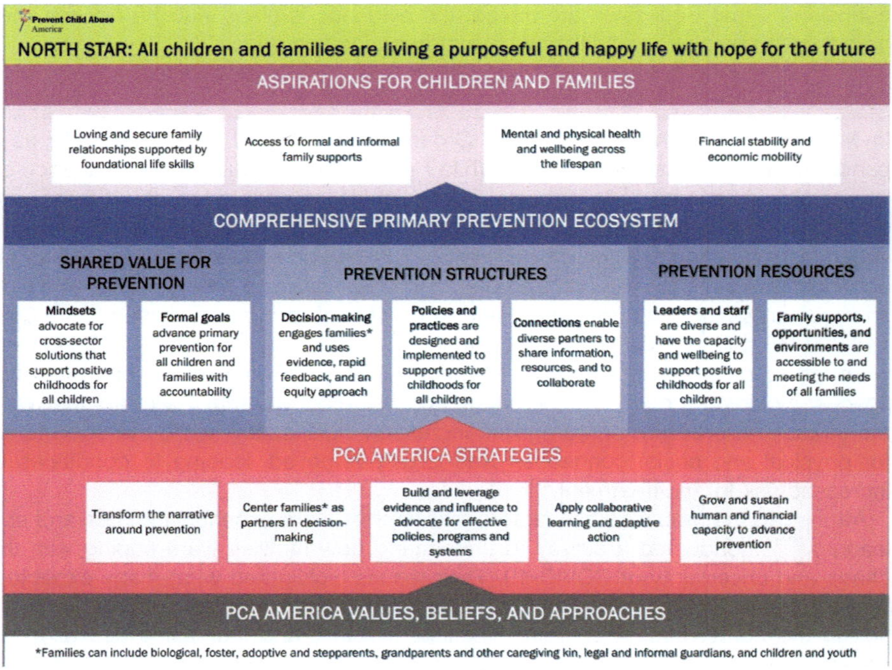

Fig. 1. Prevent Child Abuse America blueprint for family well-being. (*Courtesy of* Prevent Child Abuse America.)

Public health is focused on creating conditions for health and well-being.[51,52] Moving forward, there is a dire need to create a comprehensive system of care and support for children and families—a primary prevention ecosystem—that addresses concrete/material, physical health, and emotional needs before they become a crisis.[53] Prevent Child Abuse America codesigned a Blueprint for Family Wellbeing that calls for such a primary prevention ecosystem that includes policies and programs across sectors that can support child and family health and well-being by explicitly diminishing sources of risk and building sources of protection (**Fig. 1**).[54,55]

In terms of direct support to families, research has found robust benefits associated with approaches like home visiting[56] and family resource centers.[57] Over the past couple of decades, a growing body of research has linked family-friendly concrete and economic support policies to reductions in child abuse and neglect.[8] Specifically, paid family leave,[58,59] childcare subsidies,[60–62] earned income tax credits,[63,64] minimum wage,[65] Medicaid,[66,67] and the SNAP[68] have all been found to reduce child abuse and neglect. More recently, unconditional cash transfers have been linked to reduced child abuse and neglect.[69] In an evaluation of Rx Kids, a direct cash assistance intervention in Flint, Michigan, providing families with a modest amount of money throughout the perinatal period was associated with reductions in child abuse and neglect and child welfare involvement.[70] In noncrisis times, these programs and policies are essential for families. Once a crisis strikes, it is even more essential that families have easy, ongoing access to these supports.

DISCLOSURE

The authors have no financial disclosures or conflicts of interest to disclose.

REFERENCES

1. UNICEF. Fast facts: violence against children widespread, affecting millions globally. Available at: https://www.unicef.org/press-releases/fast-facts-violence-against-children-widespread-affecting-millions-globally.
2. Merrick MT, Ford DC, Ports KA, et al. Prevalence of adverse childhood experiences from the 2011-2014 behavioral risk factor surveillance system in 23 states. JAMA Pediatr 2018;172(11):1038–44.
3. Merrick MT, Ford DC, Ports KA, et al. Vital signs: estimated proportion of adult health problems attributable to adverse childhood experiences and implications for prevention–25 states, 2015-2017. MMWR (Morb Mortal Wkly Rep) 2019;68. Available at: https://www.cdc.gov/mmwr/volumes/68/wr/pdfs/mm6844e1-H.pdf.
4. Felitti VJ, Anda RF, Nordenberg D, et al. Relationship of childhood abuse and household dysfunction to many of the leading causes of death in adults: the adverse childhood experiences (ACE) study. Am J Prev Med 1998;14(4):245–58.
5. Gilbert R, Widom CS, Browne K, et al. Burden and consequences of child maltreatment in high-income countries. Child Maltreat 2009;373(9657):68–81.
6. National Scientific Council on the Developing Child. Excessive stress disrupts the architecture of the developing brain: working paper no. 3. 2014. Available at: www.developingchild.harvard.edu.
7. Gilbert LK, Breidling MJ, Merrick MT, et al. Childhood adversity and adult chronic disease: an update from ten states and the District of Columbia, 2010. Am J Prev Med 2015;48(3):345–9.
8. Fortson BL, Klevens J, Merrick MT, et al. Child abuse and neglect prevention resource for action: a compilation of the best available evidence. 2016. Available at: https://www.cdc.gov/violence-prevention/media/pdf/resources-for-action/CAN-Prevention-Resource_508.pdf.
9. Peterson C, Florence C, Klevens J. The economic burden of child maltreatment in the United States, 2015. Child Abuse Neglect 2018;86:178–83.
10. Belsky J. Etiology of child malteatment: a developmental-ecological analysis. Psychol Bull 1993;114(3):413–34.
11. Austin AE, Lesak AM, Shanahan ME. Risk and protective factors for child maltreatment: a review. Curr Epidemiol Rep 2020;7(4):334–42.
12. Luo Z, Chen Y, Epstein RA. Risk factors for child abuse and neglect: systematic review and meta-analysis. Public Health 2025;241:89–98.
13. Centers for Disease Control and Prevention (CDC). About violence prevention. Centers for Disease Control and Prevention. Available at: https://www.cdc.gov/violence-prevention/about/index.html.
14. Centers for Disease Control and Prevention. Risk and protective factors. Centers for Disease Control and Prevention. Available at: https://www.cdc.gov/child-abuse-neglect/risk-factors/index.html.
15. Evans GW, Li D, Whipple SS. Cumulative risk and child development. Psychol Bull 2013;139(6):1342–96.
16. MacKenzie MJ, Kotch JB, Lee LC. Toward a cumulative ecological risk model for the etiology of child maltreatment. Child Youth Serv Rev 2011;33(9):1638–47.
17. National Academies of Sciences E, and Medicine. Parenting matters: Supporting parents of children ages 0-8. 2016.
18. Klevens J, Metzler M. Bringing a health equity perspectve to the prevention of child abuse and neglect. In: Lonne D, Scott D, Higgins DJ, Herrenkohl TI, eds Re-visioning public health approaches for protecting children: Child maltreatment. Springer; 2019. Contemporary Issues in Research & Policy.

19. The Alliance for Child Protection in Humanitarian Action. Child neglect in humanitarian settings: literature review and recommendations for strengthening prevention and response. 2018. Available at: https://alliancecpha.org/en.
20. Sokol RL, Victor BG, Piellusch EK, et al. Prevalence and context of firearms-related problems in child protective service investigations. Child Abuse Neglect 2020;107:104572.
21. Child maltreatment 2023 (2025).
22. Sullivan PM, Knutson JF. Maltreatment and disabilities: a population-based epidemiological study. Pediatrics 2000;105(4):779–86.
23. Jones L, Bellis MA, Wood S, et al. Prevalence and risk of violence against children with disabilities: a systematic review and meta-analysis of observational studies. Lancet 2012;380(9845):899–907.
24. Stalker K, McArthur K. Child abuse, child protection and disabled children: a review of recent research. Child Abuse Rev 2010;21(1):24–40.
25. Rubenstein BL, Stark L. The impact of humanitarian emergencies on the prevalence of violence against children: an evidence-based ecological framework. Psychol Health Med 2017;22(S1):58–66.
26. Klika JB, Merrick MT, Jones J. Child maltreatment during the pandemic. Child Maltreat 2023;28(1):3–6.
27. Klika JB, Lee JY, Chang OD, et al. Child maltreatment during COVID-19: triangulating data across reporting sources. Child Maltreat 2025;0(0). https://doi.org/10.1177/10775595251370230.
28. Schenck-Fontaine A, Gassman-Pines A, Gibson-Davis CM, et al. Local job losses and child maltreatment: the importance of community context. Soc Serv Rev 2017;91(2):233–63.
29. Elder GH. Children of the great depression: social changes in life experience. Westview Press; 1974.
30. Conger RD, Conger KJ, Elder GH, et al. A family process model of economic hardship and adjustment of early adolescent boys. Child Dev 1992;63(3):526–41.
31. Conger RD, Elder GH. Families in troubled times: adapting to change in rural America. Aldine de Gruyter; 1994.
32. Conger RD, Conger KJ, Martin MJ. Socioeconomic status, family processes, and indivdiual development. J Marriage Fam 2010;72(3):685–704.
33. Masarik AS, Conger RD. Stress and child development: a review of the family stress model. Curr Opin Psychol 2017;13:85–90.
34. Brooks-Gunn J, Schneider W, Waldfogel J. The great recession and the risk for child maltreatment. Child Abuse Neglect 2013;37(10):721–9.
35. Schneider W, Waldfogel J, Brooks-Gunn J. The great recession and risk for child abuse and neglect. Child Youth Serv Rev 2017;72:71–81.
36. Meadows R, Sell K, Blinkoff E, Williams N, Repcheck L. The effect of the Great Recession on child well-being. 2015.
37. Lovell P, Isaacs JB. Families of the recession: Unemployed parents and their children. 2010.
38. Berger RP, Fromkin JB, Stutz H, et al. Abusive head trauma during a time of increased unemployment: a multicenter analysis. Pediatrics 2011;128(4):637–43.
39. Berger LM, Collins JM, Font SA, et al. Home foreclosures and child protective services involvement. Pediatrics 2015;136(2):299–307.
40. Lee SJ, Ward KP, Lee JY, et al. Parental social isolation and child maltreatment risk during the COVID-19 pandemic. J Fam Violence 2022;37(5):813–24.

41. Andrade C, Gillen M, Molina JA, et al. The social and economic impact of COVID-19 on family functioning and well-being: where do we go from here? J Fam Econ Issues 2022;43(2):205–12.
42. Holland KM, Jones C, Vivolo-Kantor AM, et al. Trends in US emergency department visits for mental health, overdose, and violence outcomes before and during the COVID-19 pandemic. JAMA Psychiatry 2021;78(4):372–9.
43. Russell KW, Acker SN, Ignacio RC, et al. Child physical abuse during COVID-19: trends from nine pediatric trauma centers. J Pediatr Surg 2022;57(2):297–301.
44. Sanford EL, Zagory J, Blackwell JM, et al. Changes in pediatric trauma during COVID-19 stay-at-home epoch at a tertiary pediatric hospital. J Pediatr Surg 2021;56(5):918–22.
45. Baron EJ, Goldstein EG, Wallace CT. Suffering in silence: how COVID-19 school closures inhibit the reporting of child maltreatment. J Publ Econ 2020;190:104258.
46. The hidden US COVID-19 pandemic: orphaned children. Centers for Disease Control and Prevention; 2021.
47. Lee JY, Ward KP, Chang OD, et al. Parenting activities and the transition to home-based education during the COVID-19 pandemic. Child Youth Serv Rev 2021;122:105585.
48. Katz I, Priolo-Filho S, Katz C, et al. One year into COVID-19: what have we learned about child maltreatment reports and child protective services responses. Child Abuse Neglect 2022;130(1):105473.
49. Sege R, Stephens A. Child physical abuse did not increase during the pandemic. JAMA Pediatr 2022;176(4):338–40.
50. Rostad WL, Ports KA, Merrick MT, et al. The moment is now: strengthening communities and families for the future. Child Youth Serv Rev 2023;144:106745.
51. Institute of Medicine. The future of public health. 1988.
52. Institute of Medicine. The future of the public's health in the 21st century. 2003.
53. Laraque D, Sia C. Health care reform and the opportunity to implement family-centered medical home for children. JAMA 2010;303(23):2407–8.
54. Prevent Child Abuse America. A theory of change for primary prevention in the US. 2023. Available at: https://preventchildabuse.org/wp-content/uploads/2024/04/PCA-Theory-of-Change-April262024.pdf.
55. Jones JA, Watson ER, Sutton KL. Building a primary prevention ecosystem in the United States: a model for transforming how society supports children and families. Fam Soc 2025. https://doi.org/10.1177/10443894251320216.
56. U.S. Department of Health and Human Services. New HHS study finds home visiting services improves family wellbeing (MIHOPE). 2025.
57. Bayless S, Richmond M, Pecora P, et al. Returns on investment of a family resource center to the child welfare system: estimates from a quasi-experimental study from the Western United States. Family Justice Journal 2025;4:10–6.
58. Bullinger LR. Paid family leave: an upstream intervention to prevent family violence. J Fam Violence 2022.
59. Bullinger LR, Raissian KM, Klika JB, et al. More than snuggles: the effect of paid family leave on infant maltreatment. Child Maltreatment; 2025. https://doi.org/10.1177/10775595251318939.
60. Maguire-Jack K, Park Y, Feely M, et al. Childcare subsidy employment and co-payment requirements and child maltreatment. Child Maltreat 2024;29(4):612–24.
61. Klika JB, Maguire-Jack K, Feely M, et al. Childcare subsidy enrollment income generosity and child maltreatment. Children (Basel) 2022;10(1):64.

62. Thibodeau E, Klika JB, Maguire-Jack K, et al. Childcare subsidy generosity and child maltreatment: the moderating effects of administrative burden. J Fam Violence 2024;41(1). https://doi.org/10.1007/s10896-024-00748-2.
63. Kovski NL, Hill HD, Mooney SJ, et al. Association of state-level earned income tax credits with rates of reported child maltreatment, 2004-2017. Child Maltreat 2021; 27(3):325–33.
64. Kovski NL, Hill HD, Mooney SJ, et al. Short-term effects of tax credits on rates of child maltreament reports in the United States. Pediatrics 2022;150(1): e2021054939.
65. Raissian KM, Bullinger LR. Money matters: does the minimum wage affect child maltreatment rates? Child Youth Serv Rev 2017;72(C):60–70.
66. McGinty EE, Nair R, Assini-Meytin LC, et al. Impact of Medicaid expansion on reported incidents of child neglect and physical abuse. Am J Prev Med 2021;62(1): e11–20.
67. Brown ECB, Garrison MM, Bao H, et al. Assessment of rates of child maltreatment in states with Medicaid expansion vs states without Medicaid expansion. JAMA Netw Open 2019;2(6):e1955529.
68. Austin AE, Shanahan ME, Frank M, et al. Association of state expansion of supplemental nutrition assistance program eligibility with rates of child protective services–Investigated reports. JAMA Pediatr 2023;177(3):294–302.
69. Bullinger LR, Packham A, Raissian KM. Effects of universal and unconditional cash transfers on child abuse and neglect. 2023. 31733. Available at: https://www.nber.org/papers/w31733.
70. Agarwal S, Shaefer HL, Jubaed S, et al. Cash transfers in the perinatal period and child welfare system involvement among infants: evidence from the Rx kids program in flint, Michigan. ArXiv 2025. https://doi.org/10.48550/arXiv.2511.19570.

Environmental Concerns for Children in Humanitarian Crises

Ruth A. Etzel, MD, PhD

KEYWORDS

• Air pollution • Arsenic • Lead • Tobacco • Cyanide • Pesticides • Dioxin • T-2

KEY POINTS

- Pediatric clinicians who care for children in humanitarian settings should be alert for unusual symptoms that could signal a toxic exposure.
- A thorough environmental history is needed to better understand the family's source of water, use of fuel for cooking and heating, use of tobacco and home remedies, industries located nearly, and the child's diet.
- Breastfeeding should be encouraged for at least the first 6 months of life.
- The need for laboratory testing is based on the environmental history, symptoms, and physical examination.
- Laboratories with the capability to measure specific chemicals may not be available and assistance may be necessary from international laboratories with experience measuring toxicants in human tissue.

Case study: lead poisoning among refugee children in Kosovo

An egregious example of environmental contamination affecting children in a humanitarian setting occurred after the dissolution of Yugoslavia in the late 1990s. Following Kosovo's 1998–1999 war with Serbian troops, the UN—specifically the United Nations Interim Administration Mission in Kosovo (UNMIK)—served as the de facto government of Kosovo.[1] On June 21, 1999, as the first UNMIK personnel were deployed in Kosovo, the Mitrovica Roma neighborhood was looted and burnt to the ground by Albanian mobs.[2] The neighborhood had comprised around 750 houses, with an estimated 8000 inhabitants. All were forcibly expelled and the entire neighborhood destroyed. More than half the people fled to other countries, but many stayed in Mitrovica. The UN decided to place these internally displaced people (more than 600 members of the Roma, Ashkali, and Egyptian communities) in 3 camps (Žitkovac, Česmin Lug and Kablare) in Northern Mitrovica within 3 km of the Trepca mining and smelting complex, Europe's largest lead-zinc and silver ore mine, active since the mid-1920s.[3,4] This area was known to be contaminated by toxic levels of lead, and the camps were located within 500 m of mine tailing sites. The United Nations Interim Administration Mission in Kosovo suspended lead production in 2000 because of health concerns. The camp shelters, which were

Department of Pediatrics, Georgetown University, Washington, DC, USA
E-mail address: RETZEL@GWU.EDU

Pediatr Clin N Am 73 (2026) 1007–1021
https://doi.org/10.1016/j.pcl.2026.05.002 pediatric.theclinics.com
0031-3955/26/

Abbreviations	
TEQ	toxic equivalents
TTCD	tetrachlorodibenzo-*p*-dioxin
UNMIK	United Nations Interim Administration Mission in Kosovo
WHO	World Health Organization

intended to be temporary (45–90 days) had dirt-floored dwellings and young children played on the ground, ingesting large amounts of lead. In early 2004, Romani activists notified the authorities about symptoms of probable lead poisoning among children in the camps. The death of a 4 year old girl in the Žitkovac camp prompted the World Health Organization (WHO) to conduct a health risk assessment during May through July 2004. Blood lead testing conducted using a handheld LeadCare analyzer in 2004 in children from the 3 camps indicated that all children had blood lead levels greater than 65 mcg/dL, the highest value reported by the instrument.[5] Random soil tests conducted by the WHO showed that more than 80% of soils in the camps were "unsafe" because of lead contamination. In August 2006, the WHO arranged the first of 2 distributions of oral chelation therapy to a group of about 40 children in one camp. In October 2008, the Mitrovica Institute for Health conducted blood tests on children in the camps. Out of 53 tested, 21 had life-threatening blood lead levels requiring immediate medical intervention and only 2 children had results considered to be within normal limits.[2] Lead poisoning is reported to have contributed to the death of several children although the precise cause of death in most of these cases has not been independently determined. In October 2010, the camps were finally closed after 10 years.

LEAD EXPOSURE: A WELL-KNOWN PROBLEM AMONG REFUGEE CHILDREN

This case study illustrates the importance of knowing the historical use of urban industrial land to which refugees may be relocated. The case also raises questions about the ethics of placing people directly into hazardous environments during humanitarian emergencies. This tragic situation happened despite the fact that lead poisoning has been well-understood for decades and is entirely preventable. Lead accumulates in a child's body over time; at high levels of exposure symptoms may occur within weeks or months. Children with clumsiness, agitation, or decreased activity or sleepiness (indications of CNS involvement) can rapidly progress to vomiting, stupor, convulsions and death.

Refugee children often have been documented with high concentrations of lead in their blood.[6–8] A study among 3 to 7 year old Thai children living near Burmese refugee camps found an average blood lead level of 7.71 mcg/dL (range 3–25 mcg/dL), and 26% of the children had blood lead levels of 10 mcg/dL or higher.[9] A survey of blood lead levels in 178 children aged 6 to 8 years in 3 schools in Nablus city in Palestine found a mean blood lead level of 3.2 mcg/dL; 4.5% of children had levels above 10 mcg/dL. Blood lead levels were significantly higher among children living in refugee camps near industrial/high traffic regions than among children living in residential areas of Nablus city.[10] In a representative sample of children resettled to multiple areas of the United States, 23.7% of 1 to 5 year old refugee children had blood lead levels 5 mcg/dL or greater. This was tenfold higher than the prevalence of 2.3% among all 1 to 5 year old children in the United States estimated from the 1999 to 2010 National Health and Nutrition Examination Survey.[11]

INTRODUCTION

Many environmental hazards may be encountered by children in humanitarian crises. A humanitarian crisis is defined as any circumstance where humanitarian needs are sufficiently large and complex to require significant external assistance and resources, and where a multi-sectoral response is needed, with the engagement of a wide range of international humanitarian actors.[12] Although risks from infectious diseases in humanitarian crises have been extensively recorded,[13] little attention has been paid to risk from exposure to toxicants in the water, air, food, or resulting from wartime activities. The purpose of this article is to describe some important environmental hazards to children in humanitarian settings.

WATER

Lack of Access to Water

In many humanitarian settings, water is a limited and expensive resource. Water may be brought to refugee camps on tanker trucks and then dispensed into household containers. Because of water scarcity, the frequency and quality of handwashing among adults and children may be poor. Some adults and children may wash their hands only with water, not soap. Diarrheal disease from inadequate handwashing and drinking contaminated water may be frequent in these settings.[14]

If safe water cannot be supplied, families need to treat water at home. Household water treatment is effective, simple, and inexpensive and can be done using chlorine or iodine tablets, or sachets of combined flocculant/disinfection powder. Water should be treated using the directions that come with the tablets. If household bleach or other sources of chlorine are available, water can be disinfected with a dilute chlorine solution. Solar disinfection also is an effective water treatment method. Ultraviolet rays from the sun are used to inactivate pathogens present in water. This technique involves exposing water in clear plastic bottles to sunlight for a day, for example, on the roof of a house. Empty bottles can be used that are left over from an initial shipment of drinking water.[15]

Despite water shortages and restricted sanitation facilities in emergency situations, it is critical to ensure that some of the available water supply is used for handwashing with soap (after defecation, after handling infants' feces, and before preparing food). When soap is unavailable, ash, sand, or other culturally acceptable substitutes can be used.[15]

Exposures to High Levels of Fluoride in Water

Naturally occurring fluoride concentrations in water can be a source of fluoride poisoning among refugees. Countries with high fluoride concentrations include Ethiopia, Iraq, Kenya, South Sudan, Syria and Turkey. In 2015, a 46 year old Somalia man presented with chronic, debilitating, diffuse axial bone pain, insidiously worsening over the previous 5 years, beginning with lumbar and hip pain.[16] The previous year, he could no longer rise from a chair alone and had an antalgic, shuffling gait with pronounced kyphosis. A detailed history revealed that he had lived in the Kakuma refugee camp (Rift Valley Province, Kenya) from 2009 to 2015. This camp housed 185,000 inhabitants, all of whom depended on fluoride-contaminated well water with a measured fluoride concentration of 8.4 mg/L. Naturally high fluoride concentrations in water occur in several countries with large refugee populations. For example, in the Rift Valley of Ethiopia, the pooled mean concentration of fluoride in water was 6.03 mg/L,[17] and in some areas of the country water contained a mean of 10 mg/L.[18] Drinking fluoride contaminated well water is a particular risk for children whose bones are still developing.[16]

The average fluoride concentration in water in countries with naturally high fluoride are much higher than the guideline value of 1.5 mg/L set by the WHO[19] or the level of 0.7 mg/L recommended by the Centers for Disease Control and Prevention for prevention of dental caries.[20]

Exposures to Arsenic, Manganese, Iodine and Other Elements in Water

To prevent diarrheal diseases, tube-wells were installed in Bangladesh in the 1980s and the early 1990s. Arsenic contamination was first identified in the tubewell water in 1993 in a northern district of Bangladesh.[21] Exposure to arsenic from drinking water is associated with reduced intellectual function in children, arsenicosis, and increased risk of cancer.[21,22] In Rohingya refugee camps in Bangladesh, many shallow and deep tubewells were recently installed to provide access to drinking water. A study in 2018 on manganese in groundwater in the camps found that 64% exceeded the Bangladesh standard (100 mcg/L).[23] Although no health effects were assessed, manganese exposure can impair children's cognitive development. In Saharawi refugee camps in Algeria, children's urinary concentration of vanadium, arsenic, selenium, lead, iodine, and uranium exceeded reference values, and some elements exceeded the WHO guidelines for drinking water quality.[24]

AIR

Respiratory Illness and Exposure to Air Pollution

The burden of respiratory disease in humanitarian settings has been well documented.[25] In a study of diseases among refugees in mainland Greece, respiratory infections were the most prevalent outcome. Among respiratory infections, upper respiratory infections were most common; over 46% of children under 18 years of age had at least one health care visit for an upper respiratory infection.[26] Although viral and bacterial causes of respiratory illnesses are well known, there has been little attention to the non-communicable causes of acute respiratory illnesses. A variety of environmental contaminants, including indoor air pollutants from tobacco smoke and outdoor air pollutants from open fires can result in acute respiratory illness in children. The indoor air in shelters may be polluted if people burn garbage and other items for heating and cooking. Because of inadequate access to fuel, people in humanitarian settings may use wood, clothes, tires, and plastic bags as fuel. Exposure to wood smoke has been associated with acute respiratory illness and impaired lung function.[27]

Inadequate housing is a major problem for refugee children. Cold housing, presence of dampness and molds, dust and smoke, burning of biomass fuel, crowding, poor ventilation and inadequate lighting problems were commonly reported in the houses of the al-Ama'ri refugee camp in the West Bank of Palestine.[28] Refugee families in the Gaza strip reported that the main fuels they used were wood, coal, cardboard, and a mix of wood, cardboard, and plastic. These "dirty" fuels were used for cooking, heating, baking, boiling water, and lighting. The most common symptoms they reported were nasal irritation (71.8%), followed by headache (66.4%) and dizziness (65.4%).[29] A nested case–control study of allergens and endotoxin in the Ramallah refugee camp in 2001 identified dampness as an important determinant for allergen and endotoxin but noted that other factors such as lack of mattress covers appeared unimportant.[30]

Tobacco

Rates of smoking in humanitarian crises can be high; tobacco smoke is among the most important indoor air pollutants affecting children in humanitarian crises. A study of 2500 individuals aged 15 to 24 years in the West Bank and East Jerusalem in 2018 revealed that 45.4% of male ages 15 to 19 years and 71.5% of male ages 20 to 24 years reported current tobacco use (cigarettes or waterpipes). Rates were lower for females but still significant: 21.6% for younger female ages 15 to 19 years 31.2% for female ages 20 to 24 years.[31] A cross-sectional study among 249 Rohingya refugees living in Bangladesh found that 53.4% used tobacco (including smokeless tobacco).[32]

Rates may be lower among refugees who are adolescents. One study examined patterns of smoking by tobacco product and gender among Syrian refugee youth living in host communities in Jordan. Current smoking was reported by 10.5% of refugee youth. The proportion of smoking differed significantly by gender, with 14.9% of boys and 7.0% of girls reporting current smoking.[33] Another study of Syrian adolescent refugees in South Beirut found a smoking rate of 42.3%.[34]

Because smoking is still prevalent among refugees, there is pervasive exposure to indoor tobacco smoke among young children, whose lungs are still developing. This can lead to stunting of lung growth and upper and lower respiratory illness.[35] Smoking and air pollution were linked to a delayed diagnosis of TB among Syrian refugees in Turkey in 2012 to 2018.[36] Exposure to environmental tobacco smoke is consistently associated with children's risk of TB infection.[37] Because of its harmful effects of tobacco on adolescent smokers and children living with them, efforts have been made to reduce smoking among refugee populations. Working with Syrian refugees in Lebanon, Sethi and colleagues showed that volunteer refugee health workers can implement community-based primary health activities in a complex humanitarian emergency. They demonstrated that tobacco use can be addressed alongside other common acute conditions in Syrian refugee settlements, through community health outreach, behavior change promotion, disease monitoring, and linkages to ongoing clinical care.[38] Even in countries at war, tobacco control is possible if a strong foundation has been set.[39] A recent scoping review suggested the need for more tobacco prevention and control efforts in humanitarian settings.[40]

Exposures to Carbon Monoxide

Carbon monoxide poisoning is a hazard for children in humanitarian settings. When people have been displaced from their homes, they may turn to portable generators for electricity, or unvented space heaters for warmth, or charcoal or wood for cooking. Wood, coal and charcoal fires always produce carbon monoxide. Carbon monoxide can be released from unvented space heaters that use a flammable fuel such as kerosene. Carbon monoxide is a colorless, odorless, tasteless gas that is the product of incomplete combustion. When a child breathes in carbon monoxide, it replaces oxygen on the hemoglobin molecule. The higher the carbon monoxide in the blood, the less hemoglobin available to deliver oxygen to the child's body. Symptoms may resemble the symptoms of flu, such as headaches, fatigue, nausea, dizzy spells, confusion and irritability. As levels increase, vomiting, loss of consciousness and eventually brain damage or death can occur. If carbon monoxide poisoning is suspected, it is imperative to remove the child to fresh air immediately.[41–46]

FOOD

Food Contamination and Poisoning

Cyanide in cassava

In parts of Sub-Saharan Africa, a disease called konzo has been reported among refugees and people living in areas with drought or war. Konzo is a sudden symmetric spastic paraparesis that develops in people with low protein intake who consume only insufficiently processed bitter cassava as their staple food. The condition primarily affects women and children above the age of 3, probably because in times of food insecurity, women and children eat last. Cassava contains a varying quantity of cyanogenic glucosides that protect the root against attack by animals and insects. Bitter cassava can have up to 400 mg/kg hydrogen cyanide compared with sweet cassava, which contains less than 50 mg/kg. Bitter cassava is usually prepared by soaking peeled or cut cassava roots in water for about a week, which allows for the enzymatic breakdown of cyanogenic compounds. When shortcuts are taken, larger amounts of cyanide may be consumed. Konzo has been reported in Angola, Cameroon, the Central African Republic, the Democratic Republic of Congo, Mozambique, and Tanzania. During and after the war in Mozambique (1977–1992), it was a recurring problem; more than 1100 cases were reported in 1981, over 600 cases in 1992 to 1993, and over 100 cases in 2005.[47] Even after the war ended, some people continued to depend on inadequately processed bitter cassava; the disease tends to peak during the cassava harvest.[48] Among 60,000 refugees from the Central African Republic who sought refuge in villages in eastern Cameroon between 2005 and 2007, 469 were diagnosed with konzo. Affected people typically complained about walking difficulties and weight loss and exhibit exaggerated lower limb reflexes and muscle wasting.[49] The most visible feature is the cross-legged (scissoring) gait, although the person may still be able to walk and/or run.[50] This condition can occur when timely balanced food rations are not provided to refugees.

Mushroom poisoning

Because of poverty and food scarcity, some refugees may turn to eating wild mushrooms that they harvest in the forest. A case of poisoning from *Amanita phalloides* occurred in a 28 year old refugee in Scandinavia.[51] This highly toxic mushroom can easily be mistaken for an edible wild mushroom.

Cooking utensils

Cooking vessels and utensils may also be a source of food contamination. Because of water scarcity, kitchen ware may not be washed frequently and may harbor bacterial contaminants. Some aluminum cookware brought from Afghanistan by resettled families was found to be a previously unrecognized source of lead exposure for children.[52]

Breast Milk

Pediatric clinicians should promote breastfeeding because it eliminates the use of bottles and the use of potentially contaminated water to reconstitute formula. If mother can produce milk for the infant, breastfeeding is the best option. In refugee settings, however, breast milk could be a source of infant exposure to environmental chemicals. A study that evaluated the breast milk lead levels in breastfeeding mothers in the Nablus, Ramallah, and Jerusalem regions of Palestine found that the median breast milk lead level was 4.0 mcg/L (range 2.0–12.0 mcg/L).[53] Breast milk lead levels in 19.1% of the samples analyzed were higher than the WHO's reference values of 2.0 to 5.0 μg/L for an occupationally unexposed population.[54] Breast milk lead levels were significantly higher among mothers who lived in cities and refugee camps, had lower monthly household income levels, lived close to paint shops, lived in houses with peeling or chipping paint, used eye kohl, and worked in agriculture for longer than 3 years.[53] Nonetheless, the WHO and other public health agencies continue to recommend breastfeeding for the first 6 month of life because the benefits of breast milk significantly outweigh the risks.[55,56] Steps should be taken to identify and remove the sources of chemicals to which the mother is exposed (eg, eye kohl).

Exposure to Pesticides

Harmful pesticides may be over-used in refugee camps. In 1997, a 35 year old woman from Orašje, Bosnia and Herzegovina, complained of weakness, fatigue, loss of appetite, and observed fresh blood in her stool on 2 occasions. A month later, she developed intermittent epistaxis and metrorrhagia. A careful history revealed that she had been a refugee and before she returned home the United Nations peace keeping forces in Bosnia and Herzegovina had performed mice and rat extermination in and around her house, using an unknown rodenticide. The patient was exposed to the unknown rodenticide in her cellar, where she kept potatoes. Though this occurred in an adult patient, the same exposures could happen in children.[57]

Pesticides also may be misapplied in schools for refugee children. For example, in August 2008, following an earthquake in Lixian district, China, temporary schools were erected for the children who had been evacuated from their homes. An outbreak of acute conjunctivitis associated with the spraying of alphacypermethrin insecticide occurred in a primary school in the epicenter zone, involving 136 pupils and 2 teachers. The workers responsible for pest control in the school were newly hired and due to inadequate staff training lacked knowledge of pest control. They sprayed the ground, wall and windows outside the classrooms with 10% alphacypermethrin from 8 AM to 10 AM when the children were in the classrooms. Conjunctivitis was caused by the direct irritation from insecticides in the air.[58]

MERCURY EXPOSURE

Some forms of mercury can be toxic to the nervous system of children. Skin lightning creams and soaps can contain toxic amounts of inorganic mercury. German physicians reported that the cause of an elevated mercury level in the urine of a 2 year old child living in a camp in Germany occupied by refugees from the former Yugoslavia and from Romania was traced to a cosmetic bleaching ointment containing rose oil and a mercury salt; analyses of 2 samples of the ointment indicated a concentration between 708 and 17,200 mcg Hg per gram of ointment.[59] Mercury exposure also may be an issue for children in humanitarian settings because of practices that use mercury. For example, in artisanal gold mining, liquid mercury is used to recover gold from ore. Highly toxic fumes can result when the amalgam is heated to vaporize and remove the mercury. Children in parts of Africa where these informal mining activities occur may be exposed to dangerous levels of mercury during this work.[60,61] Artisanal gold mining also may expose children to lead.[62]

WARTIME ACTIVITIES

Exposure to Contaminants Sprayed From Airplanes

Agent orange

Children fleeing from war may be the unwitting victims of aerial spraying. For example, between 1962 and 1971, 11 to 12 million gallons of Agent Orange, an herbicide contaminated with 2,3,7,8-tetrachlorodibenzo-*p*-dioxin (TCDD), were sprayed in Vietnam by the American military mainly to destroy forests where the enemy could hide, but also to deny the enemy sources of food. Agent Orange was used primarily in Vietnam, but also to a lesser extent in Laos and Cambodia. When the breast milk of women in southern Vietnam was tested in 1970, TCDD concentrations as high as 1832 parts per trillion (ppt) were found in milk lipid. Levels up to 103 ppt were found in adipose tissue in the 1980s.[63,64] Dioxins also were found as contaminants in breast milk of women in Laos.[65] Hue calculated the mean estimated PCDD/Fs infant's daily intake in a cohort of Vietnamese infants in Vietnam was about 41 to 134 pg toxic equivalents (TEQ)/kg bw/day.[66] This is much higher than the tolerable daily intake proposed by the WHO (4 pg TEQ/kg bw/day).[67] Elevated concentrations of TCDD were found in children born many years after Agent Orange spraying ended,[68] presumably from eating contaminated foods. Samples of duck, chicken, some fish, and a toad, were still contaminated with elevated TCDD, even though the original Agent Orange spraying occurred 30 to 40 years before sampling.[68] A follow-up of exposed Vietnamese children (108 boys and 77 girls) when they were 8 year old showed that heavily exposed boys had worse reading scores and lower language achievement scores; the exposed girls did not show the same problems.[69]

Very little research has evaluated the effects of TCDD exposure on children's health. In adults, occupational exposure to TCDD is associated with toxic hepatitis, peripheral neuropathy, neuropsychiatric disease, increased susceptibility to infection, abnormal lipid metabolism, and damage to the endocrine, gastrointestinal, and cardiovascular systems.[70] The US Environmental Protection Agency has classified it as a probable human carcinogen.[71] A single 6 year old child in Missouri developed acute hemorrhagic cystitis after playing in a horse arena where TCDD had been sprayed.[72]

Yellow rain

After the communist victories in Southeast Asia in 1975, campaigns were launched against Hmong tribes in northern Laos because during the war they had helped the former noncommunist governments and their principal ally, the United States. During the summer of 1975, Hmong refugees started reporting that Laotian aircraft were flying overhead and releasing a colored gas that would fall in a manner that looked, felt, and sounded like rain on the roofs. Because it was often yellow-colored, the Hmong people called it "yellow rain."[73–75] High-dose exposure to this substance resulted in bleeding from the nose and gums, cough, dyspnea, tremors, seizures, ataxia, blindness, collapse, shock, and sometimes death. Chemical analysis of samples of the yellow rain showed that it contained T-2 toxin, a potent mycotoxin.[76,77] Similar symptoms were reported by people in Kampuchea a few years later. Thousands of people reportedly died from exposure: over 6000 in Laos between 1975 and 1981, and 1000 in Kampuchea between 1979 and 1981. It is not known how many of the deaths were among children.

Depleted Uranium

Children who are refugees from war may be affected by environmental pollution from depleted uranium used for military purposes for penetrating ammunition.[78,79] During the NATO air strikes on the Federal Republic of Yugoslavia (Serbia and Montenegro) in 1999, depleted-uranium ammunition was used on over 100 locations, mainly Kosovo, in the south of Serbia, and one location in Montenegro. Depleted uranium can have toxic chemical effects (especially on the kidney), and as an α-emitter, it also has radioactive effects. Depleted uranium is about 40% less radioactive than natural uranium. Once depleted uranium munitions are fired, they form small particulate dust ranging from 0.2 to 15 microns in diameter.[80] Inhalation of dust is considered the most significant route of exposure.[81] Zunic studied children with radiological changes consistent with persistent pulmonary infiltrates during the first year after the bombing of Serbia in 1999 and described lupus erythematosus cell alveolitis as a possible nonspecific finding of radiation-induced biological response of lung tissue.[82] A study of adults from a region contaminated with depleted uranium documented some morphological changes to blood cells, in the cytoplasm, the nucleus, and chromosomes,[81] but those changes were not greater than a comparison group of X-ray workers. Another possible route of exposure to depleted uranium is dermal; this could occur if children were exposed to depleted uranium after suffering puncture wounds.[83] Pediatric clinicians can advise that children should not be playing with depleted uranium penetrators. One report from Yemen indicated that the incidence of childhood leukemia was increasing rapidly, but epidemiologic studies to determine the possible cause of the increase were not undertaken.[84] There have rarely been studies of children exposed to depleted uranium in humanitarian crises. Because of the possibility that exposure to depleted uranium may cause cancer, exposed populations should be monitored.

CLIMATE CHANGE

The changing climate may reduce access to safe drinking water and food for children in humanitarian settings.[85] Of the current 123 million forcibly displaced people in the world, three-quarters live in countries heavily impacted by climate change. Half are in places affected by both conflict and serious climate hazards, such as Ethiopia, Haiti, Myanmar, Somalia, Sudan, and Syria.[86] In mid-2024, around 90 million of the current 123 million forcibly displaced people were living in countries with high-to-extreme exposure to climate-related hazards.[86,87] Among the hazards that children in humanitarian settings experience is extreme heat. During 2007 to 2016, 108 refugee camps and settlements experienced 100 days or more of dangerous heat.[86] These camps and settlements were in Djibouti, Eritrea, Ethiopia, and Senegal. By 2050, most refugee camps and settlements are expected to endure twice as many days of dangerous heat. If current trends continue, by 2050, an estimated 614 camps and settlements will experience dangerous heat, with the top 10 hottest sites experiencing an additional 74 days of dangerous heat.[86] Recent evidence suggests that young children are disproportionately affected by extreme heat.[88]

INTERVENTIONS

There is scanty evidence on public health interventions in humanitarian crises, and of that, almost none on environmental health interventions except interventions to improve water and sanitation.[89]

Pediatric clinicians who care for children in humanitarian settings should be alert for unusual symptoms that could signal a toxic exposure. The clinician can take a thorough environmental history to better understand the child's living environment. This can include type of shelter, proximity to industrial areas, source of fuel for heating and cooking, use of tobacco, source of water, use of home remedies, and typical items in the child's diet. The need for laboratory testing should be determined based on the environmental history, symptoms, and physical examination. Laboratories with the capability to measure specific chemicals may not be available and assistance from competent international laboratories with experience measuring toxicants in human tissue may be necessary.

LONG-TERM EFFECTS

An extensive literature has documented that exposure to severe malnutrition or famine during childhood was consistently associated with increased risk of cardiovascular disease, hypertension, impaired glucose metabolism and metabolic syndrome during adulthood.[90,91] However, studies that follow children longitudinally after they have been exposed to environmental contaminants during childhood humanitarian emergencies could not be found. Significant exposures to environmental contaminants may have detrimental long-term consequences.

SUMMARY

In humanitarian crises children may be exposed to toxic substances (eg, lead, mercury, fluoride, pesticides, tobacco and carbon monoxide) through inadequate housing, polluted indoor air and water, or proximity to industrial sites. They may become ill after ingesting contaminated food (such as cassava containing cyanide) or being sprayed with chemicals dispersed from airplanes. Children who are refugees from war also may be exposed to depleted uranium used for military purposes. As the climate changes, more children in humanitarian settings will face extreme heat. Pediatric clinicians who care for these children should be aware of the potential for toxic exposures and take a thorough environmental history.

INSIGHTS TO ACTION

- Pediatric clinicians who care for children in humanitarian settings should be alert for unusual symptoms that could signal a toxic exposure.
- A thorough environmental history should include type of shelter, location of shelter near industrial areas, source of water, type of fuel for heating and cooking, use of tobacco or home remedies, and the composition of the child's diet.
- Household water treatment is effective, simple, and inexpensive and can be done by families by putting clear plastic bottles in sunlight for a day.
- Tobacco prevention and control is a priority in humanitarian settings.
- Promoting breastfeeding for at least the first 6 months of life is important.

DISCLOSURES

The author has no disclosures to report.

REFERENCES

1. Harvard Law School International Human Rights Clinic and Opre Roma Kosovo. Toxic injustice: translating UN responsibility into remedies for lead-poisoned Roma. 2022. Available at: https://humanrightsclinic.law.harvard.edu/wp-content/uploads/2022/11/HLS-IHRC-ORK-Toxic-Injustice-Final-English.pdf.
2. Rorke B. Kosovo lead poisoning: a tragic timeline of poisoned neglect. 2016. European Roma Rights Center. Available at: www.errc.org/news/kosovo-lead-poisoning-a-tragic-timeline-of-poisoned-neglect.
3. Human Rights Advisory Panel. N.M. and Others v. UNMIK, case 26/08 (26 Feb. 2016), paras 119-120. Available at: https://www.law.umich.edu/facultyhome/drwcasebook/Documents/Updates/Chapter%203%20Problem%203%20N.M.%20and%20Others%20v.%20UNMIK.pdf.
4. UN Special Rapporteur on Toxics and Human Rights. Lead contamination in Kosovo. Available at: https://www.ohchr.org/en/special-procedures/sr-toxics-and-human-rights/lead-contamination-kosovo.
5. Brown MJ, McWeeney G, Kim R, et al. Lead poisoning among internally displaced Roma, Ashkali and Egyptian children in the United Nations-Administered Province of Kosovo. Eur J Public Health 2010;20(3):288–92.
6. Plotinsky RN, Straetemans M, Wong LY, et al. Risk factors for elevated blood lead levels among African refugee children in New Hampshire, 2004. Environ Res 2008;108(3):404–12.
7. Ritchey MD, Scalia Sucosky M, Jefferies T, et al. Lead poisoning among Burmese refugee children–Indiana, 2009. Clin Pediatr (Phila) 2011;50(7):648–56.
8. Mitchell T, Jentes E, Ortega L, et al. Lead poisoning in United States-bound refugee children: Thailand-Burma border, 2009. Pediatrics 2012;129(2):e392–9.

9. Neesanan N, Kasemsup R, Ratanachuaeg S, et al. Preliminary study on assessment of lead exposure in Thai children aged between 3-7 years old who live in Umphang district, Tak province. J Med Assoc Thai 2011;94(Suppl 3):S113–20.
10. Sawalha AF, Wright RO, Bellinger DC, et al. Blood lead level among Palestinian schoolchildren: a pilot study. East Mediterr Health J 2013;19(2):151–5.
11. Pezzi C, Lee D, Kennedy L, et al. Blood lead levels among resettled refugee children in select US States, 2010-2014. Pediatrics 2019;143(5):e20182591.
12. United Nations Children's Fund (UNICEF). Core commitments for children. Available at: https://www.corecommitments.unicef.org/ccc-1-1. Accessed October 16, 2025.
13. Arcos González P, Cabria Fernández J, Gan RK, et al. The epidemiological profile of incidence and mortality from epidemics in complex humanitarian emergencies from 1990 to 2022 - a scoping review. Trop Med Int Health 2024;29(5):343–53.
14. Al Wazni AB, Chapman MV, Ansong D, et al. Climate change, fragility, and child mortality; understanding the role of water access and diarrheal disease amongst children under five during the MDG era. J Prev (2022) 2023;44(4):409–19.
15. World Health Organization. Water sanitation and health. Humanitarian emergencies. Available at: https://www.who.int/teams/environment-climate-change-and-health/water-sanitation-and-health/environmental-health-in-emergencies/humanitarian-emergenciesn.d. Accessed October 13, 2025.
16. Fabreau GE, Bauman P, Coakley AL, et al. Skeletal fluorosis in a resettled refugee from Kakuma refugee camp. Lancet 2019;393(10168):223–5.
17. Demelash H, Beyene A, Abebe Z, et al. Fluoride concentration in ground water and prevalence of dental fluorosis in Ethiopian Rift Valley: systematic review and meta-analysis. BMC Public Health 2019;19(1):1298.
18. Haimanot RT, Fekadu A, Bushra B. Endemic fluorosis in the Ethiopian Rift Valley. Trop Geogr Med 1987;39(3):209–17.
19. World Health Organization. Fluoride in drinking-water. Background document for development of WHO guidelines for drinking-water quality. Geneva: World Health Organization; 2004. Available at: https://www.who.int/docs/default-source/wash-documents/wash-chemicals/fluoride-background-document.pdf.
20. U.S. Department of Health and Human Services Federal Panel on Community Water Fluoridation. U.S. public health service recommendation for fluoride concentration in drinking water for the prevention of dental caries. Public Health Rep 2015;130(4):318–31. https://doi.org/10.1177/003335491513000408.
21. Ahmad SA, Khan MH, Haque M. Arsenic contamination in groundwater in Bangladesh: implications and challenges for healthcare policy. Risk Manag Healthc Policy 2018;11:251–61.
22. Wasserman GA, Liu X, Parvez F, et al. Water arsenic exposure and children's intellectual function in Araihazar, Bangladesh. Environ Health Perspect 2004;112-(13):1329–33.
23. Rahman MF, Mahmud MJ, Sadmani AHMA, et al. Previously unrecognized potential threat to children from manganese in groundwater in Rohingya refugee camps in Cox's Bazar, Bangladesh. Chemosphere 2021;266:129128.
24. Aakre I, Henjum S, Folven Gjengedal EL, et al. Trace element concentrations in drinking water and urine among Saharawi women and young children. Toxics 2018;6(3):40.
25. Bellos A, Mulholland K, O'Brien KL, et al. The burden of acute respiratory infections in crisis-affected populations: a systematic review. Confl Health 2010;4:3.

26. Scales SE, Park JW, Nixon R, et al. Disease burden among refugees in camps on mainland Greece, 2016-2017: a retrospective cross-sectional study. BMC Public Health 2023;23(1):1715.
27. Bede-Ojimadu O, Orisakwe OE. Exposure to wood smoke and associated health effects in Sub-Saharan Africa: a systematic review. Ann Glob Health 2020; 86(1):32.
28. Al-Khatib I, Ju'ba A, Kamal N, et al. Impact of housing conditions on the health of the people at al-Ama'ri refugee camp in the West Bank of Palestine. Int J Environ Health Res 2003;13(4):315–26.
29. Elbayoumi M, Albelbeisi AH. Biomass use and its health effects among the vulnerable and marginalized refugee families in the Gaza Strip. Front Public Health 2023;11:1129985.
30. El Sharif N, Douwes J, Hoet PH, et al. Concentrations of domestic mite and pet allergens and endotoxin in Palestine. Allergy 2004;59(6):623–31.
31. Glick P, Al-Khammash U, Shaheen M, et al. Health risk behaviours of Palestinian youth: findings from a representative survey. East Mediterr Health J 2018;24(2): 127–36.
32. Rahman A, Biswas J, Banik PC. Non-communicable diseases risk factors among the forcefully displaced Rohingya population in Bangladesh. PLOS Glob Public Health 2022;2(9):e0000930.
33. Kheirallah KA, Cobb CO, Alsulaiman JW, et al. Trauma exposure, mental health and tobacco use among vulnerable Syrian refugee youth in Jordan. J Public Health (Oxf) 2020;42(3):e343–51.
34. Rizk Y, Hoteit R, Khater B, et al. Psychosocial wellbeing and risky health behaviors among Syrian adolescent refugees in South Beirut: a study using the HEEADSSS interviewing framework. Front Psychol 2023;14:1019269.
35. Vlachou M, Kirkou G, Vivilaki V, et al. Environmental exposure to tobacco smoke and the onset of respiratory infections in neonatal, infant, and childhood stages: a systematic review. Tobacco Prevention & Cessation 2024;10(Supplement 1):A12.
36. Kurtuluş Ş, Can R. The effect of environmental exposures on the diagnosis of tuberculosis in Syrian refugees. Turk Thorac J 2021;22(6):489–93.
37. du Preez K, Mandalakas AM, Kirchner HL, et al. Environmental tobacco smoke exposure increases *Mycobacterium tuberculosis* infection risk in children. Int J Tuberc Lung Dis 2011;15(11):1490–1496.i.
38. Sethi S, Jonsson R, Skaff R, et al. Community-based noncommunicable disease care for Syrian refugees in Lebanon. Glob Health Sci Pract 2017;5(3):495–506.
39. Skipalskyi A, Habicht J, Ciobanu A, et al. Tobacco control in complex emergencies: policy case study of Ukraine. Tob Prev Cessat 2025;11. https://doi.org/10.18332/tpc/203838.
40. Gudi N, Mathias EG, Swain A, et al. Interventions for tobacco prevention and control in humanitarian settings: a scoping review. Nicotine Tob Res 2025;27(1):3–11.
41. O'Sullivan BP. Carbon monoxide poisoning in an infant exposed to a kerosene heater. J Pediatr 1983;103(2):249–51.
42. Houck PM, Hampson NB. Epidemic carbon monoxide poisoning following a winter storm. J Emerg Med 1997;15(4):469–73.
43. Daley WR, Shireley L, Gilmore R. A flood-related outbreak of carbon monoxide poisoning–Grand Forks, North Dakota. J Emerg Med 2001;21(3):249–53.
44. Centers for Disease Control and Prevention. Carbon monoxide poisoning from hurricane-associated use of portable generators—Florida, 2004. MMWR Morb Mortal Wkly Rep 2005;54(28):697–700.

45. Chen L, HuiLai M. Risk factors of nonoccupational carbon monoxide poisoning during the 2008 ice storm in Guiyang County, Hunan Province, China. Public Health Rep 2010;125(4):605–10.
46. Styles T, Przysiecki P, Archambault G, et al. Two storm-related carbon monoxide poisoning outbreaks—Connecticut, October 2011 and October 2012. Arch Environ Occup Health 2015;70(5):291–6.
47. Cliff J, Muquingue H, Nhassico D, et al. Konzo and continuing cyanide intoxication from cassava in Mozambique. Food Chem Toxicol 2011;49(3):631–5.
48. Cliff J, Nicala D, Saute F, et al. Konzo associated with war in Mozambique. Trop Med Int Health 1997;2(11):1068–74.
49. Ciglenečki I, Eyema R, Kabanda C, et al. Konzo outbreak among refugees from Central African Republic in Eastern region, Cameroon. Food Chem Toxicol 2011; 49(3):579–82.
50. Kashala-Abotnes E, Okitundu D, Mumba D, et al. Konzo: a distinct neurological disease associated with food (cassava) cyanogenic poisoning. Brain Res Bull 2019;145:87–91.
51. Smędra A, Wochna K, Zawadzki D, et al. Medical error in treatment of Amanita phalloides poisoning in pre-hospital care. Scand J Trauma Resusc Emerg Med 2022;30(1):20.
52. Fellows KM, Samy S, Rodriguez Y, et al. Investigating aluminum cookpots as a source of lead exposure in Afghan refugee children resettled in the United States. J Expo Sci Environ Epidemiol 2022;32(3):451–60.
53. Shawahna R, Zyoud A, Dwikat J, et al. Breast milk lead levels in 3 major regions of the West Bank of Palestine. J Hum Lact 2016;32(3):455–61.
54. Minor and trace elements in breast milk. Geneva: World Health Organization; 1989.
55. American Academy of Pediatrics Council on Environmental Health. Human milk. In: Etzel RA, Balk SJ, editors. Chapter 15 in pediatric environmental health. 4th edition. Itasca (IL): American Academy of Pediatrics; 2019. p. 237–55.
56. Consultation on assessment of the health risk of dioxins; re-evaluation of the tolerable daily intake (TDI): executive summary. Food Addit Contam 2000;17(4): 223–40. https://doi.org/10.1080/713810655.
57. Huić M, Francetić I, Bakran I, et al. Acquired coagulopathy due to anticoagulant rodenticide poisoning. Croat Med J 2002;43(5):615–7.
58. Xiong HY, Lin H, Xvi H, et al. Post-earthquake outbreak of insecticide-associated conjunctivitis in a primary school of Lixian district, China: an epidemiological investigation. Public Health 2010;124(6):332–8.
59. Otto M, Ahlemeyer C, Tasche H, et al. Mercury exposure. Nature 1994;367-(6459):110.
60. Bose-O'Reilly S, Lettmeier B, Gothe RM, et al. Mercury as a serious health hazard for children in gold mining areas. Environ Res 2008;107:89–97.
61. Allan-Blitz LT, Goldfine C, Erickson TB. Environmental and health risks posed to children by artisanal gold mining: a systematic review. SAGE Open Med 2022; 10:20503121221076934.
62. Dooyema CA, Neri A, Lo YC, et al. Outbreak of fatal childhood lead poisoning related to artisanal gold mining in northwestern Nigeria, 2010. Environ Health Perspect 2012;120(4):601–7.
63. Schecter A, Dai LC, Thuy LT, et al. Agent Orange and the Vietnamese: the persistence of elevated dioxin levels in human tissues. Am J Public Health 1995;85(4): 516–22.

64. Manh HD, Kido T, Tai PT, et al. Levels of polychlorinated dibenzodioxins and polychlorinated dibenzofurans in breast milk samples from three dioxin-contaminated hotspots of Vietnam. Sci Total Environ 2015;511:416–22.
65. Schecter A, Pavuk M, Päpke O, et al. Dioxin, dibenzofuran, and coplanar PCB levels in Laotian blood and milk from agent orange-sprayed and nonsprayed areas, 2001. J Toxicol Environ Health A 2003;66(21):2067–75.
66. Hue NT, Nam VD, Thuong NV, et al. Determination of PCDD/Fs in breast milk of women living in the vicinities of Da Nang Agent Orange hot spot (Vietnam) and estimation of the infant's daily intake. Sci Total Environ 2014;491-492:212–8.
67. International Programme on Chemical Safety. Assessment of the health risk of dioxins: re-evaluation of the Tolerable Daily Intake (TDI). Geneva, Switzerland: World Health Organization; 1998. Available at: https://cdn.who.int/media/docs/default-source/chemical-safety/exe-sum-final_may1998.pdf?sfvrsn=bbb9e913_1. Accessed October 16, 2025.
68. Schecter A, Quynh HT, Pavuk M, et al. Food as a source of dioxin exposure in the residents of Bien Hoa City, Vietnam. J Occup Environ Med 2003;45(8):781–8.
69. Pham T, Ngoc T, Hoang VT, et al. Effects of perinatal dioxin exposure on learning abilities of 8-year-old children in Vietnam. Int J Hyg Environ Health 2020;223(1):132–41.
70. McConnell R, Anderson K, Russell W, et al. Angiosarcoma, porphyria cutanea tarda, and probable chloracne in a worker exposed to waste oil contaminated with 2,3,7,8-tetrachlorodibenzo-p-dioxin. Br J Ind Med 1993;50(8):699–703.
71. U.S. environmental protection agency. 2,3,7,8-Tetrachlorodibenzo-*p*-Dioxin. Available at: https://www.epa.gov/sites/default/files/2016-09/documents/2-3-7-8-tetrachlorodibenzo-p-dioxin.pdf.
72. Carter CD, Kimbrough RD, Liddle JA, et al. Tetrachlorodibenzodioxin: an accidental poisoning episode in horse arenas. Science 1975;188(4189):738–40.
73. Seagrave S. Yellow rain: a journey through the terror of chemical airfare. New York: M. Evans; 1981.
74. Schneider BS. Yellow rain. Brittanica academic. Available at: https://academic-eb-com.us1.proxy.openathens.net/levels/collegiate/article/yellow-rain/439505.
75. Katz R, Singer B. Can an attribution assessment be made for yellow rain? Systematic reanalysis in a chemical-and-biological-weapons use investigation. Polit Life Sci 2007;26:1.
76. Mirocha CJ, Pawlosky RA, Chatterjee K, et al. Analysis for Fusarium toxins in various samples implicated in biological warfare in Southeast Asia. J Assoc Off Anal Chem 1983;66(6):1485–99.
77. Watson SA, Mirocha CJ, Hayes AW. Analysis for trichothecenes in samples from Southeast Asia associated with "Yellow Rain". Fundam Appl Toxicol 1984;4(5):700–17.
78. Fathi RA, Matti LY, Al-Salih HS, et al. Environmental pollution by depleted uranium in Iraq with special reference to Mosul and possible effects on cancer and birth defect rates. Med Confl Surviv 2013;29(1):7–25.
79. Marshall AC. Gulf war depleted uranium risks. J Expo Sci Environ Epidemiol 2008;18(1):95–108.
80. Briner W. The toxicity of depleted uranium. Int J Environ Res Public Health 2010;7(1):303–13.
81. Milacić S, Petrović D, Jovicić D, et al. Examination of the health status of populations from depleted-uranium-contaminated regions. Environ Res 2004;95(1):2–10.

82. Zunic S. Cytological characteristics of lung washings from children in depleted uranium stroked region. J Biol Regul Homeost Agents 2013;27(4):961–7.
83. Bleise A, Danesi PR, Burkart W. Properties, use and health effects of depleted uranium (DU): a general overview. J Environ Radioact 2003;64(2–3):93–112.
84. AlQubati AN. Childhood leukemia clusters in Yemen: the dual impact of environmental carcinogens and healthcare collapse in conflict zones. Cureus 2025; 17(4):e82396.
85. Lasater ME, Prager G, Choi YA, et al. Understanding relationships among climate change, conflict, migration/displacement and health in humanitarian settings: a scoping review. Confl Health 2025;19(1):73.
86. United Nations High Commissioner for Refugees (UNHCR). No Escape – on the frontlines of climate change, conflict and forced displacement. United Nations High Commissioner for Refugees; 2024. Available at: https://www.unhcr.org/media/no-escape-frontlines-climate-change-conflict-and-forced-displacement.
87. Laderach P, Craparo A. Protecting 90 million refugees on climate crisis frontlines. Study #GLO - 2401. 2025. Rome (Italy): Bioversity International; Cali (Colombia): CIAT, 4 p. Available at: https://cgspace.cgiar.org/items/c3f9626e-0228-40f1-a9bd-07b2c101de45.
88. Wilson AJ, Bressler RD, Ivanovich C, et al. Heat disproportionately kills young people: evidence from wet-bulb temperature in Mexico. Sci Adv 2024;10(49): eadq3367.
89. Blanchet K, Ramesh A, Frison S, et al. Evidence on public health interventions in humanitarian crises. Lancet 2017;390(10109):2287–96.
90. Grey K, Gonzales GB, Abera M, et al. Severe malnutrition or famine exposure in childhood and cardiometabolic non-communicable disease later in life: a systematic review. BMJ Glob Health 2021;6(3):e003161.
91. Ogah OS, Oguntade AS, Chukwuonye II, et al. Childhood and infant exposure to famine in the Biafran war is associated with hypertension in later life: the Abia NCDS study. J Hum Hypertens 2023;37(10):936–43.

Firearm Violence and Children

Olivia Landes, MPH[a], Sonali Rajan, EdD, MS[b,*],
Shernise Mohammed-Ali, HBSc, MPH[a], Charles Branas, PhD[a]

KEYWORDS

• Firearm violence • Minoritized groups • Low-income and middle-income countries • Children

KEY POINTS

- Firearm violence is the leading cause of death among US children and adolescents.
- Adolescents, racially minoritized youth, and children from low-income communities are disproportionately affected.
- Exposure to firearm violence has long-term effects on mental health, cognitive development, and socioeconomic outcomes.
- Evidence-based interventions at the school, community, and health care system levels can mitigate harm.
- Comprehensive firearm policy and improved data infrastructure are essential to prevention efforts.

INTRODUCTION: FIREARM VIOLENCE AS A GLOBAL PUBLIC HEALTH CRISIS

Firearm violence is widely recognized as one of the most pressing humanitarian crises of the twenty-first century, with profound implications for children's health and well-being. Around the world, communities face firearm-related mortality and morbidity that disproportionately affect the most vulnerable populations. Unlike many other large-scale health crises, firearm violence is the direct result of human behavior, weapon availability, and policy decisions, and is therefore entirely preventable. In the United States, firearms have now surpassed vehicle crashes to become the leading cause of death among children and adolescents, underscoring the urgent need for coordinated action.[1]

[a] Columbia Scientific Union for the Reduction of Gun Violence, Department of Epidemiology, Mailman School of Public Health, Columbia University, New York, NY, USA; [b] Columbia Scientific Union for the Reduction of Gun Violence, Department of Health Studies and Applied Educational Psychology, Teachers College, Mailman School of Public Health, Columbia University, New York, NY, USA

* Corresponding author. Columbia Scientific Union for the Reduction of Gun Violence, Department of Epidemiology, Mailman school of Public Health, Columbia University, New York, NY.
E-mail address: sr2345@tc.columbia.edu

Pediatr Clin N Am 73 (2026) 1023–1035
https://doi.org/10.1016/j.pcl.2026.05.003 **pediatric.theclinics.com**

Abbreviations	
CBT	cognitive behavioral therapy
HPA	hypothalamic-pituitary-adrenal
HVIPs	Hospital-based violence intervention programs
LMICs	low-income and middle-income countries
PTSD	posttraumatic stress disorder
TF-CBT	trauma-focused CBT

Recent work situates firearm violence within broader patterns of structural and political determinants of health, Analyses of firearm ownership, availability, and policy variation demonstrate that firearm violence is not random but strongly correlated with social structures and regulatory frameworks.[2] Recent modeling of firearm ownership trends across US states, revealed clear spatiotemporal patterns linked to cultural norms and legislative differences.[2] Globally, firearm violence in low- and middle-income countries is compounded by fragile health systems, a cycle of armed conflict, and access to unrestricted illegal firearms.[3] These findings expose a dual crisis of violence and inadequate data infrastructure, reflecting not only tragedies, but also structural failures in governance and prevention.[4]

Collectively, the data clearly indicate that firearm violence is more than a law enforcement or political issue: it is an urgent matter of child health that warrants mobilization of resources and expertise equivalent to other major public health emergencies. Pediatric clinicians, researchers, and policymakers share a responsibility to document, prevent, and mitigate the glaringly disproportionate impact of firearms on children.

PEDIATRIC FIREARM VIOLENCE

In the United States, firearms are the single leading cause of death among children and adolescents, surpassing motor vehicle crashes and other injuries.[5] Longitudinal analyses cataloged more than 1400 school shootings between 1997 and 2022, events that not only account for direct fatalities and injuries but also generate widespread fear, media exposure, and secondary trauma among students, families, and school personnel.[6] The frequency of such incidents has accelerated in recent years, mirroring broader societal trends of increased firearm availability and polarized debates over firearm regulation.

Geospatial studies further extend this epidemiologic lens into everyday community settings. Research in Compton, California, found that firearm-related homicides clustered along walkable routes frequently used by adolescents commuting to and from school, underscoring that pediatric firearm exposure extends well beyond high profile shootings.[7] For many children, the threat of firearm violence is embedded in the fabric of daily life.

More broadly, exposure to firearm violence during adolescence predicts heightened risks of depression, anxiety, substance use, academic disruption, and countless other poor health, learning, and developmental outcomes.[8] Such exposures contribute to the normalization of violence, shaping risk behaviors and perpetuating intergenerational cycles of disadvantage.

SUBGROUPS AT HEIGHTENED RISK OF FIREARM VIOLENCE

Firearm violence is not evenly distributed across populations. Its burden falls disproportionately on children and adolescents from low-income households, racially and ethnically minoritized groups, and communities facing structural disadvantages. These disparities underscore the role of social determinants of health in shaping vulnerability to firearm injury and exposure.

Socioeconomic disadvantage is a consistent predictor of firearm violence exposure. Children living in neighborhoods characterized by concentrated poverty, limited educational and employment opportunities, and inadequate community infrastructure are placed at high risk and far more likely to be victims or witnesses of firearm violence. Qualitative reviews of community interventions highlight how underfunded schools and limited access to health care exacerbate vulnerability.[9] Community-level analyses using measures such as the Social Vulnerability Index further demonstrate that poverty and disinvestment translate directly into increased pediatric firearm injury risk.[10]

Beyond income, race and ethnicity are powerful predictors of firearm exposure. Black and Hispanic children are disproportionately more likely than their White peers to witness or live near fatal shootings, even after accounting for neighborhood poverty.[11] Environmental racism—including exposure to poverty, segregation, and systemic disinvestmentamplifies these risks.[12] Exposure to deadly firearm violence is disproportionately concentrated among Black and Hispanic adolescents, with downstream consequences for mental health, education attainment, and broader health disparities.[13]

These vulnerabilities often intersect. Many children and teens experience overlapping risks of poverty, racial segregation, and systemic disinvestment, leading to compounded exposures. Structural inequities—such as discriminatory housing policies, underfunded schools, policing practices, and unequal and limited access to physical and mental health care—further intensify this convergence. Children who live at these intersections may face daily firearm exposure not as isolated events but as part of a broader environment of chronic adversity. For example, neighborhoods with concentrated firearm violence often overlap with areas of limited recreational space and restricted access to mental health services, creating cumulative disadvantages that undermine resilience.

Frequent exposure to firearm violence in structurally disadvantaged contexts can perpetuate intergenerational cycles of risk and constrained opportunity, not because violence is accepted as normal, but because chronic threat destabilizes developmental, educational, and economic trajectories. Importantly, children, families, and communities affected by firearm violence consistently resist narratives that frame violence as inevitable or pathologize those who live amid it, demonstrating resilience, mutual support, and sustained efforts to protect youth despite persistent exposure. Together, these realities highlight the limitations of individual-level explanations and underscore the need to shift attention upstream—toward the policies, systems, and historical decisions that have shaped inequitable environments and facilitated widespread firearm availability. Addressing these disparities therefore requires not only individual- and family-level interventions, but also structural reforms across housing, education, health care, and community investment that reduce exposure and expand opportunity.[4,13]

HEALTH AND PSYCHOSOCIAL IMPACTS OF FIREARM VIOLENCE

Beyond immediate injuries and fatalities, firearm violence imposes profound and lasting burdens on children and adolescents across mental health, cognitive development, and socioeconomic trajectories.

In line with the literature on adverse childhood experiences, it has been documented that exposure to firearm violence is consistently associated with elevated risks of depression, anxiety, and posttraumatic stress disorder (PTSD) among youth.[14] Significant declines in quality of life and increases in trauma-related symptoms have been documented among children living in neighborhoods heavily affected by firearm violence.[15] Systematic reviews further confirm that exposure to shootings—whether witnessed or directly experienced—is linked to heightened risks of emotional dysregulation, externalizing behaviors, and suicidality, with effects that persist across time.[16] Mass shootings, although far less common than community violence, exert uniquely severe psychological consequences, including elevated rates of PTSD, grief reactions, and academic disruption among child and adolescent survivors.[17]

The developmental effects extend into cognition and education. Community exposure to firearm homicide has been associated with impaired academic performance, absenteeism, and reduced concentration in school.[18] Exposure is also linked with increased handgun carrying among adolescents, reflecting maladaptive copying mechanisms and altered decision-making processes.[19] Neighborhood-level dynamics compound these risks, as environments with frequent shootings weaken trust and collective efficacy, undermining developmental processes essential for learning, cognitive growth, and social development.[20]

The biological mechanisms underlying these psychosocial outcomes are increasingly well described. Repeated trauma exposure activates the hypothalamic-pituitary-adrenal (HPA) axis, leading to chronic elevations in cortisol and toxic stress.[21] Over time, these processes contribute to structural changes in the amygdala, hippocampus, and prefrontal cortex—regions critical for emotional regulation, memory, and executive functioning.[22,23] Such neurobiological alternations highlight firearm violence as not only a social determinant of health but also an exposure with lasting neurodevelopmental implications.

The long-term socioeconomic implications are of comparable magnitude. Early exposure to firearm violence predicts disrupted educational attainment and diminished social mobility, perpetuating cycles of disadvantage and community disinvestment.[24]

For pediatric clinicians and public health practitioners alike, these findings highlight the need for proactive, trauma-informed care in clinical, school, and community settings. Validated screening tools such as the Child PTSD Symptom Scale[25] and the UCLA PTSD Reaction Index[26] can help identify at-risk children in primary care and emergency settings. Trauma-informed practice also involves creating safe clinical environments, avoiding retraumatization, and providing anticipatory guidance for families about common behavioral and environmental responses to violence exposure.[27] Evidence-based interventions such as cognitive behavioral therapy (CBT) and trauma-focused CBT (TF-CBT) remain gold standards for treating pediatric trauma, with strong support for their effectiveness in reducing PTSD symptoms and improving functioning.[28,29] Clinicians can also partner with schools, community organizations and hospital-based violence intervention programs to ensure continuity of care. Ultimately, addressing the psychosocial consequences of firearm violence requires both individualized clinical care and advocacy for structural change to foster safe environments where children can thrive.

THE AFTER-SCHOOL PERIOD AS A VULNERABILITY

Risk is not evenly distributed across the day. The after-school period—particularly between 3:00 and 6:00 PM—represents a window of heightened vulnerability when children are outside structured school supervision but may not yet be in the care of guardians. Analyses of pediatric firearm injuries by time and location demonstrate significant clustering of incidents during after-school hours in community settings such as parks, streets, and transit routes.[30] These patterns reflect broader gaps in community safety infrastructure and point to opportunities for targeted, supervised, and accessible programming to reduce exposure during predictable risk windows.

Structured after-school programs have been shown to reduce violence involvement and improve academic and psychosocial outcomes, particularly for youth who attend schools with less access to evidence-informed after-school programming.[23,31] Programs that combine academic support, mentoring, social-emotional skill development, and recreational activities not only provide safe environments but also strengthen protective factors such as connectedness, prosocial behaviors, and self-regulation. Public health frameworks emphasize that support during these hours can buffer against both victimization and perpetration of firearm violence. Partnerships between schools, community organizations, and health care systems can ensure equitable access to such programs, particularly in areas where firearm risk is highest.

SCHOOL-BASED INTERVENTIONS

Each year, dozens of K-12 schools in the United States tragically experience and must respond to intentional firearm violence. At the same time, and with the right support and resources, they are also uniquely positioned to meaningfully prevent school gun violence from occurring in the first place. In the United States, there are an estimated 90,000 K-12 schools serving nearly 51 million children and the research is very clear that investments in evidence-informed prevention would meaningfully reduce threats of firearm violence in schools.[32]

Specifically, evaluations of K-12 firearm incidents caution that purely punitive or security driven measures, such as increased surveillance or armed personnel, may foster climates of fear and disproportionately affect marginalized students.[25] In contrast, balanced approaches that integrate safety planning with mental health supports and evidence-based threat assessment strategies are more likely to prevent escalation while preserving a positive learning environment.

School communities themselves often express stronger support for interventions that build capacity rather than intensify control. Surveys of stakeholders show greater endorsement of social-emotional learning curricula, conflict resolution training, and supportive school climates compared with surveillance heavy strategies or hyper-realistic drills.[33] Trauma-informed practices—including staff training, embedded counseling, and peer-support-programs—are essential to mitigate psychological impacts of firearm exposure and promote academic continuity.

Emerging evidence also suggests that schools can play a central role in broader community firearm prevention. Programs that link schools with hospital-based violence intervention initiatives extend the continuum of care for students who have been directly injured by firearms, providing multidisciplinary rehabilitation, trauma-informed counseling, and support for academic and social reintegration.[34] These partnerships bridge medical, educational, and community systems to reduce reinjury and retaliation risk while promoting recovery and resilience. Collaboration with local behavioral health networks and restorative justice initiatives has likewise demonstrated promise in reducing recidivism and improving student outcomes.[26] Integration of firearm safety education into health curricula, when paired with parent engagement, may further support safe storage practices and reduce access among adolescents.

COMMUNITY-LEVEL INTERVENTIONS

Community-level interventions are critical for reducing pediatric firearm violence and mitigating its effects. Approaches at this level address not only immediate safety but also the structural conditions that shape exposure to violence.

Health care–based interventions are one important component of comprehensive firearm violence prevention. Hospital-based violence intervention programs (HVIPs) identify youth at the point of care following firearm-related injuries and provide wrap-around services, including case management, mental health support, and connections to education and employment.[34] Evidence shows that HVIPs can reduce subsequent injury and arrests, while also improving psychosocial outcomes among adolescents treated for violent injury.[35] Emerging data further suggest that medical-legal partnerships embedded within trauma care settings can address unmet legal and financial needs, such as access to income supports, victim compensation, housing problems, and benefits navigation, that commonly arise during recovery from violent injury.[36] Integrating pediatric providers into these multidisciplinary initiatives helps ensure that children and adolescents exposed to violence are connected with sustained medical, psychosocial, and structural support over time.

Community violence interruption models represent another pillar of prevention. Programs such as Cure Violence and Advance Peace employ trained credible messengers to mediate conflicts, promote nonviolent norms, and provide mentorship to youth at risk of perpetration or victimization. Evaluations of these models suggest reductions in shootings and improvements in community cohesion, although sustainability often depends on stable funding and policy support.[37,38]

Prevention and resilience-building extend beyond individual services. Early community-wide injury prevention efforts emphasized the creation of safe physical environments through coordinated investments in neighborhood spaces, demonstrating the feasibility and impact of place-based approaches to violence reduction.[39] Building on this foundation, contemporary studies show that investments in safe green spaces, recreational facilities, and community centers are associated with declines in neighborhood firearm violence and improved perceptions of safety among children.[40] These environmental strategies reduce opportunities for violence while fostering collective efficacy and community engagement.

Finally, support for individuals and communities after firearm violence occurs is a vital but sometimes overlooked dimension. Community-based grief counseling, school-based trauma services, and peer-support networks help buffer long-term psychosocial harm. Partnerships between health care, schools, and community-organizations can ensure continuity of care and reduce disparities in access to trauma-informed services.[41]

Together, these multi-level interventions demonstrate that preventing and mitigating pediatric firearm violence requires coordinated strategies across health care, community organizations, and policy domains.

FIREARM POLICY

Firearm policy is one of the strongest determinants of pediatric firearm exposure and outcomes. Differences in state and national regulations contribute directly to disparities in firearm mortality among children. Stronger firearm laws—particularly those related to safe storage, background checks, and child access prevention—are consistently associated with lower rates of pediatric firearm deaths.[42,43]

Recent analyses of state-level firearm policies show that states with more comprehensive firearm laws—often summarized using composite *policy grades* that reflect the strength and breadth of regulations such as background checks, permitting requirements, and child access prevention provisions—experience lower fatalities from mass shootings, including among youth.[44] Conversely, the diffusion of punitive firearm preemption laws, which prohibit local governments from enacting firearm regulations that exceed state standard, had limited the ability of communities to implement evidence-based prevention strategies tailored to local risk patterns. These constraints are particularly relevant for pediatric injury prevention, as they restrict locally driven approaches to safe storage, youth access reduction, and community-based interventions.[45] Public opinion data also reveal strong parental support for age-related restrictions and safe storage policies, suggesting broad acceptability of pediatric-centered firearm regulation.[46]

Child access prevention laws remain among the most effective at reducing unintentional firearm injuries and suicides among adolescents.[47] Universal background checks and licensing requirements further reduce rates of youth firearm homicide and suicide, with benefits extending across state lines.[48,49] While some policies, such as restrictions on high-capacity magazines and assault weapons, show mixed evidence on pediatric outcomes, international comparisons demonstrate that countries with comprehensive regulations consistently report much lower rates of firearm-related child mortality than the United States.[50]

These findings highlight firearm policy as both a clinical and public health priority. Comparative experience from other high-income countries demonstrates that comprehensive firearm regulation can substantially reduce firearm-related morbidity and mortality among children, underscoring the preventability of these outcomes.[51] Pediatric clinicians can contribute by counseling families on safe storage, supporting legislation grounded in evidence, and engaging with policymakers to reduce preventable child deaths.

GAPS IN DATA AND WHY THAT MATTER

Despite increasing recognition of firearm violence as a pediatric public health crisis, critical data gaps undermine prevention and intervention efforts. Historically, federal restrictions on firearm research funding constrained surveillance and slowed scientific progress.[52]

Recent studies emphasize the urgent need to close these gaps. Progress in pediatric firearm research has accelerated modestly in recent years, but the field still lags far behind other leading causes of child mortality.[53] Limitations include the lack of standardized national surveillance for nonfatal firearm injuries among children. Mortality data are relatively well documented, but information on emergency department visits, hospitalizations, and long-term functional outcomes remains fragmented.[54]

Disaggregated data are another deficiency. Without systematic reporting by age, race, ethnicity, and geography, disparities remain obscured, hindering the development of tailored prevention strategies.[55] Experts argue that revitalizing developmental and longitudinal research is essential to understand how firearm exposure across childhood shapes later health trajectories.[56]

Closing these gaps will require coordinated federal and state investments in surveillance infrastructure, standardized reporting mechanisms, and sustained funding. Clinicians and researchers can contribute by integrating systematic data collection into health care and school systems, strengthening the evidence base for equitable prevention.

In the global context, firearm violence and conflict-related injury represent major threats to child health and are poorly captured by existing surveillance systems, particularly in low- and middle-income countries (LMICs) where health information infrastructure is limited and conflict disrupts data collection.[57] Armed conflict and chronic exposure to violence impair children's physical and psychological development and are associated with a range of adverse health outcomes across settings.[58] Without standardized global reporting of nonfatal firearm injuries, disabilities, and long-term outcomes, these burdens remain obscured, hindering coordinated prevention and humanitarian response efforts.[57] Events such as the December 14, 2025 mass shooting at Bondi Beach in Sydney, where 2 gunmen killed at least 15 people, including at a Hanukkah celebration, despite Australia's historically strict firearm laws, underscore that firearm violence and its consequences are not unique to any one national context and that even well-regulated settings can experience sudden catastrophic events.[59] Strengthening global injury surveillance, harmonizing reporting standards across countries and conflict-affected areas, and integrating these data into international health frameworks are therefore essential to improving pediatric protection, clinical response, and equitable prevention efforts worldwide.[57]

CHALLENGES OF COLLECTING DATA ON CHILDREN

Collecting accurate data on firearm violence affecting children presents unique methodological and ethical challenges. Children may underreport exposure due to fear, stigma, or mistrust of adults, while parental reporting often fails to capture exposures occurring outside the home.[60,61] Administrative datasets such as hospital or school records rarely capture the full range of firearm experiences, particularly noninjury exposures like witnessing shootings.[62]

Linking across data systems—healthcare, education and child welfare—remains technically and legally complex because of privacy and confidentiality constraints.[63] Ethical considerations add further complexity: studies involving minors must safeguard against retraumatization, ensure informed consent, and apply developmentally appropriate measures and protocols.

Best practices include the use of validated child-focused instruments, trauma-informed approaches to data collection, and inclusion of community advisory boards to guide sensitive research.[64] Expanding infrastructure for child-centered violence research, coupled with training investigators in trauma-informed methods, will be critical to advancing an accurate and ethical evidence base.

FUTURE DIRECTIONS AND IDEAL NEXT STEPS

Future progress in preventing pediatric firearm violence will depend on integrating public health, clinical, and policy approaches. Strengthening research infrastructure remains a top priority. Dedicating funding streams are needed to support longitudinal studies, randomized trials of interventions, and improved surveillance systems capable of capturing both fatal and nonfatal firearm injuries in children.[41,50]

Expanding community partnerships is equally critical. Models that link health care providers with schools, community organizations, and local governments have demonstrated promise in addressing social determinants of health that underlie firearm risk.[25,33] Scaling these collaborations requires stable funding and integration into broader child health initiatives.

Clinicians also play an important role in advancing prevention. Normalizing firearm safety counseling—similar to seatbelt or tobacco cessation counseling—can enhance parental adoption of safe storage practices.[64] Given that firearm-related mortality includes both homicide and suicide, counseling may also include lethal means safety strategies, including the temporary removal or off-site storage of firearms during period of elevated suicide risk.[65] Evidence suggests that lethal means counseling in clinical settings can increase adoption of secure storage practices and reduce access to firearms during acute crises.[66] However, widespread implementation remains limited by training gaps, time constraints, and legal barriers in some states.[67]

Finally, addressing pediatric firearm violence requires sustained policy engagement. Evidence indicates that strong firearm laws are protective, but variability in adoption perpetuates inequities. Continued advocacy from clinicians, researchers, and communities is essential to translate evidence into policy that safeguards children's health.[41,46–48]

SUMMARY

Firearm violence represents a major threat to children's health and well-being in the twenty-first century and is increasingly recognized as a humanitarian crisis with global implications.[68] Across settings, firearm violence intersects with structural inequities, displacement, and community instability, contributing to preventable injury, disability, and psychological trauma among children. In the United States, firearm-related mortality has become a leading cause of death among children and adolescents, and its burden is not evenly distributed: children from low-income families, racially and ethnically minoritized groups, and structurally disadvantaged communities tragically bear the heaviest risks.[9–13] Beyond mortality, firearm violence disrupts mental health, cognitive development, and long-term socioeconomic trajectories.[15–20]

Evidence demonstrates that prevention is possible. School-based interventions, community partnerships, and hospital-based programs reduce risks and promote resilience.[23,25,26,32–34] Policy measures, including child access prevention laws, safe storage initiatives, and universal background checks, consistently correlate with lower rates of pediatric firearm injury and death.[41,46–48] However, data gaps and research limitations hinder the ability to fully capture the scope of the problem and to design precise interventions.[52–54]

Pediatric firearm violence is a preventable public health crisis. Reducing its toll will require coordinated action across health care, schools, communities, and policy makers, guided by a commitment to child health equity and informed by global lessons on protecting children from violence in humanitarian contexts.[68]

INSIGHTS TO ACTION

- Firearm violence is the leading cause of death among children and adolescents in the United States.[5]
- Risk is disproportionately concentrated in low-income neighborhoods and racially/ethnically minoritized communities.[11–13]
- Exposure to firearm violence is strongly associated with mental health consequences, including depression, anxiety, and PTSD, as well as adverse effects on cognition and academic performance.[15–20]
- The after-school period represents a predictable window of heightened vulnerability when pediatric firearm injuries cluster.[21]
- Trauma-informed, school-based, and community-level interventions can reduce risks and foster resilience.[23,26]
- Firearm policy—including child access prevention laws, universal background checks, and safe storage requirements—is consistently associated with lower rates of pediatric firearm injury and death.[41,46–48]

- Clinicians can contribute by integrating firearm safety counseling into routine practice and engaging in data collection to strengthen the evidence base.[64]
- Pediatric clinicians can also support prevention by partnering with schools and community organizations to expand access to safe, supervised after-school programming and other upstream supports that reduce exposure during predictable high-risk periods.[21,23]

DISCLOSURE

The authors have no relevant financial or commercial conflicts of interest to disclose.

REFERENCES

1. Snooks C, Levas M, Schultz ML. Gun violence in children: a public health crisis and an upstream approach to our response. WMJ (Wisconsin Medical Journal) 2024;123(6):543–5.
2. Barak-Ventura R, Marín MR, Porfiri M. A spatiotemporal model of firearm ownership in the United States. Patterns 2022;3(10):100546. https://doi.org/10.1016/j.patter.2022.100546.
3. Jadoon OK, Shazia S, Ullah I, et al. The global scourge of Gun violence: a call for action. J Ayub Med Coll Abbottabad 2024;36(4):14150. https://doi.org/10.55519/JAMC-04-14150.
4. Benach J, Muntaner C, et al. Arms, conventional wisdom, and public health Policy. Int J Health Serv 2022;52(4):493–510.
5. Martin SA, Bishop K, Choma EG, et al. Pediatric firearm violence in America. J Pediatr Health Care 2024;38(2):123–30.
6. Andrews AL, Killings X, Oddo ER, et al. Pediatric firearm injury mortality epidemiology. Pediatrics 2022;149(4):e2021052739. https://doi.org/10.1542/peds.2021-052739.
7. Rapa, et al. School shootings in the United States: 1997–2022. J Sch Health 2023;93(1):21–9.
8. Barboza-Salerno GE, Meshelemiah JCA, et al. Gun violence on walkable routes to and from school in Compton, California. J Urban Health 2023;100(4):567–78.
9.. Walsh CS, Sullivan TN, Kliewer W, et al. A qualitative scoping review of community firearm violence interventions. J Community Health 2025;50(2):287–305.
10. Polcari AM, Hoefer LE, Callier KM, et al. Social vulnerability index is strongly associated with pediatric firearm injury. J Trauma Acute Care Surg 2023;95(6):1203–11.
11. Kravitz-Wirtz N, Bruns A, Aubel AJ, et al. Inequities in community exposure to deadly Gun violence. J Urban Health 2022;99(3):435–47.
12. Bray-Aschenbrenner, et al. Environmental racism: associations between poverty, racism, and pediatric firearm exposure. Health Place 2022;74:102769. https://doi.org/10.1016/j.healthplace.2022.102769.
13. James, et al. Racial/Ethnic disparities in adolescent firearm exposure and outcomes. Pediatrics 2021;147(5):e2020020281. https://doi.org/10.1542/peds.2020-020281.
14. Rajan S, Branas CC, Myers D, et al. Youth exposure to violence involving a gun: evidence for adverse childhood experience classification. J Behav Med 2019;42(4):646–57.
15. Paruk, et al. Trauma exposure and mental health among South African children. Child Adolesc Psychiatry Ment Health 2019;13:32.

16. Holloway, et al. Longitudinal impacts of pediatric firearm exposure on mental health and behavior: a systematic review. Child Adolesc Psychiatry Ment Health 2021;15(1):72.
17. Cimolai, et al. Mass shootings and child/adolescent psychological outcomes: a systematic review. J Child Psychol Psychiatry 2020;61(9):1044–62.
18. Bruns, et al. Community gun homicide and academic outcomes. Educ Res 2018; 47(8):521–32.
19. Comer JS, et al. Firearm violence exposure and adolescent handgun carrying. J Adolesc Health 2017;61(6):776–82.
20. Gard AM, Brooks-Gunn J, McLanahan SS, et al. Deadly Gun violence, neighborhood collective efficacy, and adolescent development. PNAS Nexus 2022;1(5): pgac243. https://doi.org/10.1093/pnasnexus/pgac243.
21. Shonkoff JP, Garner AS, et al. Committee on Psychosocial Aspects of Child and Family Health; Committee on Early Childhood, Adoption, and Dependent Care; section on Developmental and Behavioral Pediatrics. The lifelong effects of early childhood adversity and toxic stress. Pediatrics 2012;129(1):e232–46.
22. Ordoobadi AJ, Wickard A, Heindel P, et al. Quantifying pediatric gun violence by location and time of day: a call for focused intervention. J Pediatr Surg 2024; 59(5):923–30.
23. Reeping PM, Gobaud AN, Branas CC, et al. K–12 school shootings: implications for policy and clinical practice. Pediatr Clin North Am 2021;68(2):341–53.
24. Moin ASM, Dhawan S, Shieh C, et al. Increased hormone-negative endocrine cells in the pancreas in type 1 diabetes. J Clin Endocrinol Metab 2016;101(9): 3487–96.
25. Carter PM, et al. Stakeholder acceptability of school-based firearm violence prevention strategies. J Prev 2022;43(5):657–69.
26. Purtle J, Rich LJ, Bloom SL, et al. Hospital-based violence intervention programs targeting adolescents: a systematic review. J Trauma Acute Care Surg 2015; 79(6):983–93.
27. Forkey H, Szilagyi M. Trauma-informed care. Pediatrics 2020;145(2):e20193751. https://doi.org/10.1542/peds.2019-3751.
28. Silverman WK, Ortiz CD, Viswesvaran C, et al. Evidence-based psychosocial treatments for children and adolescents exposed to traumatic events. J Clin Child Adolesc Psychol 2008;37(1):156–83.
29. Cohen JA, Mannarino AP, Deblinger E. Trauma-focused CBT for children and adolescents: treatment applications. 2nd edition. New York: Guilford Press; 2017.
30. Durlak JA, Weissberg RP, Pachan M. A meta-analysis of after-school programs that seek to promote personal and social skills in children and adolescents. Am J Community Psychol 2010;45(3–4):294–309.
31. Gottfredson DC, Cross AB, Wilson DM, et al. Effects of participation in after-school programs for middle school students: a randomized trial. J Res Educ Eff 2010;3(3):282–313.
32. Rajan S, Reeping PM, Ladhani Z, et al. Gun violence in K-12 schools in the United States: moving towards a preventive (versus reactive) framework. Prev Med 2022;165(Pt A):107280.
33. Skiba RJ, Arredondo MI, Williams NT. More than a metaphor: the contribution of restorative justice to school discipline reform. Peabody J Educ 2014;89(2): 206–28.
34. Juillard C, Smith R, Anaya N, et al. Saving lives and saving money: Hospital-based violence intervention is cost-effective. J Trauma Acute Care Surg 2015; 78(2):252–8.

35. Webster DW, Whitehill JM, Vernick JS, et al. Effects of Baltimore's Safe Streets program on gun violence: a replication of Chicago's CeaseFire program. J Urban Health 2013;90(1):27–40.
36. Tung EL, Pillai R, Sen-Gupta N, et al. Income support needs and bedside legal assistance for patients recovering from violent injuries. JAMA Netw Open 2025; 8(10):e2538044. https://doi.org/10.1001/jamanetworkopen.2025.38044.
37. McDaniel DD. Risk and protective factors associated with gang affiliation among high-risk youth: a public health approach. Inj Prev 2012;18(4):253–8.
38. Branas CC, Cheney RA, MacDonald JM, et al. A difference-in-differences analysis of health, safety, and greening vacant urban space. Am J Epidemiol 2011; 174(11):1296–306.
39. Laraque D, Barlow B, Durkin M, et al. Injury prevention in an urban setting: challenges and successes. Bull N Y Acad Med 1995;72(1):16–30. PMID: 7581311; PMCID: PMC2359423.
40. Jaycox LH, Cohen JA, Mannarino AP, et al. Children's mental health care following community violence: a review. J Behav Health Serv Res 2004;31(2): 213–36.
41. Ventura C, et al. Association of state firearm laws with firearm deaths among children. AJPM Focus 2024;3(2):100250. https://doi.org/10.1016/j.focus.2024.100250.
42. Fleegler EW, Lee LK, Monuteaux MC, et al. Firearm legislation and firearm-related fatalities in the United States. JAMA Intern Med 2013;173(9):732–40.
43. Duchesne J, Taghavi S, Toraih E, et al. State gun law grades and impact on mass shooting fatalities. J Am Coll Surg 2022;235(3):S153–4.
44. Macinko J, Cook J, Alpert A. The diffusion of punitive firearm preemption laws in the United States. Am J Prev Med 2023;65(2):197–205.
45. Jones VC, Wagner ED, Ward JA, et al. Parental support for age-related firearm policies: a national survey. BMC Pediatr 2025;25:145.
46. Monuteaux MC, Lee LK, Hemenway D, et al. Child access prevention laws and firearm fatalities among children aged 0 to 14 years. Pediatrics 2019;143(6): e20182307. https://doi.org/10.1542/peds.2018-2307.
47. Crifasi CK, Meyers JS, Vernick JS, et al. Effects of changes in permit-to-purchase handgun laws in Connecticut and Missouri on suicide rates. Prev Med 2015; 79:43–9.
48. Kaufman EJ, Morrison CN, Branas CC, et al. State firearm laws and interstate firearm deaths from homicide and suicide in the United States: a cross-sectional analysis. Lancet Public Health 2018;3(6):e323–31.
49. Grinshteyn E, Hemenway D. Violent death rates in the United States compared to those of the other high-income countries, 2015. Prev Med 2019;123:20–6.
50. Semenza DC. Addressing data deficiencies to prevent pediatric firearm violence. Am J Public Health 2024;114(2):152–4.
51. Grinshteyn E, Hemenway D. Violent death rates in the United States compared with those of other high-income countries. Prev Med 2019;123:20–6.
52. Stearns K, et al. Progress in pediatric firearm research in the United States. Adv Pediatr 2025;72:143–60.
53. Gani F, Sakran JV, Canner JK. Emergency department visits for firearm-related injuries in the United States, 2006–14. Health Aff 2017;36(10):1729–38.
54. Barber C, Azrael D, Hemenway D. Suicide mortality in the United States: the importance of attending to method in understanding population-level disparities. Annu Rev Public Health 2013;34:393–408.

55. Pardini DA, et al. Revitalizing developmental research for violence prevention. J Clin Child Adolesc Psychol 2021;50(6):893–909.
56. Turner HA, Finkelhor D, Hamby S, et al. Family structure, victimization, and child mental health in a nationally representative sample. Soc Sci Med 2013;87:39–51.
57. United Nations Children's Fund (UNICEF). Global status report on preventing violence against Children 2020. UNICEF. 2020. Available at: https://www.unicef.org/sites/default/files/2020-06/Global-status-report-on-preventing-violence-against-children-2020.pdf. Accessed January 16, 2025.
58. United Nations Children's Fund (UNICEF). Reporting on Children in armed conflict 2025. UNICEF. 2025. Available at: https://www.unicef.org/reporting-children-armed-conflict. Accessed January 16, 2025.
59. Gelineau K, Graham-McLay C, McGurk R. Father and son gunmen kill at least 15 people in attack on Hanukkah event at Sydney's Bondi Beach. Associated Press. 2025. Available at: https://apnews.com/article/australia-shooting-sydney-bondi-beach-31f711f09f677d0f88091ece25f651c1.
60. Finkelhor D, Hamby SL, Ormrod R, et al. The Juvenile Victimization Questionnaire: reliability, validity, and national norms. Child Abuse Negl 2005;29(4):383–412.
61. Vivolo-Kantor AM, Henessy KD, Holland KM, et al. Linking data systems for violence prevention: opportunities and challenges. Am J Prev Med 2016;51(5 Suppl 3):S137–45.
62. Trickett PK, Noll JG, Putnam FW. The impact of sexual abuse on female development: lessons from a multigenerational, longitudinal research study. Dev Psychopathol 2011;23(2):453–76.
63. Jaycox LH, Cohen JA, Mannarino AP, et al. Trauma-informed approaches to data collection with children exposed to violence. J Behav Health Serv Res 2004;31(2):213–36.
64. Rowhani-Rahbar A, Simonetti JA, Rivara FP. Effectiveness of interventions to promote safe firearm storage. Epidemiol Rev 2016;38(1):111–24.
65. Betz ME, Miller M, Barber C, et al. Lethal means access and assessment among suicidal emergency department patients. Ann Emerg Med 2016;67(5):584–92.
66. Runyan CW, Brooks-Russell A, Tung GJ, et al. Hospital emergency department lethal means counseling for suicidal patients. Am J Prev Med 2018;54(2):259–65.
67. Roszko PJ, Ameli J, Carter PM, et al. Clinician attitudes, screening practices, and interventions to reduce firearm-related injury. Epidemiol Rev 2016;38(1):87–110.
68. Global Burden of Violence Against Children Collaborators. The global burden of violence against children. Lancet 2024;403(10427):605–58. https://doi.org/10.1016/S0140-6736(23)02641-6.

Humanitarian Engagement by the US Military During Natural Disasters and Armed Conflict

Milissa Jones, MD, MPH[a,*], Martin Ottolini, MD, MEd[b]

KEYWORDS

• Military • Humanitarian • Natural Disaster • Armed conflict • Geneva Conventions • Engagement • Operation • Department of war (DoW)

KEY POINTS

- Military interventions providing humanitarian support can range from domestic and international responses to natural disasters, to those primarily involving armed conflict.
- Strengths of military interventions include rapidity, logistical capabilities, security, and medical support. Challenges may include costs, sustainability, and providing care for civilian populations, including pregnant women and children.
- Difficulties may arise when attempting to uphold the humanitarian ideals of impartiality and neutrality, while also being expected to resolve problems as an active combatant.

OVERVIEW AND SCOPE

This article of the role of the US military in humanitarian crises will focus primarily on the utilization of medical resources in the stabilization and care of civilian populations during complex humanitarian crises, with a concentration on the impact of such actions on the pediatric age group. Both authors bring firsthand experience as medical leaders deployed at different phases of sustained US military engagement, providing unique insights into the complexities of delivering medical and humanitarian support in conflict-affected environments. Efforts to provide clean water, nutritional support, improved housing and education, etc., were ongoing concurrently during those conflicts, though they played a larger role in the humanitarian support provided after natural disasters as discussed below.

[a] Department of Pediatrics, Pediatric Clinical Trials Unit, School of Medicine, Uniformed Services University of the Health Sciences, 4301 Jones Bridge Road, Bethesda, MD 20874, USA; [b] Capstone Student Research Program, F. Edward Hebert School of Medicine, Uniformed Services University of the Health Sciences, 4301 Jones Bridge Road, Bethesda, MD 20874, USA
* Corresponding author. 4301 Jones Bridge Road, Bethesda, MD 20874.
E-mail address: Milissa.Jones@usuhs.edu

Pediatr Clin N Am 73 (2026) 1037–1056
https://doi.org/10.1016/j.pcl.2026.05.004
0031-3955/26/Published by Elsevier Inc.

Abbreviations	
DoS	Department of State
DoW	Department of War
DSCA	Defense Support of Civil Authorities
FEMA	Federal Emergency Management Agency
FHA	foreign humanitarian assistance
JP	Joint Publication

THE PURPOSE OF US MILITARY INTERVENTION WHEN PROVIDING HUMANITARIAN SUPPORT

Natural disasters and armed conflicts exert profound and often devastating effects on children and families.[1–4] Disasters such as hurricanes, earthquakes, and pandemics disproportionately impact children, who are physiologically, developmentally, and socially more vulnerable than adults and depend on them for support.[5,6] These events can disrupt access to essential services, including health care, nutrition, education, and safe shelter, leaving children at heightened risk of injury, infectious disease, malnutrition, and psychosocial trauma. The addition of any form of armed conflict further destabilizes family units, displaces communities, and exposes children to both direct and indirect harm, including separation from caregivers, loss of family members, recruitment into armed groups, and limited access to medical care, clean water, and other critical resources.[4] Globally, children often bear the heaviest burden of disasters and conflict, with estimates suggesting that they can represent up to 50% of affected populations in many humanitarian crises.[7–9]

The US military possesses unique capabilities that enable rapid, large-scale responses to natural disasters and disease outbreaks.[10,11] These capabilities include airlift and sealift of supplies, rapid deployment of medical teams, engineering and infrastructure support, and security operations and logistical coordination in complex operational environments. While these resources are powerful tools for humanitarian relief, their employment requires careful consideration of the legal, ethical, and operational implications inherent in using armed forces in civilian contexts. Military engagement in disaster relief must balance effectiveness with sensitivity to local sovereignty and civilian needs. In addition to direct responses, the US military often supports global preparedness efforts by training local communities, governments, and additional partners in humanitarian crisis management, with the intent for this training to allow groups to develop independent capabilities. These programs aim to enhance local resilience, build sustainable capabilities, and strengthen partnerships that facilitate effective coordination during emergencies.[11]

One important difference is that military combat operations—while often aimed at stabilizing regions in crisis—can themselves be profoundly disruptive to civilian populations, and children are particularly susceptible to these effects.[12] Deliberate combat operations may result in displacement, disruption of essential services, interruption of education, and increased exposure to physical harm and psychological trauma. Children may be separated from caregivers, lose access to medical care, and experience heightened vulnerability to malnutrition, disease, and exploitative behavior, due to the breakdown of infrastructure and social support systems.[7] In recognition of these risks, US military planning incorporates specific considerations for pediatric populations, including strategies to minimize collateral damage, protect medical facilities and schools, and maintain access to essential health care.[13] Medical response planning explicitly addresses pediatric needs, with provisions for triage, age-appropriate care, vaccination, mental health support, and the protection of children in conflict zones.[13]

As a result, the experiences of the last several natural disasters and conflicts have led the US military to include pediatric considerations into both humanitarian and wartime support missions. From the lessons of experience, the US military seeks to balance operational effectiveness with the ethical imperative to safeguard vulnerable populations. This article further examines the practical and legal framework guiding US military engagement in natural disasters, disease outbreaks, and complex emergencies involving armed conflict, alongside an analysis of operational experience more than the past 25 years. It emphasizes the intersection of military activity and the welfare of children and families, exploring lessons learned, identifying strengths and weaknesses, and considering pathways for future improvement optimizing the effectiveness of US military capabilities in diverse operational settings. The following discussions refer to 2 distinct categories of interventions led by the US military: those in response to natural disasters, where rapid support of all the needs of civilian populations are paramount; and those where the US military is involved in armed conflict and is ameliorating the impact on regional populations.

NATURAL DISASTERS, DISEASE EVENTS, AND THE ROLE OF THE US MILITARY

Natural disasters—such as earthquakes, hurricanes, wildfires, floods—and major disease outbreaks pose significant threats to global stability and human health. With shifting climate patterns and increased global interconnectedness, these events have become more frequent, severe, and far-reaching.[14] Increasingly, they give rise to complex emergencies. According to United Nations doctrine, a complex emergency occurs when a natural disaster coincides with political instability, conflict, or institutional collapse, overwhelming a nation's capacity to respond.[15] In such contexts, environmental catastrophe amplifies existing vulnerabilities, disrupts governance, and exacerbates violence, displacement, and social unrest. The result is a crisis in which humanitarian needs stem not only from environmental destruction, but also from systemic political, economic, and security failures. These situations demand rapid, large-scale responses to save lives, restore essential services, and rebuild infrastructure. The US military, with its unmatched capacity for rapid deployment, logistics, medical support, security, and command and control, plays a critical role in humanitarian and disaster response operations.[16] This section examines how the US military engages in such responses—both domestically and internationally—through its doctrine, logistical framework, preparedness activities, and key missions more than the past 25 years.

Domestic Humanitarian Assistance in Response to Natural Disasters—Doctrine and Guidance

For US domestic disasters, the governing document is Joint Publication (JP) 3 to 28: Defense Support of Civil Authorities (DSCA).[10] DSCA defines the Department of War (DoW)'s role in providing assistance to civil authorities—federal, state, or local—when those authorities are overwhelmed.[10] The Stafford Act (Robert T. Stafford Disaster Relief and Emergency Assistance Act, 42 US C. § 5121 et seq.), together with Executive Order 13411, and Department of Defense (DoD) Directive 3025.18, provide legal basis for the military's domestic role.[17]

The decision to deploy military forces domestically begins with a governor's request to the President, through the Federal Emergency Management Agency (FEMA), or federal declaration under the Stafford Act. Once FEMA requests DoW support via Direct Support or Defense-Federal Emergency Support Team, the DoW provides resources under specified mission assignments. The mission ends when civil authorities regain control, or when assigned tasks are complete and terminated in writing. The steps normally followed when regional leaders request assistance within the U.S. are described in **Fig. 1**A.

Under DSCA, resources may include engineers, aviation, medical assets and logistics, but the military does not assume the lead in overall recovery—civil agencies do. Funding is typically through military appropriations for DSCA or FEMA reimbursements. Each state often signs a cost-share agreement in advance.[17] Coordination with state Emergency Management Agencies and nongovernmental organizations (NGOs) is crucial.

Even domestically, the influx of many responders means the US military must coordinate with civilian volunteer organizations, local NGOs, faith-based groups, and private contractors. Joint doctrine emphasizes the interoperability of command, communication and information systems (C3I) as essential. The DoW's Joint Task Force model and Defense Coordinating Element are used to synchronize efforts.

Foreign Humanitarian Assistance in Response to Natural Disasters—Doctrine and Guidance

The JP 3 to 29: Foreign humanitarian assistance (FHA) is the principal doctrine used to guide the conduct of the US military when engaging in foreign humanitarian crises disaster relief.[11] This publication provides the doctrinal framework for planning, executing, and sustaining US military FHA operations. It defines the purpose of FHA as "the activities conducted outside the United States and its territories to relieve or reduce human suffering, disease, hunger or privation."[11] The doctrine discusses authorities, lead agencies, roles of the military, and integration with other agencies and NGOs.

The decision to deploy the US military in response to a foreign natural disaster or disease outbreak is governed by a combination of presidential decision, Department of State (DoS) and DoW coordination, and bilateral or multilateral requests for assistance. According to JP 3 to 29, the DoW may provide FHA when specifically requested by the host nation and when the DOS determines that the US response is in the national interest, or when there is no functioning host nation government. This *request*

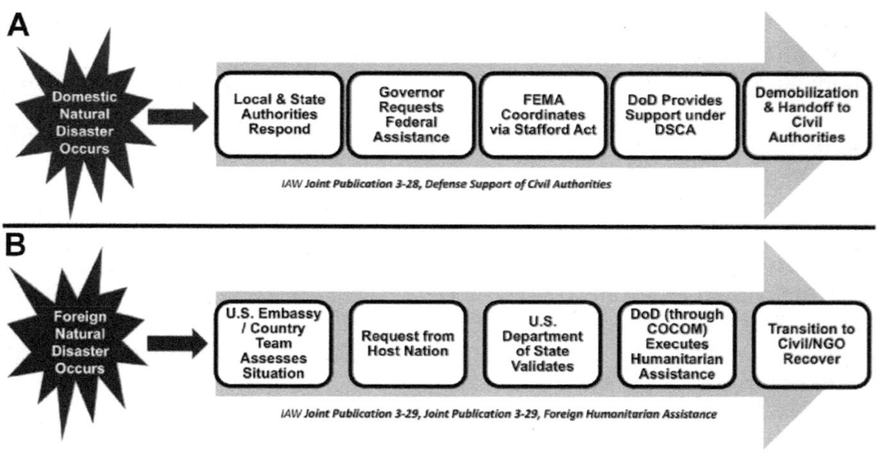

Fig. 1. (*A, B*) Activation of US military in response to domestic and foreign natural disasters. COCOM, Combatant Command; IAW, in accordance with. (*Courtesy* [*A*] IAW Joint Publication 3-28, Defense Support of Civil Authorities; and [*B*] IAW Joint Publication 3-29, Foreign Humanitarian Assistance.)

plus authorization model is crucial, and the stepwise approach is described above in **Fig. 1**B.

Once legal and diplomatic approvals are secured, DoW components may aid. The engagement ends when the host nation resumes primary responsibility, or the DoW mission transfers to a civilian lead—JP 3 to 29 describes criteria for termination of US military involvement. The scope of FHA is limited to relief and reconstruction—they cannot supplant the host nation's long-term recovery. JP 3 to 29 (Chapter IV) sets boundaries: assistance must be purely humanitarian, noncombatant, and the DoW must coordinate with other US agencies and NGO actors. The mission is terminated when specific objectives are achieved, or when the host nation requests withdrawal. Metric-based assessments, handover plans, and cost-sharing agreements often govern wrap-up.

Under US law, FHA funding is typically appropriated through DoW and DoS emergency accounts (eg, the Foreign Disaster Assistance Fund).[18] Operational costs (transportation, personnel, and sustainment) are borne by DoW budgets, while reconstruction may be supported via USAID or host nation resources. In many operations, the host nation bears local costs after initial relief. Documentation of cost-sharing is part of planning (See eg, Shearer & McGrath, 2010).

Following a disaster, a wide array of aid actors—UN agencies, NGOs, private voluntary organization (PVOs), private sector—descend on the affected area. The US military must integrate with these actors without overshadowing them. JP 3 to 29 emphasizes liaison officers, unified coordination cells, and combining military logistical capability with NGO subject matter expertise. The military provides heavy-lift, port/air-cargo operations, field hospitals, and security, while NGOs often deliver community-based, culturally specific aid.

US Military Support in Foreign and Domestic Disaster Preparedness

Effective disaster response ideally begins before the event. The US military invests heavily in preparedness through prepositioned stocks, contingency planning, joint exercises, and training at both the force and multinational levels.[19] Preparedness reduces lag time, improves coordination, and builds trust among responding entities.

Force training ensures that US personnel can operate effectively in austere, resource-limited environments where medical and logistical systems may be degraded. Programs such as the Joint Trauma System's Joint Trauma Training Program[20] and the Military Medical Humanitarian Assistance Course[21,22] prepare deploying medical teams to manage complex trauma, provide lifesaving care, and deliver humanitarian medical support in crisis settings. Training emphasizes trauma stabilization, immunization readiness, rehydration techniques, infectious disease prevention, and outbreak management. Medical readiness modules increasingly incorporate pediatric-specific content—airway management, trauma, nutrition, and care of displaced children—reflecting the demographic realities of humanitarian crises. By strengthening both clinical and preventive medicine competencies, these programs reduce morbidity and mortality while improving the overall effectiveness of military medical response.

Partner nation training and multinational exercises focus on capacity building and interoperability with allied and host nation forces. Flagship initiatives such as Pacific Partnership[23] and disaster assistance response exercises in Europe[24] and Asia provide real-world platforms for collaborative disaster planning, emergency medical response, and logistics coordination. These exercises enhance communication across military and civilian agencies, and include modules on infectious disease surveillance, vaccination campaigns, water and sanitation management, and rapid field hospital activation. Through these engagements, the US military and partner nations strengthen mutual readiness to respond effectively to both natural and man-made disasters.

Notable US Military Responses to Natural Disasters, 2000 to 2025

The US military has responded to a wide variety of crises, from abroad (tsunami in Indonesia, Haiti earthquake) to domestic (Hurricane Katrina, Wildfires in Hawaii) and global disease outbreaks (Ebola, COVID-19). **Table 1** below summarizes key operations over the past 25 years.

These responses highlight the breadth of US military capability: Navy hospital ships (US NS Comfort/US NS Mercy), Army Corps of Engineers rapid infrastructure repair, Air Force strategic airlift, Marine expeditionary forces for security, Army up-armored vehicles for rugged terrain, etc. For example, the 2004–05 Operation Unified Assistance after the Indian Ocean tsunami deployed heavy-lift aircraft, amphibious ships, and cargo handling to Indonesia and Sri Lanka.[25] Domestic responses such as Hurricane Katrina (2005) showed the military's ability to integrate with FEMA, execute search and rescue, and support evacuation.[27–29] More recently, the US military's role in Operation Warp Speed during the COVID-19 pandemic (2020–22) demonstrated rapid logistics, vaccine supply chain management, and strategic coordination with civilian health agencies.[48]

The US military's response to natural disasters has frequently encompassed pediatric-specific missions. Over the past 25 years, several large-scale events have disproportionately affected children, prompting targeted military involvement to address their unique medical and psychosocial needs. Following the Haitian earthquake in 2010, US military medical units were among the earliest organized responders, establishing field hospitals that provided trauma care, nutritional support, and sanitation infrastructure for displaced children and families.[32–34] Military personnel collaborated with local authorities and international partners in orphan reunification efforts and implemented mass immunization campaigns to mitigate the risk of secondary outbreaks of vaccine-preventable diseases in overcrowded camps.[30–32] During the Ebola outbreak in West Africa (2014–2015), US Army medical contingency teams played a central role in constructing and staffing treatment units, conducting infection prevention and control training, and coordinating vaccine delivery for children and other high-risk populations.[41,42] These actions helped restore continuity of essential health services and strengthened local health systems during a period of extreme strain. In the COVID-19 pandemic, the US military expanded its support to include large-scale logistical, operational, and clinical functions, establishing field hospitals, distributing medical supplies, and supporting vaccination site operations.[48] Military pediatricians contributed to maintaining continuity of care for military families and offered expertise in infection control and health systems resilience.

The US military holds formidable capabilities in humanitarian and disaster response missions—rapid deployment, global logistics, large-scale medical and engineering support. Doctrine such as JP 3 to 29 and JP 3 to 28 provide clear frameworks for foreign and domestic engagement.[10,11] Preparedness efforts ahead of events, and recent operational history across continents and disease outbreaks, show how these capabilities are applied. Yet, challenges remain—in coordination with civilian agencies, cost and funding mechanisms, documentation of vulnerable populations, and transition to long-term recovery. As the frequency and complexity of natural disasters and disease events rise, the US military's role in humanitarian response is likely to become even more critical—and the lessons learned from past missions will be vital in shaping future engagements.

Table 1
Key US Military engagements in response to natural disasters and disease events impacting children and families, 2000–2025

Year Military Operation Event/Location	US Military Engagement (Summary)	Total Death Toll[a]	Estimated Child Deaths[b]	Lessons Learned
2004–2005 Operation Unified Assistance Tsunami (Indian Ocean Rim Nations) Refs:[25,26]	• Air delivery of relief supplies • Cargo handling and logistics support • Medical evacuation and care • Infrastructure clearance and repair • Personnel transport and evacuation	>230,000	Between 76,000–110,000 Children	• Rapid deployment of forward-deployed forces enhances immediate response • Unified command structures improve coordination among multinational partners • Adaptability and innovation are crucial in addressing unprecedented challenges • Integration of military and humanitarian efforts maximizes relief impact
2005 Joint Task Force Katrina Hurricane Katrina (Gulf Coast, the United States) Refs:[5,6,27–29]	• Search and rescue operations • Medical assistance and evacuation • Distribution of food, water, and supplies • Infrastructure assessment and repair • Coordination with FEMA and local authorities	~1300–1800	*Specific pediatric fatality data are unpublished*	• Community preparedness enhances resilience • Timely and transparent communication is crucial • Integration of local knowledge improves response efforts • Sustained community engagement supports long-term recovery
2010 Operation Unified Response Earthquake (Haiti) Refs:[30–34]	• Air and sea delivery of relief supplies • Medical care and field hospitals • Search and rescue operations • Infrastructure assessment and repair • Coordination with U.N. and international partners for reuniting children with families	>220,000	*Specific pediatric fatality data are unpublished*	• Host nation buy-in and coordination are essential; foreign military presence should support, not supplant, local authorities • Rapid deployment of forces is critical • Integration with international partners enhances effectiveness • Civil-military coordination is essential for success

(*continued on next page*)

Table 1
(continued)

Year Military Operation Event/Location	US Military Engagement (Summary)	Total Death Toll[a]	Estimated Child Deaths[b]	Lessons Learned
2011 Operation Tomodachi Earthquake & Tsunami (Japan) Refs:[35–38]	• Search and rescue operations • Medical assistance and evacuation • Distribution of relief supplies • Nuclear disaster response support • Coordination with Japanese Self-Defense Forces and international partners	> 15,000	*Specific pediatric fatality data are unpublished*	• Prepositioned forces enable rapid response • Cultural sensitivity enhances cooperation • Joint operations with host nation forces improve effectiveness
2013 Operation Damayan Typhoon Haiyan (Philippines) Refs:[39,40]	• Air delivery of relief supplies • Cargo handling and logistics support • Medical evacuation and care • Infrastructure clearance and repair • Personnel transport and evacuation • Coordination with Philippine Armed Forces and international partners	6300	*Specific pediatric fatality data are unpublished*	• Effective coordination and liaison enable rapid multinational response • Forward deployed and scalable forces support immediate action • Heavy-lift assets and trained personnel sustain relief operations • Long-term partnerships and multilateral exercises build trust and cooperation
2014–2015 Operation United Assistance Ebola Outbreak (Liberia, *Guinea, Sierra Leone)* Refs:[41,42]	• Command and control of response effort; Construction of Ebola Treatment Units • *Strategic airlift and logistics* • Infrastructure and power • Medical clinical care training • Coordination with NGOs and CDC for and public health response	11,000 (28,500 infections)	~3500 children (>4000 infections in children)	• Clear roles and authorities enable timely response • Shared information systems *improve coordination* • Prepositioned assets support rapid deployment

2015 Operation Sahayogi Haat Earthquake (Nepal) Refs:[43,44]	• Air delivery of relief supplies • Cargo handling • Medical evacuation • Infrastructure • Personnel transport	>8000	Between 1300–2600 Pediatric deaths	• Importance of aerial transport enabling access to remote areas • Infrastructure support is critical relief efforts • Medical and casualty evacuation capacity required
2017 *No Specific Operation Name Given* Hurricanes: Harvey, Irma, Maria (Texas, US Virgin Islands, and Puerto Rico) Refs:[45–47]	• Transport of supplies • Evacuation citizens • Coordination of logistics and aid distribution, Restoration of infrastructure • Search and rescue	Harvey >100 Irma >130 Maria >2000	*Specific pediatric fatality data are unpublished*	• Importance of integrated civil-military command structure • Shared situational awareness required • Resilient infrastructure critical for response • Prepositioned resources enable rapid deployment
2020–2022 Operation Warp Speed[c] COVID-19 Pandemic (the United States) Refs:[48,49]	• Partnership with private sector and DHHS for vaccine development, logistical support, operational leadership, and vaccine distribution	1.2 million (111.8 million infections)	800–1200 children (15.5 million infections in children)	• Importance of collaborative Leadership • Flexibility • Infrastructure support
2023 Operation Ola Hou Wildfires (Maui, Hawaii) Ref:[50]	• Fire suppression • Search and Rescue • Security • Sea and Air Transportation • Temporary Power • Debris Removal	>100	*Pediatric fatality data are unpublished*	• Streamline DoD aid requests and rapid deployment of trained personnel. • Improve interagency communication and equipment interoperability. • Strengthen community preparedness and resilient infrastructure.

Abbreviations: CDC, centers for disease control; DHHS, department of health and human services.

[a] Total Death Toll refers to aggregated person estimates derived from published sources; these figures may be subject to uncertainty due to variability in reporting, methodological differences, and the range of estimates across sources for each disaster.

[b] Pediatric (Ages 0–17 y) mortality data are not uniformly reported across Natural Disaster or Disease event; the values presented represent estimates derived from available publications and demographic analyses and should be interpreted as approximate, given inherent uncertainties in the underlying data.

[c] Name later changed to *Health and Human Services (HHS)-DOD COVID-19 Countermeasures Acceleration Group, accounts for the COVID-19 pandemic from 2020 to 2022.*

THE ROLE OF THE US MILITARY IN HUMANITARIAN ASSISTANCE WHEN ACTIVELY INVOLVED IN MILITARY CONFLICT

Many of the contingencies for which the US military responds can be classified as Complex Humanitarian Emergencies. In some situations, the United States may find it necessary to use military power in its role as an active combatant. Whether primarily for the provision of immediate aid in response to a disaster, or in support of strategic objectives, the utilization of ongoing military operations involves multiple factors that impact highly vulnerable populations. Regional groups of people, often with weak or absent governance, can experience rapidly deteriorating levels of economic support for food, nutrition, housing, education, and especially medical care, often resulting in the complete loss of the ability to support basic needs. In addition, when armed conflict is a factor, these vulnerable groups are frequently physically displaced and denied their natural means of support. This may be most evident in regions where local people already are challenged to sustain their existence when not subjected to these additional pressures. **Fig. 2** below describes the complex set of factors that can play a role.[7]

The disruption and displacement caused by armed conflict dramatically increases the basic need for clean water, nutrition, shelter, safety, and ongoing education when feasible, and simultaneously increases the occurrence of trauma and emergence of infectious diseases. All these components exacerbate complex emergencies and lead to an immediate requirement for significant medical support at the individual level as well as for entire populations. These issues are further discussed as follows.

The Military Structure for Providing Responses

For centuries, military medical services have been established in a hierarchy of increasing capabilities caring for trauma and nontrauma victims, beginning with direct help from the most forward-based individuals and small facilities, and then progressing to comprehensive care provided at larger regional trauma centers. **Table 2** cites data from both a 2006 and a more recent 2022 review.[51,52] Together these accurately

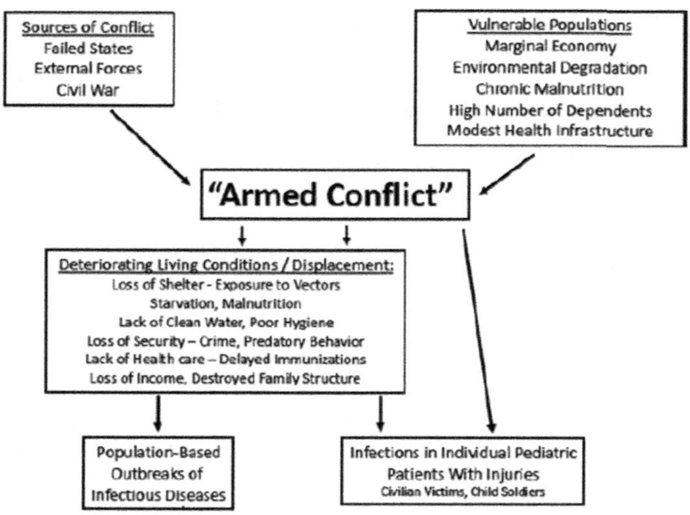

Fig. 2. The complex dynamics of armed conflict. (*Source* Ottolini M, Cirks B, Madden KB, et al. Pediatric Infectious Diseases Encountered During Wartime-Part 1: Experiences and Lessons Learned From Armed Conflict in the Modern Era. Curr Infect Dis Rep 2021;23(12):27. https://doi.org/10.1007/s11908-021-00770-1.)

Table 2
Hierarchy of care by military and civilian *role* number

US Military *Role* Number/Echelon Refs:[51,52]	Equivalent Civilian Number	Description of Duties
I	First Responders	Prehospital and enroute care (Medics and PA's in the military)
II: Battalion Aid	–	First level of Surgery in the military. Mobile and near combat activates, focus on damage control
III	III	Highest level of care near combat, limited capabilities, time-limited ICU capabilities
IV	II	Large Trauma Centers, removed from combat zones
V	I	Major Trauma Centers: Teaching and Research *Role 4 and Role 5 may involve transfer to European/US sites

Abbreviations: ICU, intensive care unit; PAs, physician assistant.
* IV and V.

describe the most commonly used terminology of the 5 echelons of care used in the long military conflicts in Iraq and Afghanistan, and note the sequentially reversed language used in the US civilian hospital system.

Of note, the potential transfer of patients to level IV and V major trauma centers back in the United States or Europe is typically reserved for US citizens, with rare exceptions. Host national and civilian trauma victims, and those suffering from other serious illnesses requiring humanitarian assistance, could be cared for at all levels (called *roles*), though often ended up requiring prolonged care at role III and role IV hospitals, which are in theater and therefore avoid challenges regarding the citizenship of the patients.

The Role of the Geneva Conventions and Principles of Humanitarian Law

When reviewing the US role in providing humanitarian assistance during natural disasters and armed conflict, one must recognize that the actions of the US military are inherently determined by American civilian leadership. The military mission is initially determined by the US government and may change in response to evolving situations. In the examples to be discussed, we see that the United States may launch humanitarian efforts, in part, to demonstrate more civilized behavior in the utilization of military power to accomplish objectives through armed interventions. Sustainability and altered circumstances may challenge and change the nature of these involvements over time. Foundationally, the US government follows the postwar 1949 Fourth Geneva Convention, especially the sections *relative to civilian persons in the time of war*.[53] This has been augmented by the additional amendments of 1977, which focus on the "Protection of Victims of International Armed Conflict," which clarifies that "In all circumstances they shall be treated humanely and shall receive, to the fullest extent practicable and with the least possible delay, the medical care and attention required by their condition. There shall be no distinction among them founded on any grounds other than medical ones."[54] In addition, in all activities the United States strives to follow the ethical priorities described in International Humanitarian Law, also summarized by the ICRC.[55] One of the more difficult implications of that body of formal guidance is that whether in primary response to emergencies, or during planned armed conflict, the provision of medical care, and support for other basic needs ideally is governed by leadership that is not involved in any inherently biased military operations. The Institute of International Law identifies the ideal as being aid and relief that is characterized as following the 3 principles of *humanity, impartiality, and neutrality*, which is an ideal to pursue, but is often impractical when situations require military operational capabilities.[56]

The History of Recent Interventions Primarily for Military Reasons

A massive outlay of military resources, including equipment and supplies, and more importantly, the dedication of vast amounts of human time, commitment, and even the lives of service members themselves, have been devoted to supporting the missions of the long 21st century conflicts in Afghanistan and Iraq. Both began with swift military invasions, followed with rapid achievement of immediate global security goals, in 2001 and 2003, respectively.[57] In most of these situations, the mission was supported by a coalition of military forces from host and partner nations, though predominantly led by the US military. Each conflict evolved into a long-term presence, consisting of the US military, host nation and coalition forces, and civilian experts, ideally working toward more democratic and legitimate forms of government. The Iraq situation eventually resulted in an initial orderly transfer of authority to local leadership, but required reintervention from coalition forces during the 2014 to 2019 time frame to reduce the influence of the Islamic state, which arose in Iraq and Syria.[57,58] Unfortunately, the earlier successes in Afghanistan led to an eventual stalemate, followed by a resurgence of the Taliban as a source of regional leadership, and a final hurried evacuation. These developments necessitated the rapid and dramatic support of the evacuees, several who were severely wounded in a final bombing of the Kabul airport.[59] The discussion of both of these 2-decade long efforts is summarized briefly in **Table 3**, which focuses on humanitarian efforts directly associated with combat operations. A recent excellent scoping review of 2 decades of pediatric humanitarian medical care focused on the patterns of pediatric civilian casualties in the countries of Iraq and Afghanistan. The authors identified 52 studies published between 2001 and 2022 that met the criteria for analysis, virtually all of which were retrospective studies.[60] Readers are directed to read this article to appreciate many of the lessons learned during 2 decades of US-led armed conflict in Iraq and Afghanistan. Some of the key representative studies are listed in **Table 3**, which includes the names and purposes of specific military operations in both countries, describes their initial and subsequent purposes, and summarizes the lessons learned through these operations.

While the table may list findings and trends of patients reviewed, with a focus on the occurrence of pediatric trauma, the summaries listed in this table and those in the scoping review report many of the lessons learned regarding the pediatric impact caused by these operations. Some of the more qualitative observations reflect the very different nature of the patterns of trauma and disease in Afghanistan and Iraq, the latter a more well-resourced nation. In Afghanistan, there was significantly less ability to rely on any local health care infrastructure. And there were high rates of non-trauma admissions, especially in younger children less than 14 years of age. Children had measurably higher injury scores and more adverse outcomes than adults. Bed utilization for pediatric patients was disproportionately high and longer. Similarly high rates of pediatric admission occurred in Iraq but fluctuated more with the tempo of ongoing combat operations, rising during the invasion and the much later *surge* of 2007 to 2008. During peak utilization in both countries, the predominance of trauma consumed up to 15% of available bed space in the well-established US hierarchal role system. In the years of 2009 to 2011, when active combat ceased, a much higher

Table 3
Notable US military engagements involving active conflict impacting children and families, 2000 to 2025

Year/US Operation/Location	US Military Engagement	Pediatric Impact	Lessons Learned
2001–2014 Operation Enduring Freedom Afghanistan Refs:[56,60–62]	Military operations to fight insurgency, establish a viable government in Afghanistan	• High % of pediatric patients, High bed days for < 17 yo • 2:1 ratio of nontrauma admissions to US hospitals in Afghanistan for <14 yo. • Pediatric casualties fared worse than adults, higher injury severity scores low Glascow Coma Scales, overall higher mortality	• High consumption of resources by pediatric trauma, often not combat-related • High rates of nontrauma admissions, possibly due to lack of civilian options • Do *humanitarian* actions by armed forces violate the precepts of impartiality and neutrality since they are involved in conflict?
2003–2006 Operation Iraqi Freedom Iraq Refs:[52,57,63]	Remove ballistic missiles and WMD's, regime change, fight sectarian warfare, establish a viable government.	• In an early Operation Enduring Freedom and Operation Iraqi Freedom analysis 10%–15% of all the United States combat support hospital admissions were children, with high rates of ICU and surgical care	• Ethical issue: the Geneva Conventions and the 1977 protocol additions required care for humanitarian injuries
2007–2011 Operation New Dawn Iraq Refs:[52,60,62,64]	Counterinsurgency strategy, reduction of sectarian warfare, develop Iraqi Security Forces	• Equal number of admissions for combat vs noncombat conditions for <14 yo. • Mortality highest for combat injuries (during 2007/8 surge) • Pediatrics fared worse than adults, higher injury severity scores, low Glascow Coma Scales, higher mortality • % of noncombat admissions rose in 2011–2013, admissions • High resources for burns, MVAs • Higher % of females, very young patients, with worse survival	• Combat-related trauma paralleled military activity, with higher morbidity and mortality for children • High rates of civilian injuries including burns and MVA accidents, and females in general • Elective surgery may be feasible, but uncertainty of long-term follow-up

(*continued on next page*)

Table 3
(continued)

Year/US Operation/Location	US Military Engagement	Pediatric Impact	Lessons Learned
2014-Current Operation Inherent Resolve Iraq, Syria Refs:[58,65]	International war against the Islamic State of Iraq and Syria: US and British forces	• Support of Iraqi Security Forces (ISF) • Islamic State defeated by 2019 • Analysis of 300 casualties from July 2015 to Jan 2016 treated by a partial *Forward Surgical Team*	• Success of specifically defined objectives • 96% > 16 yo, mainly soldiers (86%) • Pediatric cases were very rare
2014–2021 Operation Freedom's Sentinel Afghanistan Refs:[52,66]	Targeting al Qaeda leadership and infrastructure of the Taliban; assist and develop Afghan National Defense and Security Forces	• Maintain a democratic government for the whole population	• Increased focus of Afghanistan as a site for confrontation between cultures • High rates (40% of all population) of children < 14 yo in Afghanistan and Iraq. Led to high utilization of medical and surgical resources by this age group. • High resources for pediatric burns • Potential benefits of *winning the hearts and minds* of local populations • Challenges in supporting families of pediatric patients; and *transferring back* patients to less capable national systems
2021 Operations Allies Refuge and Operation Allies Welcome Afghanistan/Europe/the United States Refs:[21,59,67,68]	Withdrawal and Relocation of Host from Afghanistan	• Safety and security for more than 130,000 close partners; with 40%–60% of evacuees <17 yo	• Acute trauma and a large, displaced population (Complex Humanitarian Crisis) • Resources to stabilize and transport wounded from Kabul Airport bombing • Additional resources in supporting births, and controlling a measles outbreak • Reliance on rapid expansion of capabilities by several military facilities • Transfer Afghan support to the WHO, for dependent needs of ½ of population

Abbreviations: ISF, Iraqi Security Forces; MVA, Motor Vehicle Accident; WMD, Weapon of Mass Destruction.

rate of noncombat admissions was observed. Fortunately, when coalitions forces led by the British and the United States returned to suppress the Iraq and Syrian *Islamic State* of 2014 to 2016, there was much less need for pediatric medical support, as this was a largely regional conflict among professional soldiers.[58] Lessons to be learned continued, however, as an unexpected dramatic rise in short-term intense support was required to support Afghan allies and refugees during the fall of 2021, with both an acute trauma burden due to the bombing at the Kabul airport in late August, and the outbreak of measles that followed the large number of pediatric evacuees.[21,59] One of the bases that dealt with large numbers of Afghan nationals reported that of 10,122 subsequent health encounters, 44% were in support of pediatric patients and that 62% of these were less than 5 years of age.[67] The lessons learned from 2001 until the present time tell us that flexibility and capability in support of both pediatric trauma and nontrauma disease must be maintained for often constantly evolving situations.

STRENGTHS AND WEAKNESSES OFFERED BY THE US MILITARY IN THE PROVISION OF HUMANITARIAN ASSISTANCE IN NATURAL DISASTERS AND WAR

The US military brings significant strengths to humanitarian assistance missions in both natural disasters and armed conflicts. Rapid deployment and global logistical capabilities enable timely delivery of supplies, medical support, and infrastructure restoration when local systems are overwhelmed. In conflict settings, these capabilities are critical for stabilizing populations, securing safe corridors, and providing immediate trauma care for civilian casualties. Military medical units are equipped to deliver advanced care, including pediatric hospitalization and intensive care services, that may not be available otherwise. Military leaders, especially those providing medical capabilities, are trained to operate in high-stress, complex environments, allowing them to integrate logistics, security, and health care delivery efficiently.[69] These strengths, depicted in **Fig. 3**, demonstrate the military's ability to respond rapidly and effectively across a spectrum of humanitarian crises.

Despite these capabilities, military humanitarian operations face realistic limitations, especially in regions with ongoing conflict.[56,69] The dual role of the military—providing relief while potentially engaging in combat operations—can raise questions about neutrality and acceptance by local populations and partner organizations. Prolonged deployments are costly and resource-intensive, which can limit sustainability and long-term impact. Military medical teams, while proficient in acute adult trauma care, may struggle to address diverse civilian health needs, including chronic conditions, pediatric care, and services for the elderly or pregnant individuals. Coordination with experienced NGOs and local authorities can also be challenging, particularly when missions are politically influenced or subject to rapidly changing objectives. Moreover, the political nature and optics of using military forces in humanitarian operations during conflict can influence local and international perception, potentially complicating trust-building and cooperation with affected populations. **Fig. 3** highlights these constraints alongside the military's operational strengths, illustrating the need to balance rapid capability with ethical and logistical considerations.

The interplay of strengths and weaknesses in military humanitarian operations reflects a complex balance between capability and limitation. In natural disasters, the military excels at rapid, secure, and large-scale interventions, whereas in conflict settings, careful integration with civilian organizations is essential to maintain legitimacy and effectiveness. Lessons from past missions underscore the importance of flexibility

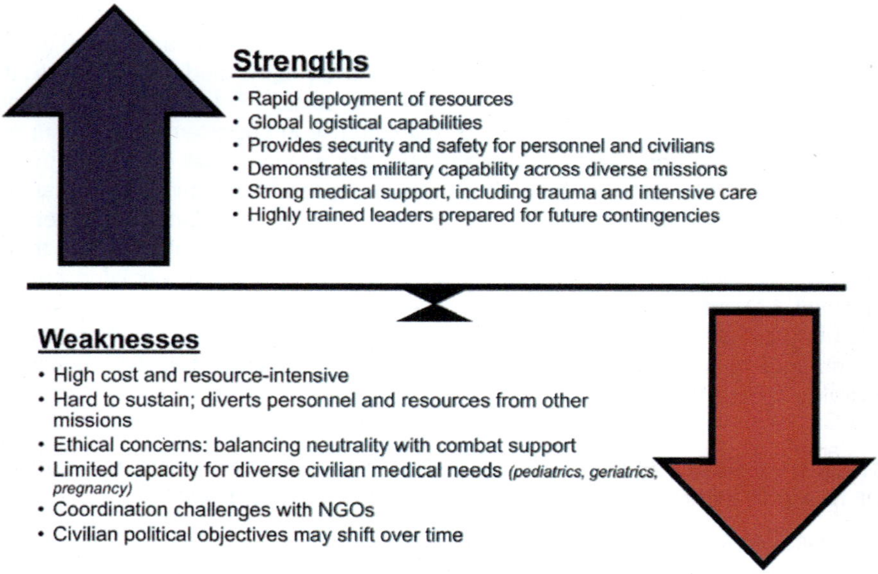

Fig. 3. Strengths and weaknesses of US military engagement in natural disasters and war.

and planning for the need to potentially support pediatric and other vulnerable populations, while integrating with local infrastructure to enhance resilience. By viewing these missions through a holistic lens that considers both operational efficiency and ethical responsibility, the military can optimize its contribution to civilian relief efforts while minimizing unintended consequences.

SUMMARY

Humanitarian crises—whether arising from natural disasters or armed conflicts—are inevitable and increasingly frequent due to global climate change, urbanization, and geopolitical instability. The US military remains uniquely positioned to respond to these crises, but effective engagement requires careful attention to sustainability, ethical considerations, and collaboration with civilian partners. Future operations will likely necessitate smaller, agile deployments, lean logistics, and prolonged field care, while maintaining the capability to care for pediatric and other vulnerable populations. By learning from past experiences and refining strategies, the military can continue to provide impactful humanitarian assistance that mitigates suffering and enhances resilience in both natural disaster- and conflict-affected populations.

DISCLAIMER

The opinions and assertions contained herein are those of the authors and do not necessarily reflect the official policy or position of the Uniformed Services University or the Department of War.

DISCLOSURE

Neither author nor their family members have a financial interest in any commercial product, service, or organization providing financial support for this article.

REFERENCES

1. Hagan JF Jr, American Academy of Pediatrics Committee on Psychosocial Aspects of Child and Family Health, Task Force on Terrorism. Psychosocial implications of disaster or terrorism on children: a guide for the pediatrician. Pediatrics 2005;116(3):787–95.
2. Peek L. Children and disasters: understanding vulnerability, developing capacities, and promoting resilience—An introduction. Child Youth Environ 2008;18(1): 1–29. Available at: https://www.jstor.org/stable/10.7721/chilyoutenvi.18.1.0001.
3. Hoffmann JA, Pergjika A, Burkhart K, et al. Supporting children's mental health needs in disasters. Pediatrics 2025;1:155.
4. Shenoda S, Kadir A, Pitterman S, et al, Section on International Child Health. The effects of armed conflict on children. Pediatrics 2018;142(6). https://doi.org/10.1542/peds.2018-2585.
5. Callaghan WM, Rasmussen SA, Jamieson DJ, et al. Health concerns of women and infants in times of natural disasters: lessons learned from Hurricane Katrina. Matern Child Health J 2007;11(4):307–11.
6. Ewing B, Buchholtz S, Rotanz R. Assisting pregnant women to prepare for disaster. MCN Am J Matern Child Nurs 2008;33(2):98–103.
7. Ottolini M, Cirks B, Madden KB, et al. Pediatric infectious diseases encountered during wartime-part 1: experiences and lessons learned from armed conflict in the modern era. Curr Infect Dis Rep 2021;23(12):27.
8. Hillers GM, Joy SC, Chatham-Stephens K, et al. Understanding natural disaster or weather-related drowning deaths among children. Pediatrics 2024;154(Suppl 3). https://doi.org/10.1542/peds.2024-067043M.
9. Harville E, Xiong X, Buekens P. Disasters and perinatal health:a systematic review. Obstet Gynecol Surv 2010;65(11):713–28.
10. Joint Publication 3-28: Defense Support of Civil Authorities (2018 Edition) (2018).
11. Joint Publication 3-29: Foreign Humanitarian Assistance (2019 edition) (2019).
12. Gewirtz AH, Muldrew L, Basha SAJ. Parenting during War. Psychiatry. Fall 2025; 88(3):262–72.
13. Joint Publication 4-02: Joint Health Services (Incorporating Change 1, September 28, 2018) (U.S. Department of Defense) (2018).
14. Ebi KL, Vanos J, Baldwin JW, et al. Extreme weather and climate change: population health and health system implications. Annu Rev Publ Health 2021;42: 293–315.
15. Nations U. UN term: complex emergency. Available at: https://unterm.un.org/unterm2/en/view/UNHQ/C5C090DE181D1B7485256A00000755B0. Accessed November 1, 2025.
16. Walters ME. The U.S. military: a reluctant humanitarian. Modern American History 2024;7(1):109–13.
17. Congress US, Robert T. Stafford disaster relief and emergency assistance act. FEMA, U.S: Government; 1988.
18. Congressional Budget Justification, Foreign Operations, Appendix 2 (United States Department of State) (2025).
19. DoD Directive 3000.05: Military support for stability, security, transition, and reconstruction (SSTR) operations (DoDD 3000.05) (2005).
20. System JT. Joint trauma SystemThe department of defense center of excellence for trauma. U.S. department of defense. Available at: https://jts.health.mil/. Accessed November 1, 2025.

21. Kiger ME, Hickey PW, Hammond CE, et al. Experiences of deployed physicians in support of operation allies refuge/operation allies welcome: lessons to inform improvements in training. Mil Med 2025;190(1–2):366–73.
22. Uniformed Services University DoP. The military medical humanitarian assistance course (MMHAC). Available at: https://medschool.usuhs.edu/ped/education/mmhac. Accessed November 1, 2025.
23. Reaves EJ, Termini M, Burkle FM Jr. Reshaping US navy Pacific response in mitigating disaster risk in south Pacific Island nations: adopting community-based disaster cycle management. Prehospital Disaster Med 2014;29(1):60–8.
24. Army Dot. Immediate response 25. Available at: https://www.europeafrica.army.mil/DefenderEurope/ImmediateResponse/dvpTag/DefenderEuropa/#:~:text=Immediate%20Response%2025%20is%20a,U.S.%20commitments%20to%20the%20Alliance. Accessed November 1, 2025.
25. Curatola JM. Lessons from “A Team of Teams” CSF-536 and tsunami relief. Mil Rev 2022;0026-4148:1–14.
26. USA U. Indian Ocean earthquake and tsunami. 2004. Available at: https://www.unicefusa.org/what-unicef-does/emergency-response/weather-disasters/tsunamis/2004-indian-ocean-earthquake #:~:text=The%20tsunami%20wiped%20away%20homes,humanitarian%20relief%20to%20the%20survivors. Accessed November 1, 2025.
27. Sariego J. CCATT: a military model for civilian disaster management. Disaster Manag Response 2006;4(4):114–7.
28. Weaver JM. The department of defense and homeland security relationship: hurricane katrina through hurricane Irene. J Emerg Manag 2015;13(3):265–74.
29. White House GWBA. Katrina lessons learned, chapter 5. George W. Bush white house archives. Available at: https://georgewbush-whitehouse.archives.gov/reports/katrina-lessons-learned/chapter5.html. Accessed November 1, 2025.
30. Hussey SM, Dukette PJ, Dunn SH, et al. The 2010 Haiti earthquake: a pathology perspective aboard the USNS comfort. Arch Pathol Lab Med 2011;135(4):417–21.
31. Galeckas K. Dermatology aboard the USNS COMFORT: disaster relief operations in Haiti after the 2010 earthquake. Dermatol Clin 2011;29(1):15–9.
32. Walk RM, Donahue TF, Stockinger Z, et al. Haitian earthquake relief: disaster response aboard the USNS comfort. Disaster Med Public Health Prep 2012;6(4):370–7.
33. Wallwork EDG, Kathy S, Morgan ML, et al. Operation unified response: air mobility command's response to the 2010 Haiti earthquake crisis. Office of History, Air Mobility Command 2010.
34. Command USS. U.S. military support to Haiti earthquake relief. Available at: https://www.southcom.mil/HaitiEarthquakeSupport/. Accessed November 1, 2025.
35. Research NBoA. Timeline of operation tomodachi. Available at: https://www.nbr.org/publication/timeline-of-operation-tomodachi/. Accessed November 1, 2025.
36. VanHorne-Sealy J, Livingston B, Alleman L. DoD's medical radiobiology advisory team: experts on the ground. Health Phys 2012;102(5):489–92.
37. Ames C, Koguchi-Ames Y. Friends in need:'Operation Tomodachi'and the politics of US military disaster relief in Japan. Natural disaster and nuclear crisis in Japan. Routledge; 2012. p. 224–36.
38. Kaczur A, Aurelio J, Joloya E. An Analysis of United States Naval Participation in Operation Tomodachi: Humanitarian and Disaster Relief in the Tsunami-Stricken Japanese Mainland. 2012.

39. Lum TM. Typhoon haiyan (Yolanda). U.S. and International Response to Philippines Disaster; 2014. Available at: https://apps.dtic.mil/sti/trecms/pdf/AD1172135.pdf.
40. Parker TC SP, Sanders G, King JE, et al. The U.S. Pacific command response to super typhoon haiyan. Joint Force Q 2016;82(3):54–61.
41. Fitzgerald F, Awonuga W, Shah T, et al. Ebola response in Sierra Leone: the impact on children. J Infect 2016;72(Suppl):S6–12.
42. Joint Forces Command – Operation United Assistance: Case study handbook (Public edition) (2016).
43. Command USIP. US Pacific command operation sahayogi haat joint after action report executive summary. 2016. Available at: https://www.pacom.mil/media/news/article/588303/nepal-earthquake-relief-effort-named-operation-sahayogi-haat/.
44. Hossain AF, Adhikari TL, Ansary MA, et al. Characteristics and consequence of Nepal earthquake 2015: a review. Geotechnical Engineering Journal of the SEAGS & AGSSEA 2015;46(4):114–20.
45. Command USN. Update: U.S. Northern Command's support to hurricane harvey response. Available at: https://www.northcom.mil/Newsroom/Press-Releases/Article/1297364/updateus-northern-commands-support-to-hurricane-harvey-response/. Accessed November 1, 2025.
46. Command USS. U.S. military support to hurricanes irma and maria relief in the Eastern Caribbean. Available at: https://www.southcom.mil/Media/Special-Coverage/US-Military-Support-to-Hurricane-Irma-Relief-in-the-Eastern-Caribbean/. Accessed November 1, 2025.
47. Garamone J. Officials detail DoD support during unprecedented hurricane season. Defense logistics agency. Available at: https://www.dla.mil/About-DLA/News/News-Article-View/Article/1362056/officials-detail-dod-support-during-unprecedented-hurricane-season/. Accessed November 1, 2025.
48. Hall JE, Packard N. Operation warp speed and the countermeasures acceleration group— A twenty-first century manhattan project: preliminary observations on the U.S. department of defense's role in the supply, production, and distribution of COVID-19 vaccines and therapeutics. Journal of Advanced Military Studies 2022;13(1):144–62.
49. Bratzler DW. COVID-19 in retrospect: public health lessons from a global crisis. Am J Med Sci 2026;371(2):107–17.
50. Defense USDo. DOD support for U.S. response to wildfires in Hawaii. Available at: https://dod.hawaii.gov/blog/2023-maui-wildfire-response/#:~:text=Maui%20Wildfire%20Response:%20Soldiers%20from,aftermath%20of%20the%20devastating%20fires https://dod.hawaii.gov/blog/2023-maui-wildfire-response/#:~:text=Maui%20Wildfire%20Response:%20Soldiers%20from,aftermath%20of%20the%20devastating%20fires. Accessed November 1, 2025.
51. Eastridge BJ, Jenkins D, Flaherty S, et al. Trauma system development in a theater of war: experiences from operation Iraqi freedom and operation enduring freedom. J Trauma 2006;61(6):1366–72 [discussion: 1372–3].
52. Gurney JM, Graf V, Staudt AM, et al. Characterization of humanitarian trauma care by US military facilities during combat operations in Afghanistan and Iraq. Ann Surg 2022;276(4):732–42.
53. Vité SJ-MH. 1949 Geneva Conventions. International Committee of the Red Cross 1949.
54. Databases IHL. Protocol additional to the Geneva conventions of 12 August 1949, and relating to the protection of victims of international Armed Conflicts

(Protocol I). 1977. Available at: https://ihl-databases.icrc.org/en/ihl-treaties/api-1977. Accessed October 20, 2025.
55. What is International Humanitarian Law? (International Committee of the Red Cross) (2004).
56. Gadler A. Armed forces as carrying both the stick and the carrot-humanitarian aid in US counterinsurgency operations in Afghanistan and Iraq. Goettingen J Int'l L 2011;3:217.
57. Defense USDo. Operation Iraqi Freedom (OIF) casualty summary. defense casualty analysis system (DCAS). Available at: https://dcas.dmdc.osd.mil/dcas/app/conflictCasualties/oif. Accessed November 1, 2025.
58. Hahn C, Staudt AM, Brockmeyer J, et al. Characteristics of Iraqi patients treated during operation inherent resolve by a forward surgical team. Mil Med 2019;184-(Suppl 1):301–5.
59. McSorley C, Shields M, Funk M, et al. Pediatric insight to humanitarian and trauma crisis response: operation allies refuge and operation allies welcome at landstuhl regional medical center. Mil Med 2026;191(1–2):e275–81.
60. Kocik VI, Borgman MA, April MD, et al. A scoping review of two decades of pediatric humanitarian care during wartime. J Trauma Acute Care Surg 2023;95(2S Suppl 1):S170–9.
61. Defense USDo. Operation Enduring Freedom (OEF) casualty summary. Defense Casualty Analysis System (DCAS). Available at: https://dcas.dmdc.osd.mil/dcas/app/conflictCasualties/oef. Accessed November 1, 2025.
62. Edwards MJ, Lustik M, Burnett MW, et al. Pediatric inpatient humanitarian care in combat: iraq and Afghanistan 2002 to 2012. J Am Coll Surg 2014;218(5):1018–23.
63. Burnett MW, Spinella PC, Azarow KS, et al. Pediatric care as part of the US army medical mission in the global war on terrorism in Afghanistan and Iraq, December 2001 to December 2004. Pediatrics 2008;121(2):261–5.
64. Defense USDo. Operation New Dawn (OND) casualty summary. defense casualty analysis system (DCAS). Available at: https://dcas.dmdc.osd.mil/dcas/app/conflictCasualties/ond. Accessed November 1, 2025.
65. Defense USDo. Operation Inherent Resolve (OIR) casualty summary. Defense Casualty Analysis System (DCAS). Available at: https://dcas.dmdc.osd.mil/dcas/app/conflictCasualties/oir. Accessed November 1, 2025.
66. Defense USDo. Operation Freedom's Sentinel (OFS) casualty summary. Defense Casualty Analysis System (DCAS). Available at: https://dcas.dmdc.osd.mil/dcas/app/conflictCasualties/ofs. Accessed November 1, 2025.
67. Koch EJ, Lopachin T, Fayos Z, et al. Humanitarian assistance lessons learned from providing acute medical care for Afghan nationals on a U.S. military base. Mil Med 2023;188(11–12):300–4.
68. Al-Mandhari A. Adapting to the events in Afghanistan: call for maintaining essential public health services and supporting critical medical supplies distribution. East Mediterr Health J 2021;27(9):855–6.
69. Bollen MK, Kalkman JP. Civil-military cooperation in disaster and emergency response: practices, challenges, and opportunities. Journal of Advanced Military Studies 2022;13(1):79–91.

The Urgency of Action: Case Studies in the 21st Century

Sudan's Protracted Humanitarian Crisis

Pediatric and Maternal Health, Trauma-Informed Continuity of Care, and the Imperative for Sustained Global Action

Maryam Elisabeth Montrichard, MD, MPH[a],
Jeffrey Goldhagen, MD, MPH[b,*]

KEYWORDS

• Sudan • Humanitarian crisis • Maternal health • Child health
• Trauma-informed care • Health disparities • Medical evacuation • Global south

KEY POINTS

- Sudan's prolonged conflict has led to a systemic collapse of maternal and pediatric health services, resulting in increased preventable mortality, malnutrition, and untreated trauma among women and children.
- Children with amputations have emerged as an underreported consequence of explosive injuries, delayed access to surgical care, and the absence of in-country rehabilitation capacity.
- Trauma-informed care is essential to address the physical and psychosocial needs of injured children.
- Sustained, child rights and Sustainable Development Goals-aligned humanitarian engagement is urgently required, as short-term emergency responses alone are insufficient to prevent lasting, intergenerational harm to Sudan's MCH outcomes.

INTRODUCTION

Armed conflict is arguably among the most enduring and powerful source of preventable maternal and child deaths globally. For all the collective decades of global commitments to equity and universal health coverage, women and children who live in

[a] Global Health Consultant, Fleming Island, FL, USA; [b] Division of Community and Societal Pediatrics, University of Florida College of Medicine-Jacksonville, International Society for Social Pediatrics and Child Health, Geneva, Switzerland
* Corresponding author. Division of Community and Societal Pediatrics, Department of Pediatrics, University of Florida College of Medicine-Jacksonville, 841 Prudential Drive, Suite 900, Jacksonville, FL 32207.
E-mail address: Jeffrey.goldhagen@jax.ufl.edu

Pediatr Clin N Am 73 (2026) 1057–1065
https://doi.org/10.1016/j.pcl.2026.05.005 pediatric.theclinics.com

Abbreviations	
ANC	antenatal care
SAM	severe acute malnutrition
SDGs	Sustainable Development Goals
UNICEF	United nations Children's Fund

conflict-affected settings face staggering inequalities in survival and access to basic health services.[1] Sudan is a particularly stark illustration of that global failure. Following escalation of armed conflict in April 2023, the nation has existed in a protracted humanitarian crisis—characterized by mass displacement, economic collapse, and near-total disruption of health and food systems. Multicountry data show that exposure to conflict is associated with lower quality maternal, neonatal, and child health care services provision and much higher mortality than nonconflict settings.[2,3]

These impacts do not end when fighting is over, but continue long after cessation or reduction of fighting has taken place resulting from ongoing damage to health systems, social infrastructure, and human capital. Extending analyses of the health impact of conflict, the current article strives to give an in-depth and comprehensive view on Sudan's maternal and child health crisis as of January 2026. Besides malnutrition and service disruption, we investigate the increasing number of children with amputations and disabilities resulting from the conflict, emphasizing the urgent necessity of trauma-informed continuity of care and long-term rehabilitation. We frame these findings in the context of the Sustainable Development Goals (SDGs), highlighting the moral and policy imperative for continual humanitarian participation with an emphasis on pediatric clinicians.[3]

HEALTH SYSTEM COLLAPSE AND STRUCTURAL BARRIERS TO CARE

Global Inequities and Sudan in Comparative Perspective

The plight of Sudan mirrors pervasive global patterns of inequity in conflict areas. Women and children from conflict countries have decreased access to critical health interventions, and higher levels of mortality relative to stable contexts, even when adjusting for income level.[1] These implications underscore that conflict is not so much a contextual issue as it is among the root causes of health inequity. Sudan's crisis is accordingly both a domestic tragedy and a worldwide failure to protect vulnerable populations in keeping with international commitments.

Sudan's health system collapse is also an inescapable result of armed conflict and critical pathways through which excess maternal and child morbidity and mortality occur. Health systems in conflict areas are vulnerable to fragmentation owing to infrastructure attacks, health worker displacement, financing disturbances and governance and accountability failures.[3,4] In Sudan, the intersection of these vulnerabilities has culminated in almost complete collapse of service delivery across all regions in the country.

Health facilities have been regularly damaged, occupied, or disabled because of insecurity and supply shortages since the escalation of violence and hostilities in 2023. As of late 2025, the World Health Organization estimates less than 50% of all health care facilities in Sudan were fully operated and some conflict affected areas of the country have functionality levels lower than 30%.[2] This reduction exacerbates the relatively weak preconflict capacity of the health care infrastructure, workforce, and system resilience. In addition to physical loss of life and infrastructure, the loss of human resources is an important impediment to care. Large numbers of doctors, nurses, midwives, and community health workers have been displaced or forced to flee, leaving other facilities inaccessible because they do not have access to fuel or funding.[5]

This exodus has affected the delivery of maternal and child health services most acutely, which are reliant on skilled midwives, obstetric providers, pediatric nurses, and community-based health workers. The resulting shortages have compromised continuity of care, referral pathways, and capacity for emergency responses, especially for obstetric complications and pediatric trauma These issues are compounded by supply chain disruption.[6] Essential medicines, vaccines, blood products, oxygen, and surgical supplies are often not available as a result of insecurity, damaged transport, and humanitarian access. Interruptions in cold chain infrastructure have threatened routine immunization programs, placing at risk vaccine-preventable disease outbreaks among displaced and undernourished children.[7]

Financial strains have also grown as a result of the conflict, which has decimated household livelihoods and public health financing.[8] The collapse of government health budgets, combined with inflation and the loss of income among displaced populations, has transferred the cost burden of care onto the families least able to afford it. Out-of-pocket payments for antenatal care (ANC), delivery, medications, and transportation have become unaffordable, forcing many women to postpone or forego care altogether.[5] Therefore, humanitarian efforts such as those by The Global Fund become lifelines for continuity of care. Studies conducted in conflict contexts provide evidence that financial barriers combined with insecurity exacerbate inequalities in service use, especially for women and children.[1]

Geographic and transportation barriers further limit access to care. Insecurity, damaged roads, fuel shortages, and checkpoints have made travel to health facilities perilous or impossible in many areas.[6] Pregnant mothers who are already in labor and caregivers of critically ill children are subject to life-threatening delays regarding access to care, which is well-documented in humanitarian settings as a source of excess mortality. Subsequently, failure of referral systems has been especially devastating for pediatric surgical emergencies who require prompt interventions before death or chronic disability set in.[7]

These structural barriers are further compounded by governance and coordination challenges. Fragmentation of health leadership, overlapping humanitarian efforts, and inadequate data availability make it difficult to plan effectively and allocate resources.[2] Without adequate national coordination mechanisms established to streamline effective multientity action, prioritizing vulnerable frontline populations falls short. Additionally, humanitarian actors frequently work in parallel systems, which may save lives in the short-term, but when not aligned to national health priorities risk leading to exacerbations of gaps in care.[9]

Crucially, the collapse of Sudan's health system affects communities differently. Women, children, and adolescents, particularly those who are displaced or in besieged areas, are hit hardest and face the harshest care barriers and adverse outcomes. As evidence from around the world demonstrates, inequalities in intervention coverage are significantly higher in conflict-affected contexts, with maternal and child health services being among the first to decline and last to recover.[6,7] This means that collapsing health systems in Sudan cannot just be considered operationally troublesome. They must be seen as a structural component of otherwise preventable maternal and child suffering. However, addressing these barriers is more than just delivering emergency care; it requires sustained investment in workforce protection, resilient supply chains, governance capacity, and equitable financing mechanisms.[5]

In the absence of systemic approaches, maternal and pediatric populations are left entangled in cycles of crisis and deprivation.

MATERNAL CHILD HEALTH IN CONFLICT SETTINGS

Disruption of Antenatal and Obstetric Care

There has been significant deterioration in maternal health indicators in Sudan from the time of conflict onset. There is a growing body of empirical evidence that armed conflict has substantial effects on ANC utilization and skilled birth attendance, and therefore on maternal morbidity and mortality.[1] In Sudan, insecurity, displacement, and the loss of health personnel have added to existing health care problems, particularly in rural and periurban areas. United Nations Fund for Population Activities (UNFPA) data has shown increasing rates of unattended births, obstetric complications, and gender-based violence, especially among displaced persons.[7]

These patterns are closely aligned with global trends in conflict-affected areas, in which maternal health outcomes are some of the first and most enduring indicators of system dysfunction. Disruption of antenatal and obstetric care is one of the most proximate and consequential pathways through which armed conflict undermines maternal and child survival. There is overwhelming evidence, in conflict settings, that coverage of crucial maternal health interventions—such as ANC, skilled birth attendance, emergency obstetric services, and postnatal follow-up—can decline dramatically.[1] In Sudan, these disruptions have grown more severe since violence escalated in 2023, exacerbating previous structural weaknesses in the health system, leaving pregnant women and newborns at extraordinary risk.

Empirical investigation of Sudan has demonstrated a significant decrease in ANC utilization in the case of conflict areas. In areas affected by armed conflict, women were less likely to visit the recommended number of antenatal visits than in more stable areas.[6] Decreased ANC attendance has been correlated to late detection of pregnancy-related difficulties such as hypertensive disorders, anemia, infections, and fetal growth restriction— conditions that are among the causes of maternal and neonatal deaths in resource-poor settings. Disruptions to maternal health care related to conflict also intersect with other wider social and gender-based vulnerabilities.[1] Displacement, food insecurity, and increased exposure to gender-based violence increase the health risks for pregnant and postpartum women. United Nations Children's Fund (UNICEF) studies show the increasing rate of sexual violence, unintended pregnancy, and insufficient family planning provision in Sudan is further exacerbating existing tension on maternal health.[10]

These are trends highlight the fact that maternal health in conflict-ridden areas cannot be separated from protection, nutrition, and social services. Crucially, the decline in antenatal and obstetric care in Sudan mirrors global developments in conflict-affected countries. Studies from 2020, comparable to current conditions, concluded that women in conflict areas continue to have a lower level of coverage of life-saving maternal health interventions after controlling for national income level, indicating that the conflict, per se, has an independent impact on maternal mortality.[1] Sudan's experience, therefore, mirrors a wider global health system failure to protect maternal and child health in politically violent contexts. Without long-term and coordinated interventions, disruptions to antenatal and obstetric care result in intergenerational poor outcomes. Maternal malnutrition, untreated infection, and complications during delivery do not only lead to neonatal mortality, but also to low birth weight, impaired child development, and long-term health disparities.[6] Early insults are linked to long-term physical and cognitive consequences and compound cycles of vulnerability for conflict-affected populations. Tackling these barriers requires further provision of services beyond isolated services.[11] Experience in humanitarian and postconflict contexts has underscored the necessity of integrated maternal–child health approaches including emergency obstetric treatment, community-based ANC delivery, coordinated pediatric care, protection, provision, and nutrition.[9] Lack of holistic solutions such as these will contribute to a Sudan in which maternal and neonatal mortality fail to meet global targets of equity, resilience, and sustainable development.

The Pediatric Health Burden

The pediatric health burden in Sudan represents the intersection of immediate life-threatening conditions and long-term developmental risks. Mortality statistics alone fail to capture the breath of underlying consequences of conflict. Millions of surviving children face lifelong consequences of undernutrition, trauma, disability, and disrupted education, in addition to increased rates of unvaccination and undervaccination.[10] At the global health level, they constitute a fundamental breach of children's rights to life and optimal health and development while also directly challenging the advancement of SDG 3 (Good Health and Well-Being), SDG 2 (Zero Hunger), and SDG 10 (Reduced Inequalities). Without sustained, child-centered humanitarian interventions that integrate nutrition, health, protection, and education, Sudan risks losing an entire generation to preventable suffering and lost potential.[9]

Food security and malnutrition

Malnutrition is the most insidious and deadly threat to child health in Sudan. Armed conflict has led to food production, markets, and humanitarian supplies being disrupted, with massive acute and chronic undernutrition in children. Sudan illustrates the correlation between exposure to armed conflict and higher rates of child wasting and stunting, especially when child populations have been internally displaced.[11] International evidence stresses that undernutrition is involved in almost 50% of all child deaths globally, acting synergistically with infectious disease and poverty.[12] The synergy is at crisis levels in Sudan. UNICEF and the World Health Organization have cautioned that the nation is confronted with among the world's largest child malnutrition emergencies, with millions of children vulnerable to irreversible developmental damage.[13,14] In Sudan, over the past 2 years, aid deliveries have been delayed amid a highly volatile security environment.

Severe acute malnutrition (SAM) acts as a barrier to immunity, increases the risk of pneumonia, diarrhea, malaria, and sepsis, and reduces the chances of survival when illness happens.[15] Malnutrition during early childhood can also be associated with long-term consequences, such as impaired cognitive development, lower educational attainment, and less economic productivity in adulthood. Such outcomes emphasize that the health burden in Sudan to children is not restricted to immediate mortality but endangers the creation of long-term human capital and postconflict recovery.[12,13]

Pediatric trauma and amputations: an emerging and underrecognized crisis

In addition to malnutrition and infectious disease, conflict in Sudan has been responsible for a rising number of children who have severe traumatic injuries, including amputations caused by explosive weapons, landmines, gunshots, severe infection, and sepsis resulting from delayed care.[7,15] Children with amputations are among the most vulnerable and least visible populations impacted by the conflict. Humanitarian surgical teams document increasing pediatric populations, predominately male individuals, requiring limb amputations due to complicated blast injuries.[16] As such, pediatric amputation affects all life stages and consequently has effects on physical mobility, mental health, education, and engagement in the economy.[11,13,17]

These children are left to suffer lifelong disability and social exclusion without access to rehabilitation and prosthetic services. Furthermore, widespread malnutrition delays wound healing.[2,14] These are not inevitable consequences, but expressions of discontinuity of care and failure of long-term humanitarian planning.[5,10] Injuries from armed conflict are an ever more significant source of the pediatric health burden in Sudan. Children are sensitive to explosive weapons and unexploded ordnance as they are at an early developmental stage while also lacking awareness of the danger associated with interacting with them. In conflict settings, injuries tend to impact multiple organ systems leading to permanent disability. As such, pediatric injuries present a complex situation requiring longitudinal care in the setting of a collapsed health system.[7]

The delayed presentation, lack of surgical capacity, and lack of rehabilitation services together make it more likely that survivable injuries will lead to long-term disability.[4,17] The lack of in-country rehabilitation exacerbates functional limitations and sabotages any successful recovery trajectories. Childhood disability has long-lasting and multigenerational legacy effects on education, work, and social life. In places where conflict reigns, such as Sudan, the impacts are exacerbated by poverty, forced dislocation, and weak national social protection mechanisms that ensure their continuation–entrenching cycles of exclusion and vulnerability.[3]

Cross-border evacuation and specialized care

Leading up to 2026, the central and urban conflict hotspots of Sudan, in and around Khartoum State and beyond, have become a focus of severe pediatric trauma, particularly amputation wounds.[10,15] Humanitarian medical records reveal that the extent of injury and length of morbidity to children with war wounds have been high, with approximately 16% of war-wounded patients treated since 2024 being children aged under 15 years referred to Bashair Teaching Hospital in south Khartoum, one of the few emergency and surgical care centers reportedly operating.[18]

Conflict intensity and civilian targeting in Khartoum, Kordofan, and surrounding North and South Kordofan and Darfur states has been accompanied by numerous acts of air and ground fire on populated zones with resultant high blast and ballistic injuries for children and caregivers.[5] These areas have long reported some of the highest volume of trauma admissions in national hospital reporting, including emergency departments flooded with consultations related to gunshot and explosive injuries. Despite limited national epidemiologic records regarding pediatric amputations due to surveillance lapses, these hospital and clinic-based observations suggest heightened war-related extremity trauma in central conflict corridors and in the greater Khartoum metropolitan area and by neighboring front line areas where amputations suffered by children occur at the highest frequency.[15]

This area-specific signal is consistent with other humanitarian reporting on ongoing violence and disruption of health care in these zones, mediating acute trauma and the requirement for referral to other local care centers outside of Sudan (eg, for reconstruction and rehabilitation in Amman, Jordan). The recent collapse of specialized surgical and rehabilitation services within Sudan has forced the evacuation of children with complicated injuries across borders.[16,17] Severely injured pediatric patients, including children with amputations, have also been evacuated to Amman, Jordan, where a multidisciplinary team of pediatricians, pediatric specialists, multinational and national humanitarian organizations, as well as rehabilitation services, provides care in which multidisciplinary partners are engaged. Such organizations are essential in providing trauma-informed child-based care that also includes psychological treatment of toxic stress symptoms, grief, and integration into education and community life. These models complement the calls for immediate measures beyond emergency actions to the promotion of integrated, multisectoral, and long-term health system resilience in a conflict context.[3]

Psychological trauma, toxic stress, and trauma-informed continuity of care

Injuries caused by conflict form an increasingly important part of the pediatric health burden in Sudan. Due to their developmental level, mobility patterns and minimal risk awareness, children are notably susceptible to explosive weapons and unexploded ordnance.[15] Injuries caused in conflict settings are commonly devastating and can involve multiple organ systems and lead to long-lasting disability.

Pediatric injuries must be viewed in relation to the collapse of health systems as a whole. Delayed presentation, lack of surgical capacity, and lack of rehabilitation services elevate the likelihood that survivable injuries will lead to chronic disabilities.[9,19] Additionally, the lack of in-country rehabilitation exacerbates functional limitations and undermines recovery trajectories. Childhood disability has life-course consequences that are more than just a matter of the body, they impact, for example, education, work, and social integration.[2] In environments such as Sudan, where conflict and instability increase these negative effects due to poverty, displacement, and inadequate social protection, cycles of exclusion and vulnerability are increased. As a result of compounded multifactorial variables, Sudanese children are subjected to deep psychological injury, in addition to physical illness.[1]

Experiencing violence firsthand and the emotional loss of family members, displacement, and living in conditions of systemic insecurity contribute to toxic stress that has well-established effects on neurodevelopment and long-term well-being. Children diagnosed with chronic stress are also more susceptible to anxiety, depression, behavioral disorders, and impaired mental development.[19] Mental health care needs in humanitarian settings are often underreported and underresourced, especially for children. Lack of school places, safe play spaces, and community support only compounds the psychological damages. These consequences are even more pronounced in children who are permanently injured or disabled, including amputees, who face additional stigma and social exclusion.[2,15]

SUMMARY

As of January 2026, the ongoing conflict in Sudan continues to exact a devastating toll on maternal and child health. Children with amputations, malnourished children, and women without access to reproductive care are not collateral outcomes rather predictable consequences of systemic neglect in conflict settings. Evidence from Sudan reinforces global findings that conflict amplifies health inequities and undermines survival across the life course.[3] Trauma-informed continuity of care, pediatric rehabilitation, and sustained humanitarian engagement aligned with the principles of human rights and the SDGs are essential to prevent irreversible generational harm.[2] Without such action, Sudan risks losing not only a generation of children but also the foundational human capital required for long-term recovery and peace.

INSIGHTS TO ACTION

- Implement screening to identify co-existing factors of health in conflict-affected children to include: missed immunizations, untreated chronic disease, malnutrition and psychological trauma, as these frequently coexist and may contribute to increased rates of morbidity than the acute presenting illness.

- Children exposed to armed conflict are at increased risk for toxic stress, anxiety, depression, and developmental impairment; utilization of trauma-informed care at every encounter, including routine assessment of psychosocial needs, should be an inclusive part of the physical evaluation.
- In humanitarian conditions, transportation barriers, insecurity and health system disruption often result in advanced disease presentations, requiring earlier escalation of care and multidisciplinary management.
- Consider rehabilitation as part of acute pediatric trauma care. Children with amputations and other conflict-related injuries need early referral for rehabilitation, prosthetic services, mental health support, and educational reintegration to optimize long-term outcomes.
- Optimal recovery for conflict-affected children requires long-term maternal-child health services, vaccination programs, nutrition support and coordination of cross-sector partnerships beyond emergency response.

DECLARATION OF ARTIFICIAL INTELLIGENCE AND ARTIFICIAL INTELLIGENCE-ASSISTED TECHNOLOGIES IN THE WRITING PROCESS

During the preparation of this article, the authors used GenAI in order to edit the article. After using this tool/service, the authors reviewed and edited the content as needed and take full responsibility for the content of the publication.

DISCLOSURE

The authors have no financial disclosures or conflicts of interest to disclose.

REFERENCES

1. Akseer N, Wright J, Tasic H, et al. Women, children and adolescents in conflict countries: an assessment of inequalities in intervention coverage and survival. Lancet Global Health 2020;8(12):e1536–47. Available at: https://pubmed.ncbi.nlm.nih.gov/32133179/. Accessed February 2, 2026.
2. Kadir A, Krishnan S, McGowan C, et al. Child public health interventions for conflict-affected populations: a systematic review. PLOS Glob Publ Health 2025;5(12):e0004880. Available at: https://pubmed.ncbi.nlm.nih.gov/41468507/. Accessed February 4, 2026.
3. Goldhagen J, Elkrail SE, Affan A. Responding to the humanitarian crisis in Sudan. BMJ Paediatrics Open 2024;8(1):1–2. Accessed February 4, 2026.
4. Omer AT, Ahmed AA, Birier AB, et al. Child health in war crisis: barriers to health-care utilization among internally displaced Sudanese caregivers. BMC Public Health 2025;25:3376. Available at: https://pmc.ncbi.nlm.nih.gov/articles/PMC12505789/. Accessed February 2, 2026.
5. The Global Fund. Sudan: delivering vital health services despite conflict and displacement. 2025. Available at: https://www.theglobalfund.org/en/stories/2025/2025-04-02-sudan-delivering-vital-health-services-conflict-displacement/. Accessed February 4, 2026.
6. Elhassan S, Osman M, Altaher A, et al. Adverse maternal and neonatal outcomes in Northern Sudan: the role of antenatal care and socioeconomic inequities in war. Reprod Health 2025;22(1):186. PMID: 41053804; PMCID: PMC12502332.

Available at: https://pubmed.ncbi.nlm.nih.gov/41053804/. Accessed February 4, 2026.
7. UNICEF. Number of children in need of humanitarian assistance in Sudan doubles as conflict enters third year amid 'perfect storm' of threats to children. 2025. Available at: https://www.unicef.org/press-releases/number-children-need-humanitarian-assistance-sudan-doubles-conflict-enters-third. Accessed February 3, 2026.
8. Doctors without Borders. Mass casualties in Sudan as warring parties strike populated areas. 2025. Available at: https://www.doctorswithoutborders.org/latest/mass-casualties-sudan-warring-parties-strike-populated-areas. Accessed February 4, 2026.
9. Save the Children International. Sudan: sharp rise in attacks on healthcare after two years of conflict with 1000 people killed this year. 2025. Available at: https://www.savethechildren.org/us/about-us/media-and-news/2025-press-releases/sudan-sharp-rise-in-attacks-on-healthcare. Accessed February 3, 2026.
10. UNICEF. 'Not the new normal' – 2024 'one of the worst years in UNICEF's history' for children in conflict. 2024. Available at: https://www.unicef.org/lac/en/press-releases/not-new-normal-2024-one-worst-years-unicefs-history-children-conflict. Accessed February 4, 2026.
11. Gooding C, Musa S, Lavin T, et al. Nutritional challenges among African refugee and internally displaced children: a comprehensive scoping review. Children 2024;11(3):318. Accessed February 4, 2026.
12. Doctors without borders. (202). Malnutrition. Available at: https://www.doctorswithoutborders.org/what-we-do/medical-issues/malnutrition. Accessed February 3, 2026.
13. UNICEF. Lives of malnourished children at risk with upsurge in violence in South Sudan. 2026. Available at: https://www.unicef.org/esa/press-releases/lives-malnourished-children-risk-upsurge-violence-south-sudan. Accessed February 3, 2026.
14. World Health Organization. Malnutrition. 2024. Available at: https://www.who.int/news-room/fact-sheets/detail/malnutrition. Accessed February 3, 2026.
15. Khalid N, Khan MA, Smith JD. Pediatric blast trauma: a systematic review and meta-analysis of factors associated with mortality and description of injury profiles. Prehospital Disaster Med 2022;37(4):492–501. Accessed February 4, 2026.
16. Hargrave J, Pearce P, Mayhew E, et al. Blast injuries in children: a mixed-methods narrative review. BMJ Paediatrics Open 2019;3:e000452. Available at: https://pubmed.ncbi.nlm.nih.gov/31548997/. Accessed February 4, 2026.
17. Mock C, MacKenzie EJ, Jurkovich GJ. Long-term disability outcomes after extremity amputation in low-resource and conflict settings. Injury 2005;54(9):2587–95. Available at: https://pubmed.ncbi.nlm.nih.gov/16085622/. Accessed February 4, 2026.
18. Doctors without Borders. Sudan: 16% of war-wounded patients at South Khartoum Hospital are children. 2024. Available at: https://msfsouthasia.org/sudan-16-of-war-wounded-patients-at-south-khartoum-hospital-are-children/. Accessed February 4, 2026.
19. Osman SHM, Nashwan AJ. Prioritizing children's mental health amidst Sudan's humanitarian crisis: policy recommendations for immediate action. Child Adolesc Psychiatr Ment Health 2023;17(1):97. PMID: 37563640; PMCID: PMC10416422. Available at: https://pmc.ncbi.nlm.nih.gov/articles/PMC10416422/. Accessed February 4, 2026.

Imperatives for Action and Impact of Humanitarian Crises Affecting Children

The Case of Haiti—Lessons and the Way Forward

Vanessa Rouzier, MD[a,b,*], Owen Robinson, MPP[c]

KEYWORDS

• Haiti • Health care • Gangs • Cholera • Displacement

KEY POINTS

- Decades of political instability, the 2010 earthquake, cholera, and gang violence have systematically weakened Haiti's governance and health system.
- Healthcare access has collapsed as hospitals close, essential services disappear, supply chains fail, and vaccination programs face disruption.
- Millions face food insecurity, widespread child malnutrition, and rising mortality driven by violence, displacement, and collapsing infrastructure.
- Nonprofits sustained essential care through service relocation, community clinics, international partnerships, and continued HIV, tuberculosis, and cardiovascular treatment.
- Long-term recovery requires stronger governance, security, health system investment, community-centered care, and sustained international support.

INTRODUCTION

Haiti's ongoing humanitarian catastrophe has had a devastating impact upon the Haitian healthcare sector that has yet to be fully quantified. The history of this small island nation in the Caribbean—the first, in 1804, to abolish slavery and obtain independence from France—has been tumultuous since its inception. A chaotic succession of *coups d'état*, dictatorial regimes, and international interventions and occupations, coupled with harmful economic and development policies from former colonial powers and allies, have led to political and economic fragility over the course of Haiti's maturation as a sovereign state. The impact of the chronic political instability and economic hardship has been compounded by recurrent natural disasters and devastating health

[a] Center for Global Health, Weill Cornell Medicine, New York, NY, USA; [b] Clinical Trials Unit, GHESKIO Centers, Port-au-Prince, Haiti; [c] International Cardiac Alliance, Burlington, VT, USA
* Corresponding author. Center for Global Health, Weill Cornell Medicine, New York, NY.
E-mail address: vrouzier@gheskio.org

Pediatr Clin N Am 73 (2026) 1067–1079
https://doi.org/10.1016/j.pcl.2026.05.006 pediatric.theclinics.com
0031-3955/26/

Abbreviations	
ART	antiretroviral treatment
CVD	cardiovascular disease
ICA	International Cardiac Alliance
NGO	non-profit organization
TB	tuberculosis
TOF	Tetralogy of Fallot

epidemics. The recent deterioration of public security and governance in Haiti, which accelerated soon after the 2010 earthquake, has had profound negative consequences upon access to quality healthcare for Haitian children and their families.

This article describes some of the ways in which Haiti's insecurity crisis has directly contributed to a severe lack of healthcare access for children living in Haiti. It argues, however, that even in an extremely challenging environment for service delivery, it is possible for pediatric healthcare organizations to continue to achieve impact. Using flexible and nimble approaches that respond to the ever-changing realities around them, organizations can adapt their strategies to continue to have life-saving impact, even in the midst of some of the world's most intractable humanitarian crises. Maintaining operations during such crises provides direct benefit to the local community by providing access to care, employment opportunities, ongoing training and capacity building and empowering local enterprises for long term sustainability. Moreover, by maintaining a baseline level of infrastructure and staff, these organizations will be better positioned to rebuild their service offerings once conditions improve. Ultimately, keeping families and children healthy in their home countries helps reduce the migration pressure to leave in search for better health or economic opportunities and preserves the hope and dignity of the most vulnerable.

HUMANITARIAN CRISIS IN HAITI: CONTEXT AND TIMELINE

The humanitarian crisis that has engulfed Haiti in recent years has roots tracing back many decades. In 1991, a military coup that ousted the popularly elected president Jean Bertrand Aristide, led to an international embargo from 1991 to 1994 that destroyed the economy and had a tremendous negative impact on health care. Childhood malnutrition increased severely in rural Haiti along with an increase in child mortality in children under 5 years of age.[1] Additionally, the sanctions led to shortages of medical supplies and disrupted hospital operations, setting the stage for a progressive yet steady deterioration of the health infrastructure. More recently, the devastating 7.0 magnitude earthquake that struck Haiti on January 12, 2010, dealt a catastrophic blow to the country (**Fig. 1**). The disaster, among the deadliest in modern history, had an estimated toll of 316,000 deaths, 300,000 injuries, 4000 to 6000 amputations, and close to 2 million internally displaced individuals.[2] Tens of thousands of homes, businesses, health facilities (including Port-au-Prince's only national teaching and tertiary hospital), and other critical infrastructure components were damaged or destroyed throughout the greater Port-au-Prince area and the neighboring city of Leogane, where the earthquake epicenter was located.[3] The earthquake's extensive damage to Haiti's already limited infrastructure crippled its ability to provide care to its population. Despite unprecedented initial support from the international community, only 1.8% of all post-earthquake reconstruction funding was directed to budgetary support of the Haitian government.[4] This resulted in the Haitian state having very weak and underfunded administrative capacity in the health sector,[5] as well as in other areas of state responsibility such as public security (**Fig. 2**). The manner in which

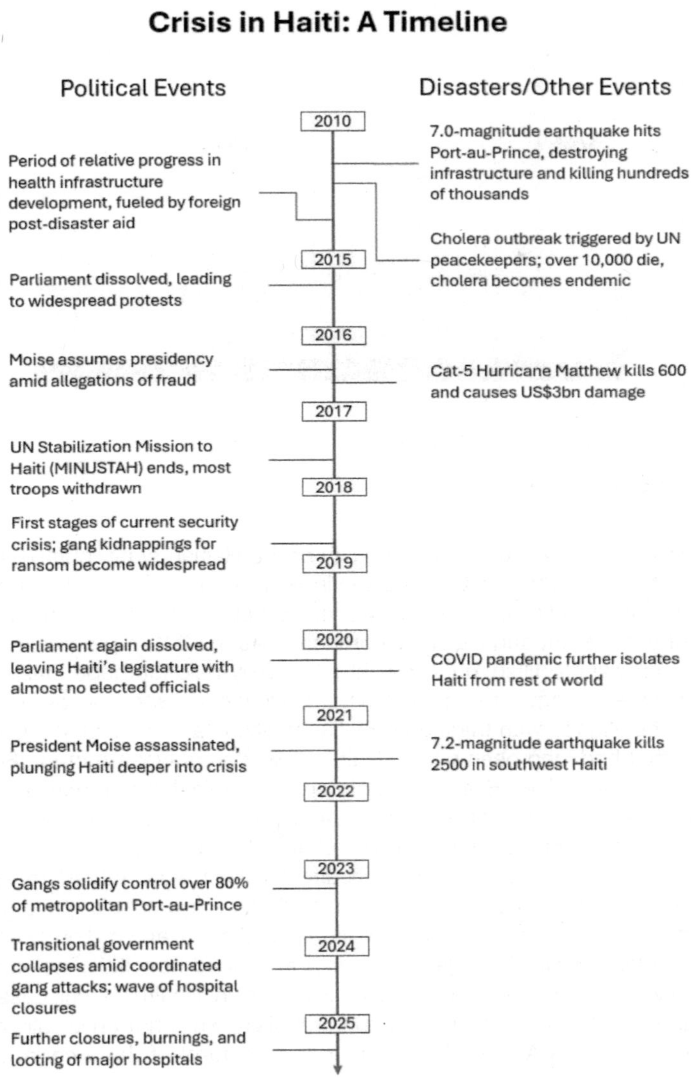

Fig. 1. Timeline of current Haiti crisis.

post-earthquake relief was administered, as well as a steady erosion in international-sector health funding from its post-earthquake peak, explains in large part the extremely deficient state of the health care system in Haiti today.[6]

That same year, Haiti experienced its first cholera epidemic that resulted in over 10,000 deaths and affected nearly 820,000 people, making it one of the deadliest cholera epidemics in recent history.[7] It overwhelmed Haiti's already fragile health care system, which was still recovering from the catastrophic earthquake earlier that year. From 2010 to 2025, Haiti was hit by recurrent epidemics including dengue, chikungunya zika, COVID-19 and resurgence of cholera as well as major natural disasters. In particular, Haiti's southern peninsula was severely impacted by category-five Hurricane Andrew in 2016,[8] and further damaged by a second 7.0 magnitude earthquake in 2021.[9]

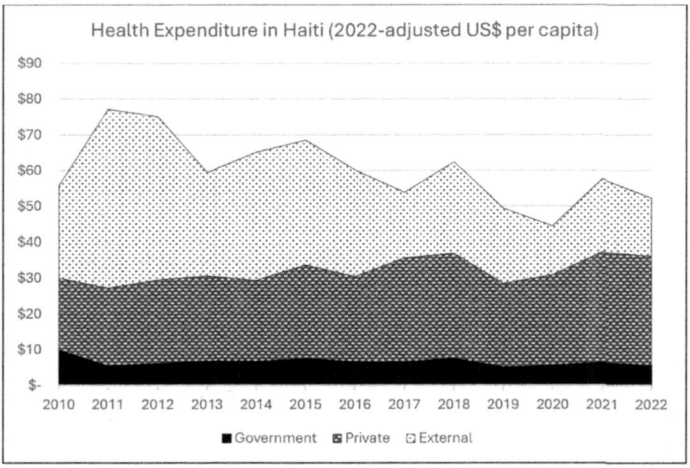

Fig. 2. Health expenditure in Haiti.[5]

In the mid-2010s, the weakened capacity of the Haitian state, combined with the withdrawal of the UN Stabilization Mission in Haiti (MINUSTAH) and an uptick in the inflow of illicit arms to Haiti, created a worsening power vacuum despite the nominal presence of a president and legislative branch.[10] As the 2010s progressed, this vacuum was increasingly filled on a neighborhood-by-neighborhood basis by street gangs that were younger, more ruthless in their tactics and use of violence, and less likely to be aligned with traditional Haitian political factions than the earlier gangs and cartels that had long been part of Haiti's unwritten power structure (**Fig. 2**).[11]

This displacement of the Haitian government by criminal organizations accelerated dramatically in 2021 following the assassination of President Jovenel Moise.[12] In early 2024, when gangs cemented physical control of 80% to 90% of metropolitan Port-au-Prince, dozens of hospitals and other health facilities were forced to close.[13] By October 2025, only one public state-run hospital and a few smaller private hospitals, clinics, and health centers remained operational to serve over 3 million people in Port-au-Prince.[14] Many of Haiti's largest and most advanced hospitals, including Hopital Bernard Mevs, were looted and burned. Partners in Health/Zanmi Lasante's 300 bed teaching and tertiary care hospital in Mirebalais, while not physically destroyed, was forced to close in April 2025 as gangs took control of the area in the Central Department.[15]

THE IMPACT OF HAITI'S CRISIS UPON HEALTH ACCESS AND OUTCOMES

Decreased Access to Health Care

Since 2018, Haiti has experienced a steady decrease in access to health care due to the increase in violence and deteriorating security situation. Gangs have progressively taken over control of neighborhoods, burning houses, attacking businesses and institutions, and kidnapping residents for ransom. The health sector has been specifically targeted: medical personnel have been kidnapped, sometimes with fatal results, and over 50 hospitals and clinics have been looted, burned or rendered non-functional.[16,17] Human Rights Watch estimates that 40,000 health personnel have left Haiti as a result of the violence.[18] Over 1200 hospital beds in intensive care unit, critical care, and trauma—representing the vast majority of all such beds nationally—have been lost as 3 of the main hospitals in Port-au-Prince and one in the Central

Department have been looted, burned, and/or forced to shut down (Hopital Bernard Mevs, the State General Hospital-HUEH, Hopital St Francois de Salles, and Hopital Universitaire de Mirebalais, respectively). In mid-October 2025, Doctors Without Borders was forced to permanently close its Port-au-Prince emergency care center, which had been a key lifeline, because of the surge in gang violence.[19] As of early 2026, only one public hospital remains open in Port-au-Prince (La Paix University Hospital), and its capacity falls far short of the needs of a metropolitan area of more than 3 million people. The blockade of major roads and destruction of hospitals and clinics has also severely disrupted supply chains for consumables and medications, as well as access to medical imaging and specialty care. Many smaller community health centers, which formed the pillar of the national vaccination program, have had to close, putting more children at risk of defaulting on their vaccines or having to travel further to obtain them. The constant risk of violence has posed particularly grueling challenges to a health care system that is near collapse.

Increased Need and Vulnerability of the Population

In addition to the reduced access to care, gang violence has restricted children's and families' access to food, leading to a nutritional crisis. According to UNICEF, in 2025, 5.7 million Haitians were living with food insecurity, including 2.85 million children; 8400 people were estimated to be facing famine-like conditions.[20] Between January and April 2025, nearly 277,000 children were suffering from acute malnutrition, and 125,000 were severely malnourished, but only 4600 children were treated for severe acute malnutrition. This represents less than 4% of the estimated need, prompting an increased risk of death for many children under 5 years of age.

In greater Port-au-Prince, gang takeovers caused a massive internal displacement of over 1.4 million people who fled their homes in fear for their lives (**Fig. 3**); by September 2025, almost 11% of the population of Port-au-Prince was forced to live in improvised shelters in schools, churches, or abandoned properties.[21] Between

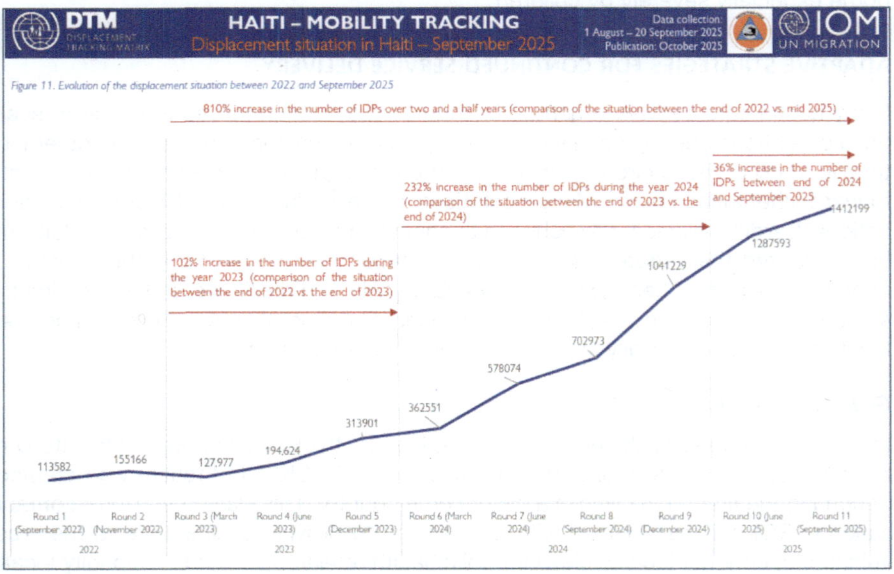

Fig. 3. Internally displaced persons in Haiti: 2022 to 2025.[24]

2022 and 2025, over 660,000 individuals were also deported back to Haiti from the Dominican Republic, United States, and elsewhere, 8% of whom were children (Siterep PAHO, Sept 2025).[22] The violence and displacement were accompanied by an alarming rise in gender-based violence and sexual assault, with young girls being the most impacted. Young men and boys were also recruited as child soldiers into gangs with the promise of relief from hunger and extreme socio-economic precarity.[23]

The burning and looting of neighborhoods by gangs was also associated with tremendous public infrastructure damage, with water and sanitation systems being further compromised from their already fragile state. Overcrowding, poor sanitation and food insecurity fueled new outbreaks of diseases, including cholera, which saw a resurgence in many neighborhoods after its near-elimination from the island in 2021. By September 2025, over 3100 suspected cholera cases had been reported by the Ministry of Health, with 37 deaths (16 in hospital, 21 in the community).[22] Tuberculosis (TB) and diphtheria outbreaks also ravaged the population in 2025, undermining progress achieved in earlier years. Increased incidence was also seen in scabies, impetigo, diarrhea, respiratory infections, and other diseases, especially among children. These developments have further compounded the vulnerability of small children, those already sick, and those who are most impoverished.

Finally, in the first 8 months of 2024, overall mortality estimates doubled compared to those of 2023, signaling an acute public health crisis.[25] This retrospective mortality survey was conducted as part of the 2024 Multi-Sector Needs Assessment to gather critical data on crude and under 5 mortality rates and their leading causes.[26] Acute and chronic illnesses were the most common causes of death, exacerbated by extreme violence, insecurity, financial precarity, and weather extremes such as flooding and droughts. Rural areas such as the Artibonite that were especially impacted by gangs showed the fastest rise in mortality.

In conclusion, widespread gang-related violence in Haiti has caused a severe humanitarian crisis with massive population displacement, significant public and health infrastructure destruction, and economic collapse that has eroded the population's access to basic needs and services. As with most such crises, the impact has been borne especially severely by children.

ADAPTIVE STRATEGIES FOR CONTINUED SERVICE DELIVERY

Many health care delivery organizations in Haiti have been forced to cease or scale back operations due to security challenges, international funding cuts, and other factors; in many of these circumstances, the organizations may have had no viable path forward other than to close. Many institutions, however, including GHESKIO and International Cardiac Alliance, have chosen to continue pursuing their missions in Haiti and have adapted their strategies to remain as impactful as possible in the context of ongoing insecurity. These examples of adaptability and resilience under dire circumstances serve as a reminder that the continued provision of care to children and their families remains especially imperative during humanitarian crises.

GHESKIO Centers

In 1982, in response to the emerging HIV epidemic, the Haitian Group for the study of Kaposi's Sarcoma and Opportunistic Infections (GHESKIO in French) was created, becoming the first AIDS clinic in a low-income country. This Haitian non-profit organization (NGO) was established with the mission to provide clinical care to the most vulnerable, conduct locally relevant public health research, and build capacity locally by training health personnel. Initially focused on HIV and its related opportunistic infections, GHESKIO led the national fight against HIV in collaboration with the Ministry of Health (MOH) and other partners, helping turn around what was a raging epidemic to a manageable chronic illness today. Collaborating with the government and other local NGOs, GHESKIO helped establish a strong foundation for HIV care in the 1980s and 1990s, combining prevention and treatment,[27–29] publishing on the epidemiology of AIDS, its risk factors, and its manifestations in the Haitian population. With this successful foundation and leadership, Haiti was one of the first countries to receive funding from the Global Fund to Fight AIDS, Tuberculosis, and Malaria in 2003 and the US President's Emergency Program for AIDS Relief in 2004, allowing for the scale up antiretroviral treatment (ART) nationally. In 2003, the GHESKIO Centers in Port-au-Prince and the Partners in Health/Zanmi Lasante clinic in Cange were the first and only two institutions in a resource-limited setting to provide ART free-of-charge to eligible patients.[30] By 2025, HIV prevention and treatment was available in over 150 facilities across Haiti's ten departments.[31] GHESKIO was instrumental in helping to set up the HIV health infrastructure model of care that was scaled up nationally.

GHESKIO is the largest medical institution providing free HIV care in metropolitan Port-au-Prince, operating 2 large outpatient centers, located respectively in downtown Port-au-Prince and the north of the city, which serve a catchment population of approximately 3 million people. The GHESKIO model of providing clinical care, conducting public-health-relevant research, and disseminating findings via training is essential to its success. Care is provided freely for the whole family in a holistic fashion with all major services offered in a one-stop option at its 2 main campuses as well as in ten community clinics throughout the city. These community clinics, put in place in 2019, are localized near patients' homes to facilitate their access to care, as they were afraid to come to the GHESKIO downtown center due to constant gang violence in the surrounding neighborhood. Over 12,000 patients receive HIV-related care with services also available for sexually transmitted infections, TB and other opportunistic infections, maternal and child health and treatment of childhood acute malnutrition.[32] Understanding that child health is often dependent on the education and economic status of the mother, programs have been developed to go beyond medical treatment to holistic packages of care. In order to support families, GHESKIO has incorporated access to microcredit loans, vocational training, nutritional support, integrated health and nutrition programs for mothers living with HIV and their infants, peer support groups for persons living with HIV, potable water distribution in immediate slum areas, and even building a primary school in the aftermath of the earthquake as well as providing over 3000 scholarships for children of patients in care.

GHESKIO's mission broadened after the devastating earthquake and cholera outbreak in 2010 to embrace global health and other pressing public health issues. It also shifted to greater partnership with the community for delivery of services in a more decentralized manner. The vision was extended from saving lives to empowering communities. In response to the shifting epidemiological context and emergence of cardiovascular diseases (CVDs) as a public health emergency, GHESKIO opened a CVD clinic in 2018 and established a longitudinal cohort study of 3005 participants to evaluate the prevalence and incidence of CVD and its risk factors in urban Haitians.[33,34] In addition to CVD-related research, clinical care is provided for our patients living with HIV for prevention and treatment of cardiovascular co-morbidity.

GHESKIO also conducts NIH-sponsored HIV, TB, and CVD-related clinical trials. Through clinical and operational research, GHESKIO seeks to define treatment and prevention models for infectious and non-communicable diseases that are appropriate and effective for Haiti. Initially focused on HIV, sexually transmitted infections, and TB, to now encompassing CVDs, the GHESKIO research program has evolved from early observational studies to large clinical trials and has been designated as an NIH clinical trials unit since 2005. In 1983, GHESKIO received its initial funding from the National Institutes of Health to define the epidemiology, natural history, risk factors, and associated co-infections of HIV/AIDS. Since then, GHESKIO's consistent research productivity, with over 350 investigator-led peer-reviewed publications, has been recognized by uninterrupted support from the NIH and successful competitive renewal grants. GHESKIO's research is conducted in collaboration with Weill Cornell Medicine (New York, NY, United States), Fondation Merieux (Lyon, France), and the Analysis Group (Boston, United States).

Research conducted at GHESKIO has been essential to improving quality of care for patients. Results from its clinical and operational studies have guided the national implementation of evidence-based strategies that are adapted to the local context.[35–38] Research efforts have also facilitated the introduction of specialized laboratory techniques in Haiti such as HIV viral load, CD4 testing, DNA PCR testing for infant HIV diagnosis, and the creation of the only biosafety level 3 (BSL-3) TB laboratory capable of doing TB cultures and drug susceptibility testing.[30] Finally, research has built capacity by training medical, laboratory, medical imaging, and pharmacy personnel to improve services available locally. GHESKIO's research has led to change WHO guidelines on TB prophylaxis,[39] earlier ART initiation and test and treat strategy for HIVAIDS,[40] and the use of oral cholera vaccine during cholera epidemics.[41]

The deteriorating security situation in Haiti has had a tremendous impact on the work done by GHESKIO. However, despite these extraordinary challenges, GHESKIO has continued to open its doors, providing thousands of people with free, high-quality health care every month. GHESKIO has not been spared from violence and insecurity, with over 20 staff members having been kidnapped by gangs in the past 2 years. All of these individuals, however, were released without having to pay a ransom because of GHESKIO's recognized long-standing work in the community. Over 250 staff members have left the country, leading to an unprecedented brain drain. This high staff turnover and loss of the best trained personnel has placed a tremendous burden on recruitment, training, and day-to-day operation in very challenging circumstances.[42] The gang takeover of many neighborhoods has forced GHESKIO to close many of its community ART distribution points, making it more challenging for patients to access care and increasing the cost and distance required to travel for medication refill or consultation. Three community centers had to be closed and patients at these sites were relocated to our closest health facility. Retention in care of patients is complicated, as many have fled to the countryside for fear of their lives as gangs burn neighborhoods and take over. In order to remain functional, GHESKIO has rapidly deployed many strategies to continue providing care to the population and supporting the staff.[43,44] Many services were relocated to safer areas, work hours were reduced for staff having to travel to dangerous areas, and GHESKIO helped fund or secure housing for many staff who had to flee their neighborhoods as gangs took over. Some community centers have been setup inside geographic areas occupied by gangs staffed with employees who live in the area. GHESKIO's contingency plan is continually being updated to ensure access to fuel, supplies, medication continues uninterrupted to allow for the continuity of services to our population. In 2025, over 10,000 patients living with HIV have continued to receive their ART, 885 patients have been treated for TB, over 1800 women have received prenatal care, 394 women have been provided emergency rape counseling and care, 1971 children have been provided vaccines, and 183 treated for severe malnutrition. In response to the humanitarian crisis, 14,675 women have received cash transfers, food and primary care, and

19,097 displaced persons in camps have been provided emergency care. Training has been intensified and is ongoing in all disciplines in order to replace essential staff. Against overwhelming odds, GHESKIO has continued not only to provide health services, but has nimbly adapted its clinical services and research activities to maintain patient care within a national health care system near collapse.[45]

International Cardiac Alliance

International Cardiac Alliance (ICA), founded as "Haiti Cardiac Alliance," is an NGO that facilitates diagnosis, surgery, and long-term follow-up for children and young adults suffering from congenital heart disease and rheumatic heart disease. Between its founding in July 2013 and the end of 2024, ICA arranged life-saving cardiac surgical and catheterization procedures for 610 Haitian patients, with a 5 year survival rate of 95.1%.[46]

While ICA's original strategic objective was to establish permanent, sustainable, Haitian-led cardiac surgical care within Haiti itself, the country's long-term unrest has forced a shift in strategy and objectives. This shift began in 2019, when it became too dangerous for visiting teams to fly into Haiti to perform cardiac surgical training visits. Over the subsequent years, ICA's team in Haiti became increasingly skilled at navigating the tasks and processes required to safely transport Haitian patients and their parents to other countries to access the cardiac procedures they needed; in parallel, ICA worked to grow its network of international placement opportunities, strengthening referral relationships with hospitals in the Dominican Republic, the Cayman Islands, the United States, and elsewhere. In 2023, ICA added a clinical social worker and a logistics specialist to its Haiti team to help patients and families navigate the complexities of medical examinations, passport applications, visa appointments, medication refills, and travel logistics in the context of ever-worsening crisis and instability.

Although ICA can no longer treat as many patients each year as it did prior to Haiti's current crisis, its resilient and flexible approach has helped it to preserve Haitian patients' access to cardiac surgical care against all odds. A recent case illustrates how several elements of this approach came together.

In October 2024, a rural ICA partner clinic in southwest Haiti first emailed ICA about "Jean," a 27 month old boy presenting to them for the first time. This child had never been formally diagnosed with a cardiac condition, but was underweight, experienced frequent dyspnea, and had baseline blood oxygen saturations of 80%, frequently dropping to 30% to 40% during cyanotic crises. It was clear from the initial description that Jean likely had an urgent heart defect; but he had no access to echocardiography, no passport, and no cardiac medications.

At the time, it was physically impossible for Jean and his father to reach Port-au-Prince for diagnosis due to gang-imposed roadblocks on the only route connecting their region to the capital. ICA arranged for a US-based pediatric cardiologist to consult remotely with Jean's primary care physician and review bedside imaging, in the hopes of keeping him as stable as possible until road conditions improved enough for him to reach the capital.

After 5 weeks of impenetrable roadblocks, security improved enough for Jean and his father to make a risky attempt to reach Port-au-Prince, which they managed to do on the back of a motorcycle in close coordination with ICA's social work and logistics team. Jean was soon diagnosed with severe Tetralogy of Fallot (TOF) requiring urgent surgery, and ICA was able to quickly transmit the echocardiogram images to a hospital in Dominican Republic capable of performing the surgery Jean needed. Meanwhile, ICA worked with Haitian government officials to expedite emergency passports for

Jean and his father. With passports and hospital approval in hand, ICA then leveraged high-level diplomatic relationships to obtain the medical visas that Jean and his father would require to enter the Dominican Republic, and finally partnered with Haiti's leading medical transport organization, which generously donated a direct medevac helicopter flight to the Dominican Republic. Within just several weeks of formal diagnosis, Jean reached the Dominican Republic and was admitted directly to the hospital, where he soon underwent successful surgical TOF repair. He is now back home in Haiti in excellent health.

Not all of ICA's patients in Haiti are able to obtain surgical care so quickly, or at all—some must wait months or years before receiving the heart surgeries they urgently need, and others pass away while waiting. Jean's case, however, underscores that even in an extremely resource-limited, politically unstable environment, it is possible to achieve life-saving impact through a flexible, multifaceted approach that encompasses clinical care, logistical navigation, and social work accompaniment.

SUMMARY

In conclusion, child health outcomes cannot be separated from the broader context of national security, governance, and the rule of law, as these structural factors fundamentally shape access to health care and long-term well-being. Long-term investments in security, governance, and the rule of law can therefore be as crucial to child health outcomes as more targeted investments in health care delivery. Even amid severe humanitarian crises, whether natural, manmade, or both, pediatric health care organizations demonstrate that adaptable, innovative strategies can sustain essential services and save lives despite extraordinary constraints. These organizations must be able to continually evolve to achieve impact, using creative and resourceful approaches to overcome obstacles as they arise. Moreover, organizations that prioritize the preservation of their personnel and infrastructure during times of crisis not only maximize their immediate impact but also strengthen their capacity to rebuild and expand care delivery once stability returns.

INSIGHTS TO ACTION

- Pearl: Flexible care models that combine clinical services, social support, logistics coordination, and community engagement can maintain life-saving care even in highly unstable environments.
- Pitfall: Rigid program designs that cannot adapt to changing security conditions are less likely to sustain impact.
- Pearl: Decentralized service delivery models (community clinics, mobile outreach, local distribution points) can preserve access to care when transportation routes and centralized facilities become inaccessible.
- Pitfall: Measuring success solely by facility-based service delivery may underestimate the value of community-based and cross-border care solutions.
- Pearl: Child health outcomes cannot be separated from the broader context of national security, governance, and the rule of law, as these structural factors fundamentally shape access to healthcare and long-term well-being.

DISCLOSURES

The authors have no financial disclosures or conflicts of interest to disclose.

REFERENCES

1. Gibbons E, Garfield R. The impact of economic sanctions on health and human rights in Haiti, 1991-1994. Am J Publ Health 1999;89(10):1499–504 [Erratum appears in Am J Public Health 2000;90(1):140]. PMID: 10511830; PMCID: PMC1508819.
2. Arnaouti MKC, Cahill G, Baird MD, et al. Haiti disaster response–junior research collaborative (HDR-JRC). Medical disaster response: a critical analysis of the 2010 Haiti earthquake. Front Public Health 2022;10:995595. https://doi.org/10.3389/fpubh.2022.995595.
3. United Nations Office for the Coordination of Humanitarian Affairs. UNDAC mission report: Haiti earthquake, January 2010. Published 2010. Available at: https://www.unocha.org/publications/report/haiti/undac-mission-report-haiti-earthquake-january-2010. Accessed October 7, 2025.
4. Macdonald I, Doucet I. The NGO Republic of Haiti. The nation. 2015. Available at: https://www.thenation.com/article/archive/ngo-republic-haiti/. Accessed October 7, 2025.
5. World Bank. Health expenditure by sector, Haiti. *Health, Nutrition, and Population Statistics Database*. Available at: https://databank.worldbank.org/source/health-nutrition-and-population-statistics (Accessed 12 December 2025).
6. Fatton R Jr. Crisis and institutional collapse in Haiti. Curr Hist 2025;124(859):48–53.
7. Pape JW, Rouzier V. Embracing oral cholera vaccine–shifting response to cholera. N Engl J Med 2014;370(22):2067–9.
8. Marcelin LH, Cela T, Shultz JM. Haiti and the politics of governance and community responses to Hurricane Matthew. Disaster Health 2016;3(4):151–61. PMID: 28321361; PMCID: PMC5351817.
9. Daniels JP. Earthquake compounds Haiti's health challenges. Lancet 2021;398(10304):944–5. PMID: 34509222.
10. Global Initiative Against Transnational Organized Crime, *Gangs of Haiti Timeline* (October 2022), PDF. Available at: https://globalinitiative.net/wp-content/uploads/2022/10/GITOC-Gangs-of-Haiti-Timeline.pdf. Accessed December 12, 2025.
11. Office of the United Nations High Commissioner for Human Rights. Haiti's criminal markets: mapping trends in firearms and drug trafficking. ReliefWeb. Available at: https://reliefweb.int/report/haiti/haitis-criminal-markets-mapping-trends-firearms-and-drug-trafficking. Accessed December 12, 2025.
12. Porter C, Crowley M, Méheut C. Haiti's president assassinated in nighttime raid, shaking a fragile nation. New York Times, 2021. Available at: https://www.nytimes.com/2021/07/07/world/americas/haiti-president-assassinated-killed.html.
13. US Committee for Refugees and Immigrants. Country conditions in Haiti. 2024. Available at: https://refugees.org/wp-content/uploads/2024/05/USCRI-Haiti-Country-Conditions.pdf. Accessed December 12, 2025.
14. Associated Press. Doctors without Borders permanently closes its emergency center in Haiti's capital. 2024. Available at: https://apnews.com/article/haiti-msf-doctors-without-borders-center-closes-violence-68595071309e258e9c67ca233eb31822. Accessed December 12, 2025.
15. Charlier P. Mirebalais: last bastion before the total collapse of the Haitian healthcare system. Ethics Med Public Health 2025;33:101096. https://doi.org/10.1016/j.jemep.2025.101096.

16. Medeus AJR, Pierre CJ, Merilan LLS, et al. Impact of gang violence in Haiti on healthcare delivery and medical education. Lancet Reg Health, Am 2024;36: 100811. https://doi.org/10.1016/j.lana.2024.100811.
17. United Nations Office at Geneva. Haiti gangs crisis: top rights expert decries attacks on hospitals. 2025. Available at: https://www.ungeneva.org/en/news-media/news/2025/01/101893/haiti-gangs-crisis-top-rights-expert-decries-attacks-hospitals. Accessed December 12, 2025.
18. Human Rights Watch. Haiti. In: World Report 2025. New York, NY: Human Rights Watch; 2025. Available at: https://www.hrw.org/world-report/2025/country-chapters/haiti. Accessed January 19, 2025.
19. Integrated Food Security Phase Classification. Haiti: IPC acute food insecurity snapshot. 2025. Available at: https://www.ipcinfo.org/fileadmin/user_upload/ipcinfo/docs/IPC_Haiti_Acute_Food_Insecurity_Mar_Jun2025_Snapshot_English.pdf. Accessed December 12, 2025.
20. UNICEF USA. Crisis in Haiti escalates—endangering children's lives. 2025. Available at: https://www.unicefusa.org/stories/crisis-haiti-escalates-endangering-childrens-lives. Accessed December 12, 2025.
21. International Organization for Migration. Displacement in Haiti reaches record high as 1.4 million people flee violence. 2025. Available at: https://www.iom.int/news/displacement-haiti-reaches-record-high-14-million-people-flee-violence. Accessed December 12, 2025.
22. Pan American Health Organization. Sitrep humanitaire—Haiti: rapport de situation Cluster Santé no. 25 (31 August–6 September 2025). 2025. Available at: https://www.paho.org/sites/default/files/2025-09/sitrep-n25-haiti-humanitariansituation-healthcluster-epiweek36-2025-frpdf.pdf. Accessed December 12, 2025.
23. Amnesty International. Haiti: children suffering gang recruitment, attacks and sexual violence amid escalating crisis. 2025. Available at: https://www.amnesty.org/en/latest/news/2025/02/haiti-children-suffering-gang-recruitment-attacks-sexual-violence/. Accessed December 12, 2025.
24. International Organization for Migration. Displacement situation in Haiti: round 11. 2025. Available at: https://dtm.iom.int/sites/g/files/tmzbdl1461/files/reports/DisplacementsituationinHaiti-Round11-September2025.pdf. Accessed December 12, 2025.
25. REACH Initiative. Haiti: a deepening public health crisis. 2025. Available at: https://reliefweb.int/report/haiti/haiti-deepening-public-health-crisis-january-2025. Accessed October 7, 2025.
26. REACH Initiative. MSNA 2024 en Haïti: note méthodologique. 2024. Available at: https://repository.impact-initiatives.org/document/impact/069ddef2/REACH_MSNA_2024_Note-Methodologique_Haiti_FR_.pdf. Accessed December 12, 2025.
27. Pape JW, Liautaud B, Thomas F, et al. Characteristics of the acquired immunodeficiency syndrome (AIDS) in Haiti. N Engl J Med 1983;309(16):945–50.
28. Pape JW, Liautaud B, Thomas F, et al. Risk factors associated with AIDS in Haiti. Am J Med Sci 1986;291(1):4–7.
29. Pape JW, Liautaud B, Thomas F, et al. The acquired immunodeficiency syndrome in Haiti. Ann Intern Med 1985;103(5):674–8.
30. Rouzier V, Farmer PE, Pape JW, et al. Factors impacting the provision of antiretroviral therapy to people living with HIV: the view from Haiti. Antivir Ther 2014;19-(suppl 3):91–104.
31. Monitoring, evaluation and surveillance interface. Haiti. Available at: https://www.mesi.ht/Questionnaire/Monitoring. Accessed December 12, 2025.

32. Pape JW, Severe PD, Fitzgerald DW, et al. The Haiti research-based model of international public health collaboration: the GHESKIO centers. J Acquir Immune Defic Syndr 2014;65(suppl 1):S5–9.
33. Yan LD, Sufra R, St Sauveur R, et al, Haiti Cardiovascular Disease Cohort Study Team. Spectrum of prevalent cardiovascular diseases in urban Port-au-Prince, Haiti: a population-based cross-sectional study. Lancet Reg Health Am 2024; 33:100729. https://doi.org/10.1016/j.lana.2024.100729.
34. Lookens J, Tymejczyk O, Rouzier V, et al. The Haiti cardiovascular disease cohort: study protocol for a population-based longitudinal cohort. BMC Public Health 2020;20(1):1633.
35. Severe P, Juste MA, Ambroise A, et al. Early versus standard antiretroviral therapy for HIV-infected adults in Haiti. N Engl J Med 2010;363(3):257–65.
36. Koenig SP, Bang H, Severe P, et al. Cost-effectiveness of early versus standard antiretroviral therapy in HIV-infected adults in Haiti. PLoS Med 2011;8(9): e1001095. https://doi.org/10.1371/journal.pmed.1001095.
37. Leger P, Charles M, Severe P, et al. Five-year survival of patients with AIDS receiving antiretroviral therapy in Haiti. N Engl J Med 2009;361(8):828–9.
38. George E, Noël F, Bois G, et al. Antiretroviral therapy for HIV-1–infected children in Haiti. J Infect Dis 2007;195(10):1411–8.
39. Pape JW, Jean SS, Ho JL, et al. Effect of isoniazid prophylaxis on incidence of active tuberculosis and progression of HIV infection. Lancet 1993;342(8866): 268–72. PMID: 8101302.
40. Koenig SP, Dorvil N, Dévieux JG, et al. Same-day HIV testing with initiation of antiretroviral therapy versus standard care for persons living with HIV: a randomized unblinded trial. PLoS Med 2017;14(7):e1002357. https://doi.org/10.1371/journal.pmed.1002357. PMID: 28742880; PMCID: PMC5526526.
41. Rouzier V, Severe K, Juste MAJ, et al. Cholera vaccination in urban Haiti. Am J Trop Med Hyg 2013;89(4):671–81. https://doi.org/10.4269/ajtmh.13-0171.
42. Chan M. A story of Haiti that is too often untold: GHESKIO's resilient model of community-based healthcare. Harvard Center for International Development. 2024. Available at: https://www.hks.harvard.edu/centers/cid/voices/story-haiti-too-often-untold-gheskios-resilient-model-community-based-healthcare. Accessed October 7, 2025.
43. Joseph P, Sun R, Guiteau C, et al. Continuity of care during severe civil unrest with a model of community-based HIV care in Haiti. Lancet Reg Health, Am 2024;37:100847. https://doi.org/10.1016/j.lana.2024.100847.
44. Marc JB, Pierre S, Ducatel O, et al. Early initiation of fast-track care for persons living with HIV during civil unrest in Port-au-Prince, Haiti. J Int AIDS Soc 2025; 28(2):e26419. https://doi.org/10.1002/jia2.26419.
45. Metz M, Sufra R, Ogyu A, et al. Improvements in blood pressure control and the hypertension care continuum over 2 years in urban Haiti amidst civil unrest. J Clin Hypertens 2025;27(9):e70153. https://doi.org/10.1111/jch.70153. PMID: 40991240; PMCID: PMC12459303.
46. International Cardiac Alliance. Annual report. 2024. Available at: https://www.intlcardiac.org/annual-report. Accessed October 7, 2025.

Children Are Victims in the War on Ukraine

Mariia Kiselova, MD[a], Yuriy Antipkin, MD[b],
Oleksandr Volosovets, MD[c],
Bruce K. Rubin, MEngr, MD, MBA, FRCPC[d,e,*]

KEYWORDS

• War in Ukraine • Children's health • Education • Humanitarian aid

KEY POINTS

- The full-scale invasion of Ukraine has affected the physical and mental health of mothers and children. Both those in active war zones and those across the country subject to air raids show signs of physical and psychological fragility.
- Health care services are stretched thin due to an increased need for medical services for those injured by war, attacks on health care facilities with loss of life, difficulty obtaining medical supplies, and sustaining preventive services like immunizations.
- The Russian Federation has abducted more than 35,000 Ukrainian children for indoctrination and abuse.
- Educational opportunities have been severely compromised especially among displaced children and those in the occupied territories. As well, medical education has suffered under the strain.

INTRODUCTION

When North Americans say "supporting children's lives and futures," they mean well-being, opportunities, and health. In Ukraine, we are now talking about physical survival, and we often narrow the meaning of the future to survive until tomorrow. "Children are its most vulnerable hostages," said the First Lady of Ukraine, summarizing the gap between peacetime expectations and our daily struggle for survival.[1]

[a] Department of Health of the Lviv Regional State Administration, Faculty of Postgraduate Education, Danylo Halytsky Lviv National Medical University, Lviv, Ukraine; [b] All-Ukrainian Center for Motherhood and Childhood of the National Academy of Medical Sciences of Ukraine, National Academy of Medical Sciences of Ukraine, Kyiv, Ukraine; [c] Department of Pediatrics 2, Bogomolets National Medical University, Kyiv, Ukraine; [d] Department of Pediatrics, Virginia Commonwealth University, Richmond, VA, USA; [e] Danylo Halytsky Lviv National Medical University, Kyiv, Ukraine

* Corresponding author. Department of Pediatrics, Virginia Commonwealth University, Richmond, VA.

E-mail address: bkrubin@outlook.com

Pediatr Clin N Am 73 (2026) 1081–1090
https://doi.org/10.1016/j.pcl.2026.05.007 **pediatric.theclinics.com**
0031-3955/26/

Abbreviations	
COVID-19	coronavirus disease 2019
DTP	diphtheria tetanus pertussis
IDP	internally displaced persons
PTSD	posttraumatic stress disorder
TB	tuberculosis
UN	United Nations
UNICEF	United Nations Children's Fund
WHO	World Health Organization

The upended and threatened lives of Ukrainian children is a consequence of the conflict of Russia's full-scale invasion of the country with all the horrors of war.[1–4]

BACKGROUND UKRAINE AND THE WAR—A CHRONOLOGY OF EVENTS

The History of Ukraine and the War—A Timeline of Events

Ukraine is one of the poorest countries in Eastern Europe, with a steadily declining population but a large territory. Before the coronavirus disease 2019 (COVID-19) pandemic and the war, morbidity and mortality rates in Ukraine were among the highest in Europe, including infant mortality, but were decreasing due to the introduction of perinatal technologies and evidence-based medicine in pediatric practice.[5,6] Since gaining independence in 1991, the focus of the Ukrainian government's public policy has been to enhance the life, education, and health of every child, and to involve local authorities and private partnerships in this endeavor.[7]

For more than 3.5 years, Ukrainian cities and villages have been under constant rocket fire from Russia. According to the monitoring portal Alerts, since the start of the full-scale war, there have been over 71,485 air raids on Ukrainian cities due to missile and drone attacks (https://alerts.in.ua), especially in the Donetsk, Kharkiv, and Zaporizhzhia regions. More than 10,000 civilians have been killed and 20,000 wounded. As of December 27, 2025, crimes against children, not including active combat operations, amounted to 677 dead and 2312 wounded children (https://www.gp.gov.ua). However, these are only the cases that have been reported and reliably verified.

"The injuries and deaths of families and children are a predictable and tragic consequence of the use of high explosive weapons against targets in major cities," said the head of the Monitoring Mission, Danielle Belle.[8] The United Nations (UN) Human Rights Monitoring Mission in Ukraine has expressed alarm at the intensification of Russian missile and drone attacks and the growing number of civilian casualties. Most civilian casualties and damage to educational and medical facilities due to Russian aggression continue to occur in government-controlled territory.

According to the World Health Organization (WHO) Representative in Ukraine, Jarno Habicht, since the beginning of the full-scale invasion, 1971 medical facilities have been damaged, and about 300 have been destroyed, of which 40% were on primary health care facilities, approximately 200 ambulances are lost annually, and 157 doctors have been killed while providing care to patients.[9] These attacks have made it difficult for people to access medical care, forcing them to postpone medical care. During the targeted missile attack on July 8, 2024, when the country's largest children's hospital, OKHMATDYT, and a maternity hospital were bombed in Kyiv, 34 adults and 3 children were killed and 170 people were injured. Direct hits to 5 buildings of OKHMATDYT have made it difficult to receive trauma, rehabilitation, and psychiatric care. In 2025 alone, the WHO recorded 2254 attacks on health care facilities (**Fig. 1**).

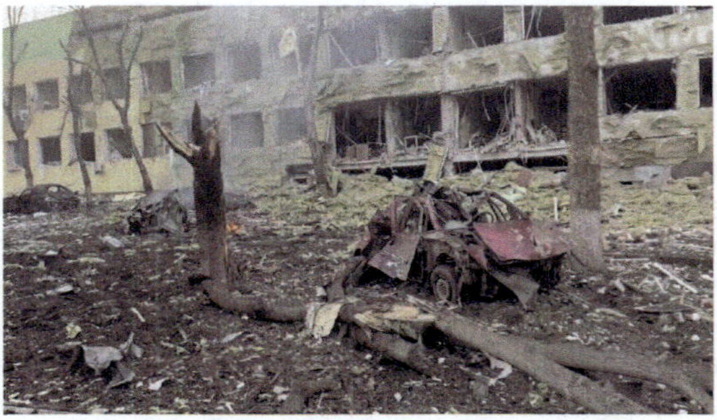

Fig. 1. A children's hospital in the city of Mariupol was destroyed as a result of a Russian airstrike. (*Source* This file is taken from the website of the information agency of the Ministry of Defense of Ukraine and is distributed under the Creative Commons Attribution 4.0 International license. https://armyinform.com.ua/2022/03/26/francziya-vymagatyme-vid-rf-znyaty-oblogu-mariupolya/.)

Since the beginning of the invasion, about 4.8 million Ukrainians have been displaced to Russia including 19,546 children forcibly deported from Ukraine to Russia since February 24, 2022 (**Fig. 2**). Again, these are only those cases that were officially reported it to the National Information Bureau of Ukraine. The Russian Commissioner for Children's Rights, Maria Lvova-Belova, against whom a criminal case has been opened by international courts, openly admits that up to 700,000 children have been abducted from Ukraine.[10]

In 2023, President Zelenskyy of Ukraine said, "We don't know the exact number ... of our children are like this (abducted). But we know that we must return them all. We know that we must restore the rights and security of all Ukrainian children." As the

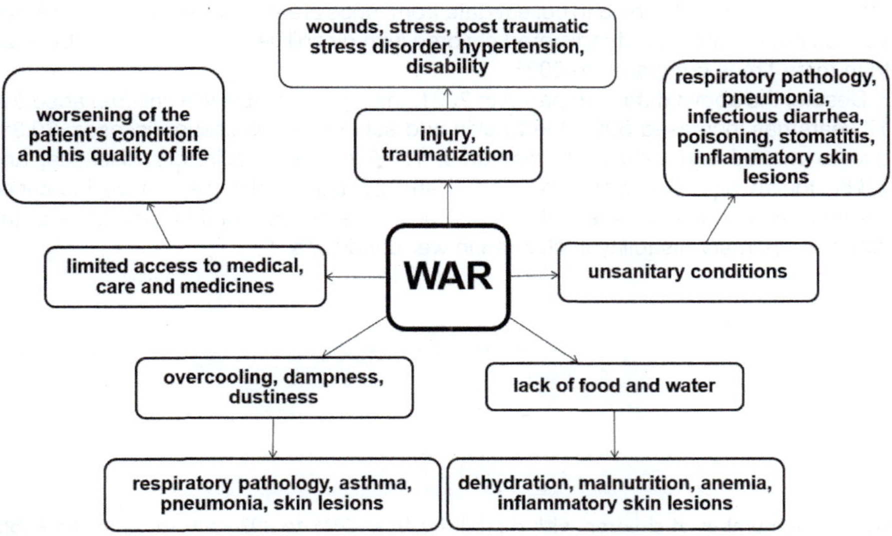

Fig. 2. The impact of the consequences of war on children's health. (*Source* Volosovets OP, Vyhovska OV, Kryvopustov SP, et al. Wojciech Feleszko Problems of providing medical care to children of Ukraine as a result of Russian aggression. Child Health. 2023;18(3):9–13 https://doi.org/10.22141/2224-0551.18.3.2023.1578.)

Ukrainian Parliament Commissioner for Human Rights notes that during the Russian invasion of Ukraine, almost 70% of Ukrainian children were forced to leave their homes and move within the country or abroad. The war has separated children from their parents, who defend their homeland or were unable to leave Ukraine with their children under martial law, and more than 2 million children and their families have fled Ukraine. Children staying in Ukraine remain in danger. During air raids, children are forced to study and often spend the night in bomb shelters in crowded conditions, lacking fresh air. This increases the risk of developing respiratory diseases.[11]

Russia has destroyed half of Ukraine's power-generating capacity, which during peak times, especially in winter, leads to emergency power outages of electricity, communications, heating, and water supply throughout the country. This makes it difficult to provide children with an education and contributes to an increase in respiratory illness. Refugee children and their families (internally displaced persons: IDP), who often live in temporary dormitories, are in a particularly difficult situation.

Access to medical care for children is difficult in the frontline and deoccupied territories of Ukraine, primarily due a lack of medical professionals, which, together with extremely difficult living conditions, affects access to and quality of medical care for children and adults, including emergency medical care, medical examinations, and vaccinations.

Currently, the situation in the frontline regions has worsened due to the relocation of medical workers to other regions of Ukraine and their emigration. This requires special measures to ensure medical care for children in these areas, namely volunteering and using medical workers from other regions to work temporarily in these regions.

Against the backdrop of the war and the COVID-19 pandemic, general and primary disability among children has increased in Ukraine. Thus, in 2015, 153,547 children with disabilities were registered in Ukraine, and in 2023, there were 158,901 children despite fewer children remaining in Ukraine and difficulty with reporting (**Figs. 3–5**). The lowest rates of disability are in the temporarily occupied and recently liberated regions, since it is challenging to collect data from these areas. For example, in the Kherson region, the number of registered children with disabilities has decreased by more than three times compared to 2021.

Despite the above data, compared to 2021, the rate of disability in children aged 0 to 17 years has increased 30% due to skin and subcutaneous tissue diseases, 20.3% due to mental and behavioral disorders, 7.1% due to respiratory diseases, and 3.3% due to digestive diseases. Mental and behavioral disorders have increased the most among school-age children and adolescents, accounting for 33.1% of the causes of primary disability in children in war conditions.[12]

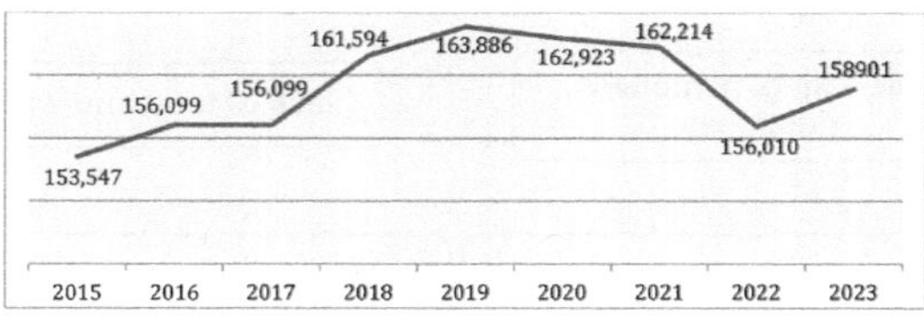

Fig. 3. The number of children with disabilities from 2015 to 2023 according to the Public Health Center of the Ministry of Health of Ukraine. (*Source* Polyanska L, Sazonova I. Total disability of children aged 0 - 17 years in Ukraine». Information and statistical guide for 2021 – 2023. State Institution "Public Health Center of the Ministry of Health of Ukraine". Kyiv. 2024. p. 32.)

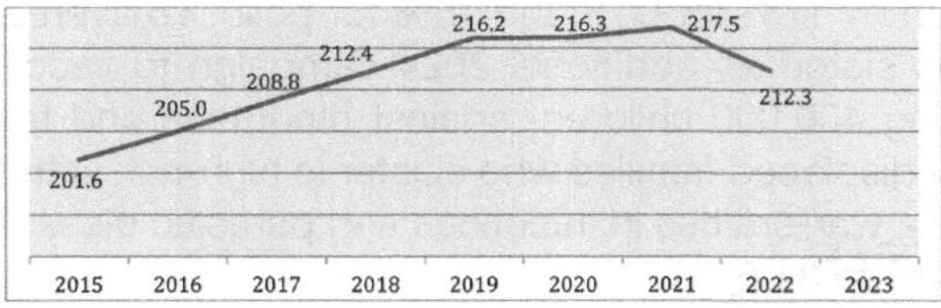

Fig. 4. The rate of general disability of children from 2015 to 2023 according to the Center for Public Health of the Ministry of Health of Ukraine (per 10 thousand people). (*Source* Polyanska L, Sazonova I. Total disability of children aged 0 - 17 years in Ukraine. Information and statistical guide for 2021 – 2023. State Institution "Public Health Center of the Ministry of Health of Ukraine". Kyiv. 2024. p. 32.)

TREATMENT OF CHRONIC DISEASES

Assessing the true burden of chronic illness among Ukrainian children in 2022 to 2024 is hampered by incomplete surveillance. Nonetheless, available figures reveal troubling upward trends. In 2023, the tuberculosis (TB) incidence among children aged 0 to 14 years reached 10.4 per 100,000 marking a 40.5% rise from 2022 and accounting for 3.2% of all registered TB cases. Adolescents aged 15 to 17 years had an even sharper increase of 55.3% from 10.3 to 16.0 per 100,000. Coinfection of active TB with human immunodeficiency virus climbed by 5.1%, reaching 8.2 per 100,000 in 2023.[12] The 2023 to 2024 respiratory-virus season underscored children's vulnerability: influenza, acute respiratory viral infections, and COVID-19 together affected young patients in more than half of all reported cases. Beyond TB and viral pathogens, global patterns point to rising asthma, pediatric diabetes, childhood obesity, and cancer, trends that Ukraine's strained health care funding may soon be unable to monitor, let alone manage.[11]

ACCESS TO IMMUNIZATION

Routine childhood vaccination once formed a robust shield against 10 diseases including TB, poliomyelitis, diphtheria, pertussis, tetanus, measles, hepatitis B, *Haemophilus influenzae* type b, rubella, and mumps. These were provided for free under Ukraine's public-procurement program. However, war has frayed these defenses. In 2023, diphtheria tetanus pertussis (DTP) coverage plunged 16% below prewar baselines and lagged by 37% behind European Union (EU) averages; polio immunization fell by 22%. Only 83.4% of infants aged under 1 year received the 3 dose DTP series, and just 84.9% had their polio immunization. The war decreased the percentage of

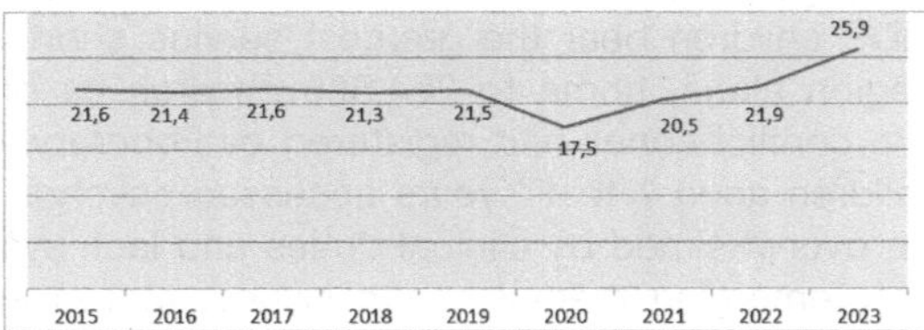

Fig. 5. The rate of primary disability among children from 2015 to 2023 according to the Center for Public Health of the Ministry of Health of Ukraine (per 10 thousand people). (*Source* Polyanska L, Sazonova I. Disability of children aged 0 - 17 years in Ukraine. who first became disabled in 2021 - 2023»»». Information and statistical guide for 2023. State Institution "Public Health Center of the Ministry of Health of Ukraine". Kyiv. 2024. p.28.)

immunized children by 17% for DTP and 15% for polio. To avert outbreaks, the Ministry of Health has slated an additional 2024 campaign to vaccinate over 1 million Ukrainians including 400,000 children, against diphtheria and tetanus, with special focus on internally displaced families who cluster in high-risk settings.[12] This urgency is underscored by a war-era rise in infectious and parasitic disease incidence among infants from 22.64% to 31.68%.

HUMANITARIAN IMPACT OF MARTIAL LAW ON CHILDREN'S HEALTH

Since February 2022, violence has displaced nearly two-thirds of Ukraine's children. Widespread loss of income and an energy crisis have compounded nutritional, housing, and health care insecurities. A United Nations Children's Fund (UNICEF) survey reported that 80% of families see their finances deteriorating, and child poverty has soared from 43% to 82%, not just for war regions or for IDP. Among the 5.9 million IDP, access to essential services is severely disrupted, while the destruction of nearly 300 medical facilities by late 2023 has decimated pediatric care capacity in frontline regions.[9,12]

MENTAL HEALTH CRISIS AMONG UKRAINIAN CHILDREN

Since February 2022, the mental well-being of Ukraine's children has been shattered. An estimated 1.5 million children now face heightened risks of depression, anxiety, and posttraumatic stress disorder (PTSD); normal reactions to abnormal events that without timely support, foster long-term physical, psychological, and social maladjustment. According to the WHO, roughly 10% of trauma survivors develop significant psychological trauma and another 10% manifest behavioral or psychiatric disorders that affect daily life.[13,14] In 2023, the Ukrainian Children's Fund surveyed 2000 mothers of 3 to 17 year olds, excluding occupied Crimea and Donbas. Key findings were that 60% of children had directly endured war-related events, most frequently separation from family or friends (28%), relocation (25%), shelling (24%), and prolonged stays in shelters (17%). As well 11% fled abroad with their mothers; 8% lived under occupation; 6% witnessed deaths; 5% faced hunger or water scarcity. Among adolescents aged over 16 years, anxiety (fear of the future, insomnia, nightmares, and concentration problems) was most common; in children aged 3 to 9 years, traumatic reenactments appeared in play and art. However, only 13% of mothers believed their children required professional support, and just 5% had sought it in the preceding 3 months. Of those who did seek help, 93% obtained services, 78% in person, 8% online, and 7% by phone.[15]

Despite high levels of distress, many families reported that their children did not need medical care; 40% had sought general medical services in the past quarter (most often for those aged under 5 years), and 98% of those requests were fulfilled either in person. IDP children bear the greatest service shortfall. In the western Ivano Frankivsk region alone, home to 264,566 children as of November 2024, 30,640 arrivals from conflict zones had registered by February 2024, yet only 458 (2.5%) of these children aged 7 to 17 years accessed psychological support that year. Clinicians are overwhelmed by clinical duties and lack systematic screening protocols to identify emerging mental health issues. Moreover, the absence of any national register for displaced children thwarts coordinated monitoring and timely intervention.[16,17]

Without swift, coordinated action, the unseen wounds of war will scar Ukraine's children long after the last shell falls. Their recovery, and the nation's future, depends on our collective resolve to protect and heal the most vulnerable.

THE STATE OF EDUCATION DURING MARTIAL LAW IN UKRAINE

Under martial law, access to education varies significantly depending on the place of residence. In urban areas, the organization of the educational process is better due to more stable infrastructure and better provision of technology. In contrast, in villages, the war has exacerbated long-standing problems: lack of equipment, unreliable Internet, teacher shortages, and lack of safe shelters.

Among children from low-income families, 32% in urban areas and 46% in rural areas do not have regular access to education. At the same time, among IDP, schoolchildren in urban areas have 86% enrollment and 80% in rural areas. This indicates significant, but still insufficient, support from the state and international organizations in meeting the educational needs of IDPs. The monitoring of school readiness for the 2024 - 2025 academic year revealed that 57% of students planned full-time education, 21% mixed (full-time + distance), 22% only distance. Despite frequent air alerts, 89% of principals, 84% of teachers, and 84% of students consider the current learning format safe. The main criteria for choosing the school's mode of operation are the availability of shelter (90%), security in the region (70%), and the opinion of parents (45%). The institutional audit for 2023 to 2024 showed that 74% of schools have basic shelters, 17% do not have them at all, and 14% to 26% of institutions cannot accommodate the number of children needing shelter. Seventy-one percent of students complain that classes are interrupted during the alarms, and the premises are unsuitable for classes. The loss of logistical support has also exacerbated inequality.[15]

Twelve percent of schools do not have Internet access, especially in villages, where it is often the only option for remote learning. Only 46% of high school students have access to desktop computers or tablets, and 63% to 74% use smartphones. Among younger students, these figures are even lower. In 40% of primary school families and 23% of secondary school families, children share 1 device. Although the number of teachers with computers has increased compared to 2021 to 2022, 25% of teachers still do not have their own workplace, and 20% of schools do not have Internet.[18]

Despite the destruction and economic difficulties, the Ukrainian education system has shown impressive resilience. Thanks to the efforts of educators, the government, and international partners, conditions are being created to support learning, address the psycho-emotional needs of students, and gradually overcome educational losses. However, every lack of communication, every malfunctioning shelter, and every unreached child is a risk of irreversible gaps in the knowledge that will shape their future.

Helping children during the war in Ukraine requires coordination between the international humanitarian community, local organizations, the government, and volunteers. Providing basic needs, psychosocial support, and access to health care and education are key aspects of preserving the health and future of Ukrainian children. Only in close cooperation between the Government of Ukraine and civil society, with the support of the international community, and through the decisive and effective actions of the UN, WHO, UNICEF, the World Bank, other international institutions, and volunteer organizations, will we be able to overcome the unprecedentedly devastating consequences of the war.[19]

MEDICAL EDUCATION

Medical education of future pediatricians, both students and residents, has also been challenging during war. War affects both education and daily life. At the fall of the Soviet Union in 1991, Ukraine had 14 medical institutes aimed at teaching medical and pharmaceutical sciences. In 2022, Ukraine had 23 medical institutions with both Ukrainian nationals and medical students from around the world.[20] Many students, especially international students, have left Ukraine, and some medical educators have moved to field hospitals in or near the war zone, some have left, and others face stress of an increased workload. Much of this burden falls on residents and fellows.

A cross-sectional study of 776 Ukrainian medical students in years 2 to 5 at I. Horbachevsky Ternopil National Medical University to evaluate the emotional well-being and academic achievement of these students.[21] Following the first 18 months of the war, 62.5%, 59.6%, and 58.8% of Ukrainian medical students self-reported signs of stress, anxiety, and depression, respectively. Severe and extremely severe depressive symptoms were reported in 25.6% of students, anxiety in 31.9%, and stress in 29.7%, with a higher prevalence among female students, and 44.2% of responders had significant symptoms of PTSD. Academic performance in 2023 was significantly lower compared to the prewar period in 2019.

Medical schools from around the world have stepped up to the challenge of helping these students continue their studies. As an example, during the summer of 2022, the School of Clinical Medicine, University of Cambridge hosted 20 medical students from Kharkiv National Medical University for a 7 week intensive clinical elective program to provide an immersive clinical placement that would help students to attain the necessary knowledge and experience to become competent and confident practicing doctors.[22–24]

HOW CAN YOU HELP?

Childhood in war is a horror that cannot be forgotten. To ensure children's resilience and resistance to emotional and physical suffering, comprehensive assistance is needed—from providing all the basic support for a stable life to constant, uninterrupted attention to mental health with the development and implementation of individualized rehabilitation and education programs that have already found their place in the lives of children of war. Resources are also always needed to provide hospital care and training for Ukrainian pediatricians.

You can make donations to well-known organizations such as UNICEF, Save the Children, Voices of Children, The Children of Ukraine Foundation, and GlobalGiving to help children in Ukraine with nutrition, medical care, education, and psychological support. Other reputable organizations include the International Rescue Committee, which helps refugees, Nova Ukraine, a nonprofit organization that focuses on humanitarian aid and building a stronger democratic society, and United Help Ukraine (https://unitedhelpukraine.org/), a 501c3 nonprofit organization that supports children's health and education. For additional information, please contact Prof Mariia Kiselova (maria.kiselova@hotmail.com), Prof Bruce Rubin (bkrubin@outlook.com), or Prof Oleksandr Volosovets (avolosovets@gmail.com).

DECLARATION OF ARTIFICIAL INTELLIGENCE AND ARTIFICIAL INTELLIGENCE-ASSISTED TECHNOLOGIES IN THE WRITING PROCESS

During the preparation of this article, the authors used ChatGTP in order to comprehensively cover the topic and to prepare a first draft of the article. After using this tool/service, the authors reviewed and edited the content as needed and take full responsibility for the content of the publication.

ACKNOWLEDGMENTS

The authors acknowledge the contributions of Halyna Beketova, MD, Oksana Vygovska MD, Tatiana Mavropulo, MD, Iryna Redko, MD, Roman Gan, PhD, Kateryna

Savinova, PhD, Lesia Sakalosh, PhD, Khrystyna Slivinska-Kurchak, PhD, and Roman Kizyma.

DISCLOSURE

The authors all report no conflicts of interest related to this article.

REFERENCES

1. Олена Зеленська: МаєМо дати дітяМ гідне дитинство всупереч російській агресі. Available at: https://www.president.gov.ua/news/olena-zelenska-mayemo-dati-dityam-gidne-ditinstvo-vsuperech-99141. Accessed September 23, 2025.
2. Anjum G, Aziz M, Hamid HK. Life and mental health in limbo of the Ukraine war: how can helpers assist civilians, asylum seekers and refugees affected by the war? Front Psychol 2023;14:11292–9.
3. War in Ukraine pushes a generation of children to the brink, warns UNICEF. UNICEF Ukraine. Available at: https://www.unicef.org/ukraine/press-releases/war-ukraine-pushes-generation-children-brink-warns-unicef. Accessed September 23, 2025.
4. Acute reaction to stress. Post-traumatic stress disorder. Disorder of adaptation. Evidence-based clinical practice guideline. 2024. Available at: https://www.dec.gov.ua/wp-content/uploads/2024/07/kn_2024_ptsr.pdf. Accessed March 18, 2025.
5. Mortality rate in Ukraine exceeded birth rate almost three times last year—Ministry of justice. Available at: https://www.ukrinform.ua/rubric-society/3955261-v-ukraini-torik-smertnist-perevisila-narodzuvanist-majze-vtrici-minust.html. Accessed March 15, 2025.
6. Antipkin YG, Volosovets OP, Maidanik VG, et al. The state of health of the child population—the future of the country (part 1). Child Health 2018;13(1):1–15.
7. Volosovets OP, Abaturov OE, Beketova GV, et al. Fertility, perinatal mortality and infant mortality in Ukraine: evolution from 1991 to 2021 and current risks. Zdorovia Dytyny 2022;17(7):6–17. Available at: http://www.mifua.com/media/uploads/arhiv/zr/2022/7(tom%2017)/ZR_7(Tom17)(zak125)_2022.pdf.
8. United Nations in Ukraine. Statement from Danielle Bell, the head of the United Nations Human rights monitoring Mission in Ukraine. 2025. Available at: https://ukraine.un.org/en/301207-statement-danielle-bell-head-united-nations-human-rights-monitoring-mission-ukraine. Accessed December 27, 2025.
9. WHO reports on 1,940 confirmed attacks by Russians on healthcare facilities in Ukraine. Available at: https://www.who.int/ukraine/news/item/19-08-2024-grim-milestone-on-world-humanitarian-day–who-records-1940-attacks-on-health-care-in-ukraine-since-start-of-full-scale-war. Accessed September 25, 2025.
10. Institute for the Study of War. Russia is turning deported Ukrainian children into bargaining chips. Washington, DC: Institute for the Study of War; 2023. Available at: https://www.understandingwar.org. Accessed September 23, 2025.
11. Volosovets OP, Vyhovska OV, Kryvopustov SP, et al. Wojciech Feleszko Problems of providing medical care to children of Ukraine because of Russian aggression. Child Health 2023;18:9–13.
12. Polyanska L., Sazonova I. Disability of children aged 0 - 17 years in Ukraine. who first became disabled in 2021 - 2023. Information and statistical guide for 2023. State Institution “Public Health Center of the Ministry of Health of Ukraine”. Kyiv. 2024.
13. Agulnik A, Nogovitsyna Y, Kizyma R, et al. Strategies to promote sustainable care for children with cancer in Ukraine. Lancet Oncol 2024;25(3):285–8.

14. Additional round of immunization against diphtheria and tetanus: how to check your vaccine status and get vaccinated free of charge. Available at: https://moz.gov.ua/uk/dodatkovij-raund-z-imunizaciyi-proti-difteriyi-ta-pravcya-yak-pereviriti-svij-vakcinalnij-status-i-otrimati-sheplennya-bezoplatno. Accessed September 23, 2025.
15. World Health Organization. Three years of war: rising demand for mental health support, trauma care and rehabilitation. Geneva: WHO; 2025. Available at: https://www.who.int/europe/news/item/24-02-2025-three-years-of-war-rising-demand-for-mental-health-support-trauma-care-and-rehabilitation. Accessed September 23, 2025.
16. 18 months of war for Ukraine's children. UNICEF Ukraine. Available at: https://www.unicef.org/ukraine/documents/18-months-of-war-for-ukraines-children. Accessed September 30, 2025.
17. Bürgin D, Anagnostopoulos D, Vitiello B, et al, Board and Policy Division of ESCAP. Impact of war and forced displacement on children's mental health—multilevel, needs-oriented, and trauma-informed approaches. Eur Child Adolesc Psychiatry 2022;31:845–53.
18. Anjum G, Aziz M, Hamid HK. Life and mental health in limbo of the Ukraine war: how can helpers assist civilians, asylum seekers and refugees affected by the war? Front Psychol 2023;14:1129299.
19. UNICEF. 5.3 million children in Ukraine have limited access to education. 2023; 14:1129299. Available at: https://www.unicef.org/ukraine/press-releases/war-has-hampered-education. Accessed September 23, 2025.
20. Education in Ukraine under the conditions of the state of martial information and analytical compilation. Kyiv 2022. Available at: https://mon.gov.ua/static-objects/mon/sites/1/zagalna%20serednya/serpneva-konferencia/2022/Mizhn.serpn.ped.nauk-prakt.konferentsiya/Inform-analityc.zbirnOsvita.Ukrayiny.v.umovakh.voyennoho.stanu.22.08.2022.pdf (in Ukrainian).
21. War in Ukraine pushes a generation of children to the brink, warns UNICEF. Available at: https://www.unicef.org/ukraine/press-releases/war-ukraine-pushes-generation-children-brink-warns-unicef. Accessed September 23, 2025.
22. Srichawla BS, Khazeei Tabari MA, Găman MA, et al. War on Ukraine: impact on Ukrainian medical students. Int J Med Stud 2022;10(1):15–7.
23. KordaM SA, Shevchuk O, Shulhai O, et al. Psychological well-being and academic performance of Ukrainian medical students under the burden of war: a cross-sectional study. Front Public Health 2025;12:1457026.
24. Hodkinson J, Lillicrap M, Wilkinson P, et al. Medical education through an invasion: insights from an elective programme for Ukrainian medical students at the University of Cambridge. Front Med 2023;10:1211526.

Latin American Children of the US Immigration Crisis

The Essential Roles that All Pediatric Health Care Professionals Must Play

Janine Young, MD[a,*], Marsha Rae Griffin, MD[b], Jose Ignacio Santos, MD, MS[c], Bruce Lesley, MA[d], Eric A. Russell, MD[e], Fernando Sanchez Mendoza, MD, MPH[f]

KEYWORDS

- Advocacy • Pediatric health care • Immigrant children
- Unaccompanied immigrant children • Latin America • Deportation • Legal status
- Undocumented

KEY POINTS

- Current US immigration policy negatively impacts the health and wellbeing of immigrant children, their families and the communities where they live.
- Pediatric health care professionals have been at the forefront of advocating for immigrant children who currently make up 26.5% of all US children.
- Advocacy for immigrant children comes in many forms including *clinical advocacy,* community *advocacy*, and *advocacy through U.S. legal and policy efforts.*
- The health of immigrant children moving through Latin America to the United States is a long-standing humanitarian crisis in need of a coordinated multinational response.
- Multinational data sharing of real-time public health needs of migrating children is essential to allow for collaborative positive child health responses.

[a] Division of Academic General Pediatrics, Department of Pediatrics, University of California San Diego School of Medicine, 7910 Frost Street, 345, San Diego, CA 92123, USA; [b] Community for Children, Inc., 1527 47th Street, Sacramento, CA 95819, USA; [c] Experimental Research Unit, National Autonomous University of Mexico, Torre de Investigacion, 5to piso, Facultad de Medicina, UNAM/Hospital General de Mexico, Dr. Balmis No. 148, Col. Doctores, Alcaldia Cuauhtemoc, C.P. 06726, Mexico City, Mexico; [d] First Focus on Children, 1400 I Street, NW, Washington, DC, 20005, USA; [e] Division of Pediatric Emergency Medicine, Baylor College of Medicine, 6621 Fannin Street, A2210, Houston, TX 77030, USA; [f] Division of Academic General Pediatrics, Department of Pediatrics, Stanford University School of Medicine, 453 Quarry Road, Mail Code 5660, Palo Alto, CA 94304-1419, USA

* Corresponding author.

E-mail address: jay028@health.ucsd.edu

Pediatr Clin N Am 73 (2026) 1091–1116

https://doi.org/10.1016/j.pcl.2026.05.009 **pediatric.theclinics.com**

Abbreviations	
AAP	American Academy of Pediatrics
CBO	community-based organization
CBP	Customs and Border Protection
CHIP	Children's Health Insurance Program
EBLL	elevated blood lead level
IMSS	Instituto Mexicano de Seguro Social
LTBI	latent tuberculosis infection
NBS	newborn screening
PAHO	Pan American Health Organization

BACKGROUND

We live in unprecedented times with the US federal government enacting dracionian and questionably legal immigration policies without any concern for their impact on immigrant and US children's welfare and wellbeing. Historically and in present day, pediatric health care professionals and child health advocates have been and are at the forefront of providing essential support to these children and, today, we must also do so.

US immigration policies directly affect the well-being of immigrant children and therefore, pediatric health care professionals need to understand immigration terms and definitions (**Table 1**).[1–8] Limiting entry of specific groups is a prominent feature of US history, as exemplified by the *1924 Immigration Act*, which excluded people from Ireland, Italy, and China.[9,10] Specific focus on Latin American children began in earnest in 1929 with the *Undesirable Aliens Act*, that targeted Mexican immigrants and made undocumented migration illegal.[11] In 1929, President Hoover ordered the repatriation of Mexican and Mexican–Americans (US-born) and deported approximately 2 million people, with 60% thought to be US citizens, most of them children.[12] It was in this environment and time that the American Academy of Pediatrics (AAP) was founded,[13] when 23% of US children were immigrants primarily from the United Kingdom, France, Germany, and Ireland,[10] and when the AAP began its efforts to enhance the health and well-being of all children by addressing the social determinants of health, child health, and public health services.[14]

The US has always been made up of significant numbers of immigrants. This includes during our more recent history; in fact, data comparing the percentage of children in immigrant families in 1990 versus 2023 show an increase in the number of children in immigrant families throughout all US states from 13.4% to 26.5%, with a median increase of 200%.[3]

Throughout US history, immigration policies have directly impacted immigrant children by (1) determining eligibility for US entry and placing barriers to achieving naturalization, thereby limiting access to resources[12] (ie, refugee status, asylum status, Trafficking or Special Immigrant Juvenile visas) (see **Table 1**); (2) defining and modifying a child's deportation risk; (3) creating deportation risks for undocumented guardians; and (4) influencing the perception of safety in immigrant communities, thereby impacting children's lives. Most children migrating to the US, whether with families or as unaccompanied children, come from Mexico and Central America[15]; other immigrants come from South America, the Caribbean, Africa, China, India, and other less-represented countries.[16,17]

With the current administration's border immigration enforcement efforts, border crossings have significantly decreased; in fact, as November 2025 there were 154,991 attempted border crossings compared to 1,456,019 in 2024.[18] This drop in

Table 1
Key terms and definitions

Term	Definition
Undocumented immigrant child	Without legal authority and legal documents to remain in the US
Unaccompanied immigrant child; Unaccompanied minor	Children who have migrated to the United States alone, have been trafficked there, and/or who arrived at the US border with a nonlegal guardian (eg, grandmother, adult sibling, uncle, aunt) and separated from that adult by US Department of Homeland Security or Customs and Border Protecation
Refugee status	Legal status granted overseas to populations deemed admissible to the US by the sitting US President with a pathway to citizenship; must prove a well-founded fear of persecution in home country[2]
Immigrant child; Child in immigrant family	A general term for any child who either immigrated to the US, or who is US-born to at least 1 immigrant parent[3]
Migrant child	A general term for a child who has or is migrating from their home country due to a desire to reunite with a US legal guardian or other relative, to escape persecution, abject poverty, abuse, neglect, abandonment, and/or natural disasters[4]
Asylum seeker status	Someone who has a well-founded fear of persecution in home country (refugee definition) and presents at a US border or port of entry, including a US consulate or embassy overseas[5]
Asylee	Someone granted legal status after claiming asylum seeker status; pathway to citizenship[5]
US Department of Homeland Security	The US federal agency that oversees Customs and Border Protection and Immigration Customs Enforcement
Customs and Border Protection	Overseen by the US Department of Homeland Security, CBP has authority to secure US borders, apprehend people crossing US borders, detain people in CBP-run detention centers at the US border, and deport or release into the US pending judicial review by an immigration judge; CBP is granted legal guardianship of unaccompanied children until these children are relinquished to the US Office of Refugee Resettlement custody
Immigration and Customs Enforcement	Overseen by the US Department of Homeland Security, Immigration and Customs Enforcement is a federal law enforcement agency and has the authority to enforce immigration laws, including the arrest, detainment and deportation of undocumented immigrants
US Department of Health and Human Services	The US federal agency that oversees the Office of Refugee Resettlement
Office of Refugee Resettlement	Overseen by the US Department of Health and Human Services, the Office of Refugee Resettlement has been funded to oversee housing and medical screening of unaccompanied immigrant children until released to a US legal guardian or nonlegal guardian sponsor

(*continued on next page*)

Table 1
(*continued*)

Term	Definition
Trafficking Visa	A legal status provided to children (and adults) who are able to prove that they were subjected to extreme forms of trafficking including labor and sex trafficking[6]
Special Immigrant Juvenile Visa	A legal status provided to children who are able to prove that they were abandoned, abused, and/or neglected in their home country[7]
Naturalization	Process to obtain US citizenship through requirements set by Congress[8]

crossings has led to a focus on undocumented immigrants far from the border and has put greater emphasis on immigration enforcement throughout the US, where the majority of non–US-born immigrant children are established in their communities. The resulting social disruption for these children has negatively impacted access to essential health care, mental health, social, and educational services; this toxic stress negatively affects their physical and mental well-being.[19–21] Not only are pediatric health care professionals concerned about the deportation of undocumented children, but they are also concerned about the deportation of undocumented parents who may have US-born children, who can then be faced with being left parentless.

This article will address the needs of immigrant children, provide examples of advocacy efforts, and make policy recommendations. Below, we discuss essential ways in which pediatric health care professionals can make a difference.

Note, immigrant children include (1) undocumented unaccompanied immigrant children, (2) undocumented children of immigrant families, and (3) US-born citizen children of an undocumented parent (see **Table 1**). The latter consists of approximately 4.5 million children in the US,[22] and for those whose parents are deported, can be further categorized into US citizen children removed with parents to the parents' country of origin and US citizen children who lose their parents and remain with relatives or in US child protective service custody (**Fig. 1**).[23]

CLINICAL ADVOCACY FOR IMMIGRANT CHILDREN

Immigrant child advocacy comes in many forms. Most immigrant children born in low- and middle-income countries who now live in the US (approximately 2.5 million making up 3.5% of all children living in the US)[24] (see **Fig. 1**) did not have access to routine well child examinations (including assessments of growth, development, hearing, vision, blood pressure), or systematic serologic screening for medical issues in their home countries, including for latent tuberculosis (TB) or strongylodiasis.[25–28] The support for and provision of evidence-based medical care to screen for and address health issues is one direct way in which pediatric health care professionals can advocate.

Advocacy also includes ensuring that state requirements and curricula are developed to provide medical providers with training in immigrant health. Some academic medical centers have begun to offer formal training in immigrant health; others have developed electives that teach about issues that are unique to immigrant children.[29] **Table 2**[30–33] presents key training topics needed to deliver evidence-based care to immigrant children.

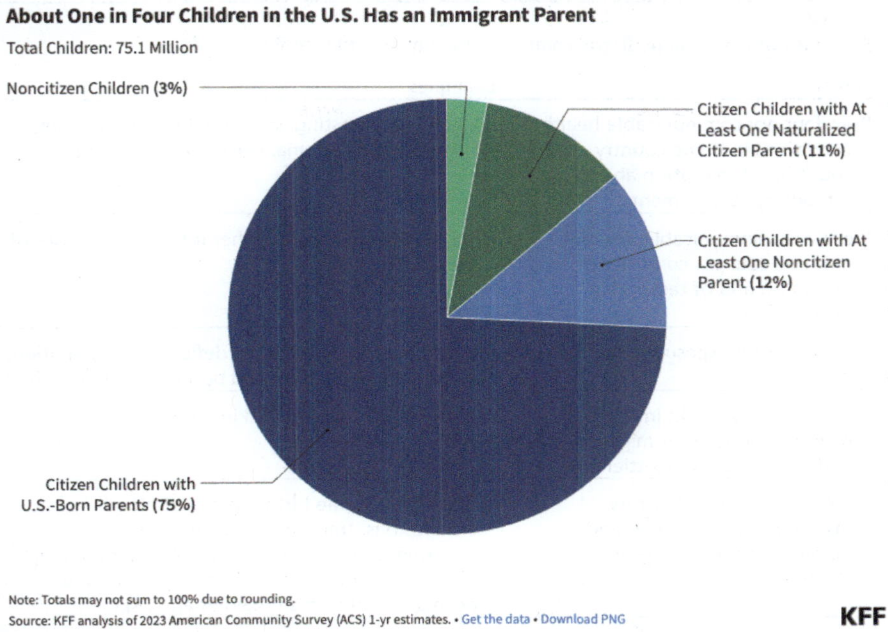

Fig. 1. Numbers of US children in immigrant families, 2023.[23] (*Source* Drishti Pillai, Akash Pillai, and Samantha Artiga, Children in Immigrant Families: Key Facts on Health Coverage and Care, KFF, May 19, 2026. URL: https://www.kff.org/racial-equity-and-health-policy/children-of-immigrants-key-facts-on-health-coverage-and-care/. Accessed December 10th, 2025.)

Below is a brief overview of other important aspects of clinical care that includes a summary of recommended laboratory screening for Latin American non–US-born immigrant children based on available disease prevalence. Screening should be provided when caring for these children, whether recently arrived in the US or have been living there for years.

Of note, when provision of medical care is discussed, cost of this care for children and caregivers also needs to be considered. As of 2025, 14 states and Washington, DC have Medicaid coverage for all children, including immigrant children without legal status.[34] However, in states without Medicaid coverage for all children, this is yet another area requiring advocacy on the part of health care professionals. In fact, it is with health care provider advocacy that current states with Medicaid coverage for all children passed this essential legislation.[35]

AN ESSENTIAL UNDERSTANDING OF LATIN AMERICAN CHILD AND ADOLESCENT HEALTH

Compared to US-born children, Latin American–born infants, children and adolescents have higher rates of anemia, an increased risk of exposure to active TB, and variable rates of acute malnutrition, with higher rates in children in Haiti (5.0%) and Barbados (6.8%). Coverage for the first 3 DTP vaccines at 1-year of life is highly variable in Latin America, ranging from 54% in Venezuela and Haiti, to 99% coverage in multiple other countries (**Table 3**).[36–42]

The impact of violence on children and adolescents in Latin America cannot be overstated with staggering homicide rates in multiple countries, including the highest

Table 2
Examples of essential pediatric immigrant health curricular topics

Topics	Examples
Prevalent noncommunicable health conditions in home country, countries of migration and of temporary resettlement	malnutrition, wasting, stunting, obesity, diabetes, hypertension, asthma, chronic lung disease
Prevalent communicable diseases in home country, countries of migration and of temporary resettlement	tropical medicine topics, other infectious diseases of significance
Environmental exposure risks	mercury, lead, arsenic, iodine deficiency, air pollution, exposure to open fires and burning of biomass fuel
Trauma exposure risks in home country, countries of migration and of temporary resettlement	risk of assault, rape, trafficking, injury
Approach to medical history taking of newly arriving and longer-standing immigrant children	birth weight, home birth, history of blood transfusions, traditional cutting, surgeries, assessment of risk for vertically and horizontally transmitted infections, cultural practices and beliefs, use of home remedies and risks
Approach to obtaining a social history	migration history, education history, literacy, numeracy, home supports, family structure, separation for siblings, parents, history of US Office of Refugee Resettlement shelter custody as proxy for unaccompanied immigrant child status
Approach to comprehensive physical examination	performing a head-to-toe examination looking for missed diagnoses including dental caries, congenital heart disease, rhematic heart disease, renal disease, goiter, malnutrition, rickets, undescended testicles
Recommended laboratory screening for immigrant children	Centers for Disease Control Domestic Refugee Screening Guidelines[30] CareRef[31]
Legal status as a social determinant of health	Legal status types and linkage to immigration supports; medical/legal partnerships, local and national resources
Pediatric anticipatory guidance for immigrant children and families	Education laws, labor laws (including limit to hours worked and type of work allowed),[32] immigration enforcement and safety of children in families at risk of deportation, medication dosages and measuring, literacy of family and best ways to provide medical information, antibiotic use, preventive care and frequency, ER use, 911, dental visits; nutrition
Travel to visit friends or relatives	Vaccines and prophylactic medications prior to travel;[33] Laboratory screening recommended on return to the US
Vicarious trauma/moral injury	Mental health and well -being supports for health care providers

Table 3
Latin American health data by country of origin compared to US health data[36–39]

	Health Expenditure, % of GDP, 2021[a]	Anemia[40](6–59 mo) <11 g/dL 2019 Data %	Active TB[41] Per 100,000 Population, all Ages, 2023	DTP3 Coverage at 1-Year-Old, %, 2023	Pediatric Obesity, 5–19 y, %, 2022	Wasting at <5 y, %
Argentina	9.71	19	35	66	20.3	1.7
Barbados	8.09	20	0.81	85	23	6.8
Belize	4.98	23	27	85	21.8	1.8
Bolivia	8.16	37	105	67	16.3	2.0
Brazil	9.89	12	49	90	15.5	3.4
Chile	9.32	20	18	96	27.5	0.3
Colombia	9.02	22	46	90	10.6	1.6
Costa Rica	7.57	19	9.9	99	13.8	1.8
Cuba	13.79	18	7.9	99	17.1	2.0
Dominican Republic	4.92	28	42	90	15.5	2.2
Ecuador	8.29	24	58	70	12.6	0.7
El Salvador	9.72	25	84	96	11.6	2.9
Guatemala	6.90	10	33	88	7.7	0.8
Haiti	3.48	60	149	54	11.4	5.0
Honduras	9.16	26	31	73	12.6	1.9
Jamaica	7.19	23	3.2	99	15.5	3.2
Mexico[42]	6.08	22	29	85	17.7	1.0
Nicaragua	9.68	21	43	n/a	12.8	2.2

(*continued on next page*)

Table 3
(continued)

	Health Expenditure, % of GDP, 2021[a]	Anemia[40](6–59 mo) <11 g/dL 2019 Data %	Active TB[41] Per 100,000 Population, all Ages, 2023	DTP3 Coverage at 1-Year-Old, %, 2023	Pediatric Obesity, 5–19 y, %, 2022	Wasting at <5 y, %
Panama	9.68	16	58	71	14.3	1.1
Paraguay	8.03	28	62	71	14.5	1.0
Peru	6.15	30	173	84	17	0.6
Suriname	5.68	39 (2014)	29	72	18.2	5.5
Uruguay	9.36	25	42	95	17.7	1.4
Venezuela	4.01	28	45	54	14.9	4.1
US (comparison)	17.36	6	3.1	94	20.6	0.1

Note: No data available for new HIV infections (as of 2023) and prevalence of hepatitis B (as of 2020), by country; no data available for stunting of children less than 5 y.

Abbreviation: n/a, not available.

[a] Health expenditure percentages of gross domestic product are noted to provide context of investment in health by country and return on investment and include US data as a comparison.

Data compiled, unless otherwise noted, by J Young from https://data.who.int/countries/.

noted in El Salvador (86.98 deaths/100,000 population); prevalence of intimate partner violence (ages 15–49 years) and associated stress to children is also a significant issue in multiple countries, with Peru (38%) having the highest rate of violence. Access to effective family planning for adolescents and women also impact children and families, with Haiti (45.4%) having low access rates. High neonatal and under 5 year child mortality rates include Haiti, the Dominican Republic, and Venezuela (*neonatal*: 23.72, 22.31, 15 per 1000 live births; *<5 years*: 56.87, 32.25, 24.26 per 1000 live births, respectively); and maternal mortality per 100,000 live births is also staggeringly high for Haiti (327.6), Venezuela (226.7), and Bolivia (146.4) (**Table 4**).[42]

Table 5[43–46] summarizes the Centers for Disease Control and other public health agencies' recommended approach to laboratory screening of immigrant children from Latin America, based on available prevalence data. It is recommended that pediatric health care professionals follow these guidelines for both newly arriving children and select testing for those who have resided in the United States for years.

Newborn Screening

Only 16 of 33 Latin American countries have newborn screening (NBS) programs. Expanded NBS panels have been adopted in some countries; however, disease testing varies by region with rural areas having limited access to appropriate testing. As of 2021, only 6 countries have greater than or equal to 90% coverage and 12 have greater than or equal to 70% coverage. The 16 countries that have active NBS programs screen for congenital hypothyroidism, 14 for phenylketonuria, 12 for congenital adrenal hyperplasia and cystic fibrosis, and 8 for galactosemia.[45] NBS for hemoglobinopathies, including sickle cell disease, occurs in Brazil, Costa Rica, Panama, and Uruguay, however, also has limited access in remote areas.[47] This has resulted in children with missed diagnoses that must be considered.[48] Immigrant infants 12 months and younger should have NBS performed as well as thyroid function testing through age 5 years.[49]

Anemia and Lead

Screening occurs in all of Latin America, particularly for children under age 5.[50] However, prevalence of anemia and elevated blood lead levels (EBLL) varies by sociodemographic and economic status, with indigenous children and those living in rural areas noted to have higher rates than other children and in areas with specific lead-exposure environmental risks (eg, battery disposal sites). A 2021 pooled mean blood lead level study (**Fig. 2**)[51] notes a lack of data available in all of Central American and some South American countries.[51] Known lead exposures include the use of lead-tainted paint, spices, cosmetics, home remedies, and wrappings on candies.[52,53] Given high prevalence of anemia and EBLL and variable screening, all infants and children should have a complete blood count, differential and lead level sent.

Tuberculosis

Screening for latent tuberculosis infection (LTBI) has not been widely adopted across Latin America. The focus is on identifying and treating patients with active TB disease.[25] As such, it is essential to test for both active TB and LTBI in all immigrant infants and children from Latin America.[54]

Prenatal Infectious Diseases

Access to screening and what is included in testing varies across Latin America and depends on country, region, rurality of residence, and socio-economic status. For

Table 4
Pediatric-relevant health statistics by Latin American country and the US

Country	Proportion of Childbearing-Aged Females with Satisfied Needs for Effective Family Planning, %, 2022	Lifetime Physical and/or Sexual Intimate Partner Violence, Ages 15–49 y, 2018, %	Under 5 Mortality per 1000 Live Births, 2022	Births Attended by Skilled Health Worker, %, 2022	Neonatal Mortality per 1000 Live Births, 2022	Maternal Mortality per 100,000 Live Births, 2023	Homicide Rate per 100,000 Population, 2019
Argentina	80.3	5	9.85	99 (2020)	5.49	33.2	6.05
Barbados	70	n/a	10.38	98 (2020)	7.09	34.88	11.45
Belize	64.9	24	12.82	95 (2020)	9.36	66.8	37.89
Bolivia	50.3	18	23.94	72 (2022)	12.71	146.4	9.29
Brazil	89.3	23	14.59	98 (2021)	8.29	66.91	32.35
Chile	n/a	21	6.82	100	4.5	9.88	3.91
Colombia	86.6	30	12.42	98	6.77	59.4	38.87
Costa Rica	80.8	27	10.1	99 (2021)	6.93	24.12	12.36
Cuba	86.9	14	7.94	100 (2021)	3.99	34.8	5.07
Dominican Republic	77.4	19	32.25	99 (2019)	22.31	124.5	17.58
Ecuador	82.5	33	13.2	96 (2020)	7.16	55.4	6.96
El Salvador	73	21	10.82	99 (2021)	4.57	39.11	86.98
Guatemala	66.1	21	22.1	70 (2017)	10.36 (2021)	93.7	25.76
Haiti	45.4	23	56.87	42 (2016–2017)	23.72	327.6	20.88
Honduras	79	17	16.03	94 (2019)	9.15	46.7	64.08
Jamaica	78.7	24	19.26	100 (2021)	14.5	130.1	53.6
Mexico[42]	83.2	24	12.87	88 (2022)	7.87	42.11	30.07

Nicaragua	89.8	23	13.93	94 (2017)	8.89	60.3	9.25
Panama	65.2	16	13.88	93 (2021)	6.88	37	17.33
Paraguay	78.9	18	17.57	91 (2021)	9.41	58.27	8.68
Peru	67.2	38	16.13	95 (2023)	7.92	51.4	7.01
Suriname	57.5	28	16.79	100 (2021)	10.25	83.6	5.63
Uruguay	n/a	18	6.8	100 (2021)	4.33	15.31	8.61
Venezuela	n/a	19	24.26	99 (2018)	15	226.7	62.83
US	78.4	26	6.47	99 (2021)	3.44	16.63	5.78

Data compiled and adapted by J Young from https://data.who.int/countries/ unless otherwise noted.

Table 5
Essential US laboratory screening for immigrant children from Latin America[43–46]

	0–12 mo	13 mo-<12y	13y-<18y	Pregnant	Breastfeeding
Newborn screen	y	–	–	–	–
Thyroid function testing	y	y (some experts recommend testing through age 5 y)			
Venous Lead	y	y	y	y	y
Complete blood count and differential	y	y	y	y	y
Interferon gamma release assay (serum TB testing)	y	y	y	y	y
Hepatitis B Surface Antibody	y	y	y	y	y
Hepatitis C Antibody	y	y	y	y	y
HIV Antibody	y	y	y	y	y
Syphilis Enzyme Immunoassay or Rapid Plasma Reagin	y	y	y	y	y
Chagas disease, *T. cruzi* IgG serology (if resided >6 mo in Latin America)[46]	y	y	y	y	y
Strongyloides Immunoglobulin G	y	y	y	y	y
Stool ova and parasites x 2, collected 12–24 h apart (if <12 mo in US, eosinophilia, or symptoms suggesting a soil-transmitted helminth infection)	y	y	y	y	y
Giardia stool Antigen or stool polymerase chain reaction (PCR) for giardia	y	y (some experts recommend testing through age 5 y)	–	–	–
Urine gonorrhea/ chlamydia PCR	–	–	y	y	y
Urine pregnancy test	–	–	females: y	–	y

Adapted by J Young from the CDC Domestic Refugee Screening Guidelines and Care Ref, unless otherwise noted.

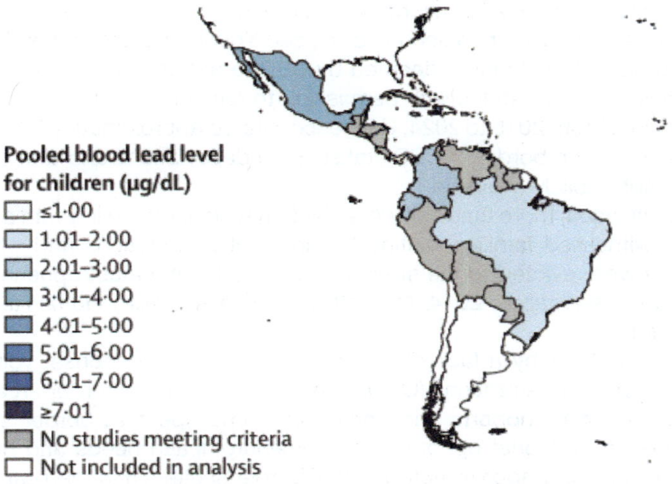

Fig. 2. Latin American children ages 0 to 14 years and pooled mean blood lead levels.[50] Map lines delineate study areas and do not necessarily depict accepted national boundaries. (Reprinted with permission from Elsevier. The Lancet Planetary Health, March 2021, 5 (3), e145-e153.)

example, in Mexico, pregnant females who present for prenatal care are universally screened for hepatitis B, C, HIV, and syphilis. However, prenatal Chagas disease screening has not been widely adopted.[46] Indigenous populations and those living in rural areas far from clinics tend to have decreased access to prenatal care and prenatal lab screening.[46,55–57] Based on lack of universal and comprehensive screening access across Latin America, infants and children of all ages whose mothers have no copies of records of prenatal lab testing results should be tested for all vertically transmitted infections, including hepatitis B, C, HIV, and syphilis.

THE EMERGENCE OF A HUMANITARIAN CRISIS LEADING TO GRASS ROOTS ADVOCACY

Pediatric health care providers and child advocates along the US–Mexico border have long been confronted with the needs of immigrant children. Below is a summary of children arriving at the border starting in 2014 who were granted permission to remain in the US pending immigration hearings (ie, asylum seekers), as these children have become the focus of heightened enforcement actions.

Large-scale migration of people across the southern border has been variously characterized as *a flood*, *an invasion*, or *a surge*. Those working with immigrant children at the border recognized increasing arrivals and raised the alarm through advocacy, finally capturing national attention in 2014.[58] US Customs and Border Protection (CBP) began releasing thousands of immigrant families at bus stations throughout the border region without providing food, shelter, or transportation assistance,[59] given that federal oversight and coordination ended at release.

Until 2025, when the Trump Administration terminated most legal pathways for entering the US, children crossed the southern US border by traveling with parents, relatives, family friends, alone or with smugglers. All children and families apprehended at the US border (as well as the limited number still permitted entry currently) are initially held in US CBP processing centers. CBP officers *process* both unaccompanied children and children with families. For a comprehensive explanation of procedures for unaccompanied children, see Young and colleagues.[1]

Until February 2025, families deemed by CBP to not pose a danger were typically granted asylum-seeker status with permission to remain in the US pending an immigration hearing. From 2019 to 2024, CBP encountered approximately 2.7 million family units at the southern border.[60] CBP statistics on deportations and turn-aways at the border are not publicly available.

Of those released, more than half were children typically traveling with a lone parent. Volunteers witnessed families waiting for hours at bus stations and when stations closed, they were evicted to the streets—a humanitarian catastrophe in the making (*unpublished observations, 2014, M. Griffin, Rio Grande Valley Humanitarian Respite Center Clinic*).

Filling the void left by a lack of a coordinated federal response, volunteers and community-based organizations (CBOs) from border and nonborder areas mobilized to provide essential supports and services.[61] Time spent at border shelters was limited, allowing only brief opportunities to identify health needs and provide care. At time of writing, only approximately half of border shelters had medical triage capabilities with similar gaps at nonborder shelters.

An example of local advocacy is demonstrated here. In 2014, local pediatric healthcare providers and child advocates created an immigrant clinic in a Rio Grande Valley Humanitarian Respite Center and founded a nonprofit, Community for Children, to address critical gaps in pediatric care. Community for Children raised funds through the AAP and others to purchase needed medications for children arriving at the Respite Center (*unpublished expert experience, M. Griffin*) Clinicians from across the country volunteered, with faculty from several academic centers bringing residents.

The team cared for many families, yet it became apparent that the most vulnerable patients needed additional support and expedited follow-up, including children with serious medical conditions, pregnant/postpartum women, and newborns. Medical providers recognized the need for a sustainable system to assure linkage of children to medical care upon arrival at destinations across the US.

By 2018, the team created a collaborative partnership to address these issues and founded Pediatric Specialty Care Access Network (PediSCAN) which developed into a national network of general pediatricians affiliated with medical centers and subspecialists who urgently linked children to primary/subspecialty care at arrival. Families were enrolled at the border and received health navigation until care was established. Community for Children covered costs of medications and transportation to first visits (and cost of that visit, if needed). The destination community/clinic was then responsible for identifying resources (See **Box 1** for a PediSCAN case example). PediSCAN now has champions in 50 cities, successfully linking hundreds of children to care. Through PediSCAN, partnerships have been fostered at major shelters along the border (**Fig. 3**).

In 2024, team members visited border communities to speak with partners, including CBOs and international humanitarian medical organizations, psychologists, physicians, religious leaders, trusted CBP agents, and county/city government and public health officials. The team sought to learn from their experience and unique perspectives. Each shelter and community developed a collaborative model based on local resources and trusted partnerships.

Through these shared experiences and collaborations, border-wide innovative solutions were developed (**Box 2**).[1,62–64] Many of these solutions can be extrapolated to similar struggles faced throughout the US.

Box 1
Pedi SCAN case example

Pedi SCAN Case, Late 2024: At 2:00 AM, we received urgent text messages and calls from Lulu, who operates a shelter for medically fragile immigrants, requesting assistance with a critically ill 20-year-old male. Luis (pseudonym) was traveling by ambulance from Mexico City to Reynosa accompanied by his physician, Dr Martinez, a third-year surgical resident in Mexico City. Multiple calls were made to a cooperative CBP agent who arranged the ambulance transfer at the bridge. Hours later, another frantic call came from Lulu, who was at the ED in McAllen. Despite the patient's dire condition—his entire abdominal cavity was exposed—the hospital was refusing to admit the young man and told him that he had no rights in the United States. Throughout the night, we made subsequent calls to the charge nurse to monitor Luis's status and to ensure that at least someone was monitoring his vital signs. The hospital social worker explicitly refused assistance, stating that we would NEVER find any hospital to accept Luis nor secure air transport. He needed to go back to "wherever he came from."

The new director of the ED arrived the next morning. Reviewing the case, he lamented the treatment of immigrants he had witnessed in border hospitals. He admitted Luis to his own ED service and personally managed Luis's care while hospitalized.

The Pedi SCAN Champions in Boston consulted trauma surgeons at Massachusetts General Hospital who accepted the patient. While medical air transport from the border would have cost thousands of dollars. Dr Martinez determined that Luis could fly commercially in a seated position if accompanied by an experienced clinician with necessary supplies to manage complications. Last minute first class tickets from McAllen, Texas to Boston cost $740. Dr Martinez obtained permission from his attending physicians to return from Mexico City and escort Luis to Boston. The ED doctor and floor nurses gathered all the needed supplies. Pedi SCAN Champions in Boston and other cities contributed to the cost of the tickets. The Pedi SCAN Champions in Boston met them at the airport at midnight and drove him to the hospital. Dr Martinez remained with Luis throughout the night in the ED until he could personally sign out to the trauma surgeons.

Abbreviation: ED, emergency department.

PEDIATRIC SERVICES FOR CHILDREN OF DEPORTED PARENTS IN MEXICO AND OTHER LATIN AMERICAN COUNTRIES

Since a large proportion of parents being deported or who are self-deporting are Mexican with US- or Mexican-born children, it is important to understand the pediatric services offered there.[65] For more information about health resources in Latin

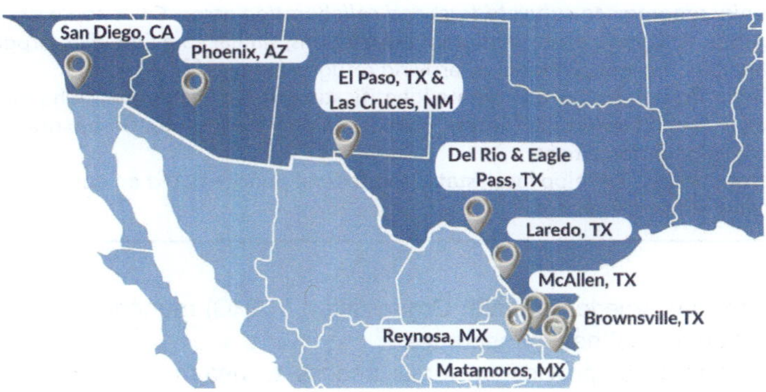

Fig. 3. Location of select major shelters along the US–Mexico border referring to SCAN. Map lines delineate study areas and do not necessarily depict accepted national boundaries. (*Created using* Canva.)

Box 2
Immigrant children and families—gaps in care and systems solutions at the Southern US Border and Throughout the US

Current Gaps in Municipal, State, and National Efforts

- *The absence of coordinated infrastructure*: No interstate, border-wide or national system exists to support migrants once released from CBP custody and no state or federal agency provides formal oversight.
- *Institutional fragmentation:* Schools, CBOs, faith-based organizations, hospitals, universities, state and municipal governments often operate in silos with limited and variable resources available to function
- *Lack of standardized processes:* No border-wide or national protocols exist to welcome newcomers or identify medically high-risk individuals upon release from CBP custody
- *Information silos:* No mechanism facilitates sharing of issues, emergencies, stressors, innovations, or resources across the border region.
- *Inadequate public health infrastructure:* Border and nonborder health departments were neither designed nor adequately funded to address daily health challenges of newly arriving immigrant children and families.
- *Absent care coordination*: Once high-risk immigrants are identified, no coordinated follow-up system or portable medical record system currently exists for this population.
- *Health care access barriers:* Upon arrival at destinations, families face confusing and overwhelming health care systems. Federal policy provides inadequate support for health care access for resource-limited populations.

Solutions and Recommendations

Develop and coordinate:

- *Centralized welcoming system:* Develop a unified data entry system across all border and nonborder shelters enabling multiple facilities to share information and resources. Provide medical support at the border and at all shelters throughout the US for rapid triage and treatment, as needed.
- *Refugee status consideration:* Grant all newly released families and unaccompanied children refugee status with time-limited benefits associated with that status, similar to the Office of Refugee Resettlement–led Unaccompanied Refugee Minor Program.[61]
- *Portable electronic medical records;* Build a secure international electronic medical record system accessible to hospitals, clinics, and shelters on both sides of the border[1] similar to the refugee Electronic Disease Notification System.[62]
- *Mental health infrastructure*: Provide mental health triage and support at the border and throughout migration to final US destinations, including psychological first aid and trauma-informed training for all CBOs, federal immigration enforcement agencies, and faith-based organizations.
- *Addressing social barriers*: Develop medical legal partnership models or other integrated systems in border shelters and nonborder destination clinics.
- *Community programs to cultivate trust and collaboration* across CBOs and within communities with newcomer immigrant populations, similar to a Canadian program that links Canadian sponsors with newly arriving refugee families.[63]
- *Family reunification support*: Facilitate identification of family members who may be detained in federal detention centers, were lost along the journey, or separated by current US immigration enforcement.
- *Data driven policy* – Develop local, state, and federal policies based on data gathered at the border and nonborder states.

America, the Pan American Health Organization (PAHO) monitors and provides updates about countries' health resources.[66]

Mexico attempts to provide universal access to health services for all children through health programs, employment-linked social security, and public and private clinics and hospitals.[67] The Mexican constitution provides all citizens with access to health care through a network of public health facilities and public health services that offer programs focused on child health, such as breastfeeding and immunization promotion. Similarly, foreign-born children have a right to free public health care under Mexico's General Health Law, including access to preventive health services and more common medications. Children of legal residents whose parents have employment-based insurance through the Instituto Mexicano de Seguro Social (IMSS), are eligible for this health insurance that provides coverage for $500 per year.

For repatriated Mexican adults and their children, one 2018 study estimated the health care access for the approximately 550,000 US-born minors living in Mexico (defined as children <18 years) versus that of Mexican-born children.[68] The US-born group had the highest uninsured rate, 39% versus 12.8%, and they also had the highest private insurance rate, 11.7% versus 2.8%, respectively, even though they were all eligible for public insurance. Logistic regression demonstrated that a >5 year transition period is needed for US-born children to achieve health insurance coverage rates comparable to Mexican-born children. US-born children were more likely to live in smaller communities in Mexico (<2500 residents), and their parents were less likely to be enrolled in IMSS, suggesting that parents were employed informally and outside of formal employment-linked health insurance. The study suggests that while health insurance is obtainable for US-born Mexican children, there is a transition time to achieve integration and that institutional barriers, lack of Spanish language fluency and essential Mexican documents, limit access; for children with chronic illness and who live in smaller communities, limited access to pediatric subspecialty care also is an area of concern.

Other Latin American countries' citizens have been repatriated with their undocumented and US-born children. These children, like those deported to Mexico, need time to transition back into the sociocultural environment, including gaining access to governmental and pediatric programs. US pediatric providers who see children of immigrant parents with risks for deportation, particularly those children with complex medical conditions, should investigate health care system access in their country of origin and use resources, including PAHO information sites, to help to link these children to care.

POLICY RECOMMENDATIONS FOR PROTECTING THE HEALTH OF CHILDREN CROSSING AND DISPLACED ACROSS THE US–MEXICO BORDER

As noted above, US immigration policy has long affected the health and well-being of children. Thus, US immigration policy should be child- and family-sensitive and humane in its actions. Children who cross or are displaced across the US–Mexico border experience layered health and developmental risks that neither country's existing systems are designed to absorb.[69–74] A coherent policy response should treat migrant and transnational children as rights-bearing subjects in health, immigration, and international law, with coordinated reforms in binational governance structures in the US, Mexico, and other nations.[75–78]

CHILD CENTRIC RIGHTS AND CROSS-BORDER RISK

The immigration and health systems that govern children at the US–Mexico border remain fundamentally adult-centric, with health, immigration, and international legal barriers that are misaligned with children's unique needs.[76] Child centric policlies are needed Immigrant children on both sides of the border often confront adversarial legal restrictions as adults do, but more often lack legal counsel, developmentally appropriate accommodations, or meaningful opportunities to participate in decisions affecting their health and future.[70,76,78]

US POLICY: UNIVERSAL CHILD COVERAGE AND DECOUPLING FROM ENFORCEMENT

The US should move toward universal health coverage for *all* children, irrespective of immigration status. This requires including undocumented and mixed-status children in Medicaid, the Children's Health Insurance Program (CHIP),[79] and the Affordable Care Act[80]–based plans and adopting multi-year continuous eligibility to reduce churn for children in immigrant families. Evidence from states that have expanded Medicaid-like programs for all children shows significant improvements in preventive care access and early connection to primary and specialty services.[1,75,81]

Federal agencies and Congress can support these efforts by the following methods:

- Facilitating state plan amendments and waivers to expand eligibility for immigrant children;
- Investing in culturally and linguistically appropriate outreach and enrollment pathways; and
- Reducing administrative barriers that disproportionately burden mixed-status households.[81–83]

Equally important is decoupling immigration enforcement from health, education, and child-welfare systems. Immigration enforcement in or near child-serving institutions produces chilling effects that deter families from seeking necessary care.[84] Policies should prohibit enforcement actions in clinical, school, and child-welfare settings; limit information-sharing between service agencies and immigration authorities; and reinforce confidentiality protections for children and caregivers.

Language access is central to equitable pediatric care. Encounters without trained interpreters are consistently associated with increased medical errors and poorer comprehension among limited-English-proficient families. Federal and state regulators should treat interpreter services as an essential benefit within Medicaid and CHIP and require health systems to provide them consistently.[83]

Given the parallel rise in adolescent deaths from homicide, suicide, and firearms in both countries, these protections should be coupled with cross-border violence prevention, firearm safety, and youth mental health strategies that prioritize border communities.[63]

Care standards for children in CBP custody must be strengthed so that all children, not just those under 12 or with acute symptoms, receive timely, in-person evaluations by pediatric-trained clinicians.[1] Discharge processes from both CBP and the Office of Refugee Resettlement should include translated instructions, necessary medications and equipment, and funded medical case management to ensure safe transition to community care.[1,70] Academic centers and community health systems can formalize *fast-track* pathways for high-risk conditions, building on successful cross-border oncology collaborations.[85]

Recognizing immigration status as a modifiable social determinant of health, major immigration and border-security actions should be accompanied by child health impact assessments, with a presumption against policies known to cause trauma, such as family separation for deterrence purposes.[1,76,84]

MEXICAN POLICY: UNIVERSAL ACCESS AND DOCUMENTATION FOR TRANSNATIONAL CHILDREN

Mexico should prioritize US-born and other transnational children for employment-independent health coverage and guaranteed access to comprehensive pediatric services.[69] Many of the more than half-million US-born children living in Mexico remain uninsured or encounter documentation barriers that impede school enrollment and affiliation with health services.[72]

Policies could include automatic or school-based nationality registration for eligible children; mutual recognition of US and Mexican birth certificates as proof of binational status; consulate-supported efforts to simplify and subsidize documentation and enrollment; and, targeted investment in adolescent mental-health services, injury-prevention programs, and trauma-informed care, especially in high-violence regions.[69,71–74]

For US-born children living in Mexican border municipalities, US federal policy should guarantee access to essential health services in US regardless of documentation status, reflecting their binational status and heightened vulnerability.[69,72]

REESTABLISHING A BINATIONAL GOVERNANCE

A reestablished or substantially reformed US–Mexico Border Health Commission could coordinate binational pediatric strategies, harmonize clinical pathways, monitor cross-border child-health indicators, and support emergency responses during migration surges or public-health crises. The commission could also pilot cross-border Medicaid/CHIP portability for US-citizen children living in Mexican border municipalities and expand binational specialty networks to ensure that residence near an international border does not determine access to life-saving care.[1,69,72,77]

A RIGHTS-BASED CHILD HEALTH AGENDA

A rights-based approach affirms that children on either side of the border are rights holders whose health, safety, and development cannot depend on citizenship or parental status. Core elements include the following:

1. Treating immigration policy within a structural public-health policy;
2. Ensuring universal, nondiscriminatory access to essential medical and mental-health services; and
3. Supporting children's participation in decisions affecting their care, safety, and family unity.[76,78,81,82,86]

Implementing these principles requires federal, state, local, and binational action, as well as collaboration across health, education, justice, and social-service sectors.

SUMMARY

Although the immigration landscape remains in constant flux, the needs of immigrant children, historically and in present day, are enduring and must remain a priority. The health of immigrant children moving through Latin America into the US has become a chronic humanitarian crisis due to ongoing climate change, increasing natural disasters, associated regional food scarcity, lack of secure housing, political instability, war, and abject poverty; thus, migration of children will continue whether any given countries' borders are officially open or closed. Based on this stark reality, multinational Latin American and US public health monitoring, data sharing, and collaborative responses need to be built and maintained with ongoing funding invested in this work to allow for nimble, real-time responses to the health needs of migrating communities' children and adolescents. Innovative solutions must incorporate multinational partners—including hospitals, professional pediatric organizations, and CBOs throughout the US and Latin America. Pediatric health care professionals and child rights experts must advocate to support the health of immigrant children.

ACKNOWLEDGMENTS

The authors thank immigrant patients, their families, and new and long-existing immigrant communities throughout the United States for continuing to educate us about their health, well-being, and barriers to accessing care. SCAN was developed by Drs Marsha Griffin, Eric Russell, Paul Wise, Lisa Chamberlain, Karla Fredricks, Robert Nelson, Lazlo Madaras, and Del Garcia and Karen Mountain from Migrant Clinician Network. Community for Children was created by Drs Marsha Griffin, Stan Fisch, and Minnette Son, Judith Livingston, Catherine Monserrat, and Mike Seifert. They thank and acknowledge Rita Cedeño Carpio for her valuable assistance with organizing, verifying, and managing the references used in this article. The authors highlight that all their relatives emigrated to the US and were allowed entry (or excluded/deported) due to US immigration policies of those times.

DISCLOSURE

J. Young is funded as a site PI by the Minnesota Department of Public Health/Centers for Disease Control Division of Global Migration from 2017-9/2026 to research/write/edit the Centers for Disease Control Domestic Refugee Screening Guidelines, write/edit content for CareRef, and to develop the Minnesota Centers of Excellence in Newcomer Health.

REFERENCES

1. Young J, Binford W, Bochenek MG, et al. Health risks of unaccompanied immigrant children in federal custody and in US communities. Am J Public Health 2024;114(3):340–6.
2. UHNCR. The 1951 Refugee convention and 1967 protocol relating to the status of refugees. UHNCR. Available at: https://www.unhcr.org/us/about-unhcr/overview/1951-refugee-convention (Accessed 11 December 2025).
3. Ruggles S, Alexander JT, Genadek K, et al. Children in U.S. immigrant families. Migration Policy Institute; 1990. Available at: http://migrationpolicy.org/programs/data-hubhttps://www.migrationpolicy.org/programs/data-hub/charts/children-immigrant-families.
4. Migration Data Portal, Child and young migrants, *Migration Data Portal*, 2024, Available at: https://www.migrationdataportal.org/themes/child-and-young-migrants#definition (Accessed 11 December 2025).
5. American Immigration Council. Asylum in the United States. Fact sheet. 2025. Available at: https://www.americanimmigrationcouncil.org/fact-sheet/asylum-united-states/#:~:text=An%20asylee%E2%80%94that%20is%2C%20a,Be%20Barred%20from%20Obtaining%20Asylum. Accessed December 11, 2025.
6. U.S. Citizenship and Immigration Services. Victims of human trafficking: t nonimmigrant status. USCIS. Available at: https://www.uscis.gov/humanitarian/victims-of-human-trafficking-t-nonimmigrant-status. Accessed December 11, 2025.
7. U.S. Citizenship and Immigration Services. Special immigrant juvenile status. USCIS 2025. Available at: https://www.uscis.gov/working-in-US/eb4/SIJ#:~:text=You%20are%20dependent%20on%20the,of%20you%20or%20your%20parents. Accessed December 10, 2025.
8. U.S. citizenship and immigration services. Citizenship and naturalization. USCIS. 2025. Available at: https://www.uscis.gov/citizenship/learn-about-citizenship/citizenship-and-naturalization. Accessed December 11, 2025.

9. Chinese exclusion act (1882). 1882. Available at: https://www.archives.gov/milestone-documents/chinese-exclusion-act. Accessed December 11, 2025.
10. Chishti M, Gelatt J. A century later, restrictive 1924 U.S. immigration law has reverberations in immigration debate. The Online Journal of the Migration Policy Institute; 2024. Available at: https://www.migrationpolicy.org. Accessed December 11, 2025.
11. Immigration and Ethic History Society. Undesirable aliens act of 1929. Blease's Law); 2019. Available at: https://immigrationhistory.org/item/undesirable-aliens-act-of-1929-bleases-law/. Accessed October 22, 2025.
12. Minian AR. 1930: repatriation of Mexicans - ana minian. Stanford University Department of History; 2020. Available at: https://history.stanford.edu/news/1930s-repatriation-mexicans-ana-minian. Accessed October 22, 2025.
13. Baker JP, Pearson HA. Dedicated to the health of all children. American Academy of Pediatrics 2005. Available at: aap.org/en/about-the-aap/gartner-pediatric-history-center/aap-history/aap-founding/?srsltid=AfmBOoKSVB1aOsCleklKy2iA90i2H0_yNzpbUiuh_FmbLZsHeicLyZN. Accessed November 6, 2026.
14. United States Government. 42 U.S.C. § 701 et Seq. (Subchapter V – Maternal and Child Health Services Block Grant); Available at: https://www.uscod.house.gov/view.xhtml?req=(title:42%20section:701%20edition:prelim (Accessed 11 June 2026).
15. As school systems receive growing numbers of recently arrived immigrant students, better data are needed on characteristics of this group. Migration Policy Institute; 2023. Available at: https://www.migrationpolicy.org/news/recently-arrived-immigrant-students. Accessed December 11, 2025.
16. Sugarman J. Recent immigrant children: a profile of new arrivals to U.S. schools. 2023. Available at: https://www.migrationpolicy.org/sites/default/files/publications/mpi-recent-immigrant-children-2023_final.pdf. Accessed December 11, 2025.
17. Office of Refugee Resettlement. Unaccompanied alien children by country of origin, 2021-2024. Administration for children & families. Available at: https://acf.gov/orr/uac/country-origin. Accessed December 11, 2025.
18. Wu J, Strickler L, Murphy J, et al. US deportation tracker: counting Arrests, deportations. NBC News; 2025. Available at: https://www.nbcnews.com/data-graphics/us-immigration-tracker-follow-arrests-detentions-border-crossings-rcna189148. Accessed December 1, 2025.
19. Kim J, Nicodimos S, Kushner SE, et al. Comparing mental health of US children of immigrants and non-immigrants in 4 racial/ethnic groups. J Sch Health 2018;88(2):167–75.
20. Heinrich C, Hernández M, Shero M. Repercussions of a raid: health and education outcomes of children entangled in immigration enforcement. J Pol Anal Manag 2022;42(2):350–92.
21. Acevedo-Garcia D, Joshi PK, Ruskin E, et al. Restoring an inclusionary safety net for children in immigrant families: a review of three social policies. Health Aff 2021;40(7):1099–107.
22. Gelatt J, Ruiz Soto AG, Bachmeier JD. Changing origins, rising numbers: unauthorized immigrants in the United States. 2025. Available at: https://www.migrationpolicy.org/sites/default/files/publications/mpi-unauthorized-immigrants-fact-sheet-2025_FINAL.pdf. Accessed December 11, 2025.
23. Pillai D, Pillai A, Artiga S. KFF analysis of 2023 american community survey (ACS) 1-yr estimates. KFF; 2025. Available at: https://www.kff.org/racial-equity-and-health-policy/children-of-immigrants-key-facts-on-health-coverage-and-care/. Accessed December 10, 2025.

24. Haley JM, Gonzalez D, Bernstein H, et al. Children of Immigrants in 2022–23: National and State Patterns; The Urban Institute, 2025. Available at: https://www.urban.org/research/publication/children-immigrants-2022-23 (Accessed 11 June 2026).
25. World Health Organization. Latent tuberculosis infection : updated and consolidated guidelines for programmatic management. World Health Organization, Global TB Programme; 2018. Available at: https://iris.who.int/handle/10665/260233. Accessed December 11, 2025.
26. Venturini E, Fusani L, Mantella A, et al. Strongyloidiasis in children outside the tropics: do we need to increase awareness? Microorganisms 2021;9(9). https://doi.org/10.3390/microorganisms9091905.
27. Centers for Disease Control and Prevention. Intestinal parasites (refugee health domestic guidance). CDC (U.S. Department of Health & Human Services); 2025. Available at: https://www.cdc.gov/immigrant-refugee-health/hcp/domestic-guidance/intestinal-parasites.html.
28. American Academy of Pediatrics. Recommendations for preventative pediatric health care (periodicity schedule). American Academy of Pediatrics 2018;142. https://doi.org/10.1542/peds.2018-1218.
29. Refugee Health Residency Program. Society of refugee healthcare providers. 2025. Available at: https://refugeesociety.org/resources/residency-programs/#brxe-lwlhlu. Accessed December 11, 2025.
30. Centers for Disease Control and Prevention. Domestic immigrant and refugee health guidance for health care professionals. CDC Immigrant and Refugee Health 2024. Available at: https://www.cdc.gov/immigrant-refugee-health/hcp/domestic-guidance/index.html. Accessed December 11, 2025.
31. Minnesota Department of Health. CARE ref - Community assessment and referral for everyone. Minnesota department of health. Available at: https://careref.web.health.state.mn.us/. Accessed December 11, 2025.
32. Greenbaum J, Kaplan D, Young J, et al. Exploitation, labor and sex trafficking of children and adolescents: health care needs of patients. Pediatrics 2023;151(1). https://doi.org/10.1542/peds.2022-060416.
33. Global TravEpiNet. Available at: https://gten.massgeneral.org/. Accessed December 11, 2025.
34. Broder T. Health care coverage (Maps). National Immigration Law Center 2025. Available at: https://www.nilc.org/resources/healthcoveragemaps/. Accessed December 11, 2025.
35. Kusma JD, Raphael JL, Perrin JM, et al. Committee on child health financing. Medicaid and the children's health insurance Program: optimization to promote equity in child and young adult health. American Academy of Pediatrics 2023; 152(5). Available at: http://publications.aap.org/pediatrics/article-pdf/152/5/e2023064088/1548748/peds.2023-064088.pdf. Accessed December 11, 2025.
36. Zijlmans W, Stuursma A, Roelofs A, et al. Anemia in young children living in the Surinamese interior: the influence of age, nutritional status, and ethnicity. Res Rep Trop Med 2017;8:21–4.
37. Jamaica JM. Prevalence of anemia among children: % of children aged 6-59 months. CEIC. Available at: https://www.ceicdata.com/en/jamaica/social-health-statistics/jm-prevalence-of-anemia-among-children–of-children-aged-659-months. Accessed December 11, 2025.
38. Belize: prevalence of anemia among children. The Global economy. Available at: https://www.theglobaleconomy.com/Belize/anemia_among_children/. Accessed December 11, 2025.

39. Barbados. Prevalence of anemia among children. The Global economy. Available at: https://www.theglobaleconomy.com/Barbados/anemia_among_children/. Accessed December 11, 2025.
40. Global Health Observatory Data Repository, World Health Organization. Prevalence of anemia among children (% of children ages 6-59 months). The World Bank Group; 2025. Available at: https://data.worldbank.org/indicator/SH.ANM.CHLD.ZS. Accessed December 11, 2025.
41. World Health Organization. Guatemala country health data overview. World Health Organization Data; 2025. Available at: https://data.who.int/countries/320. Accessed December 11, 2025.
42. Marie E. 2023 ENSANUT report findings on lead levels in Mexico. Pure Earth Pollution Blog 2024. Available at: https://www.pureearth.org/2023-ensanut-report-lead-levels-in-the-population-of-mexico/. Accessed December 11, 2025.
43. Centers for Disease Control and Prevention. Refugee health domestic guidance. CDC Immigrant and Refugee Health 2024. Available at: https://www.cdc.gov/immigrant-refugee-health/hcp/domestic-guidance/index.html. Accessed December 11, 2025.
44. Minnesota Department of Health. CareRef clinical assessment tool. Minnesota Department of Health - Refugee Health Resources; 2025. Available at: https://careref.web.health.state.mn.us/. Accessed December 11, 2025.
45. Borrajo GJC. Newborn screening in Latin America: a brief overview of the state of the art. Am J Med Genet C Semin Med Genet 2021;187(3):322–8.
46. Lynn MK, Rodríguez Aquino MS, Buendía Rivas CA, et al. Prenatal Chagas disease screening in Latin America: the current policy landscape and potential utility of an expanded maternal-familial Trypanosoma cruzi testing framework. The Lancet Regional Health 2025;47. https://doi.org/10.1016/j.lana.2025.101139. Americas.Elsevier Ltd.
47. Pimentel dos Santos H, Bonini Domingos C, Martins de Castro S. Twenty years of neonatal screening for sickle cell disease in Brazil: the challenges of a Continental country with high genetic heterogeneity. J Inborn Errors Metab Screen 2021;9. https://doi.org/10.1590/2326-4594.
48. Gaikwad S, Ganvir S, Uke P. Newborn screening in developing countries: the need of the hour. Cureus 2024;5. https://doi.org/10.7759/cureus.59572.
49. Centers for Disease Control and Prevention. Laboratory Testing (Domestic Guidance). CDC Immigrant and Refugee Health; 2025. Available at: https://www.cdc.gov/immigrant-refugee-health/hcp/domestic-guidance/laboratory-testing.html.
50. Vázquez LI, Valera E, Villalobos M, et al. Prevalence of anemia in children from latin America and the Caribbean and effectiveness of nutritional interventions: systematic review and meta–analysis. Nutrients 2019;11(1). https://doi.org/10.3390/nu11010183.
51. Ericson B, Hu H, Nash E, et al. Blood lead levels in low-income and middle-income countries: a systematic review. Lancet Planet Health 2021;5(3):e145–53.
52. Centers for Disease Control and Prevention (CDC). Lead poisoning associated with use of traditional ethnic remedies–California, 1991-1992. MMWR Morb Mortal Wkly Rep 1993;42(27):521–4.
53. Centers for Disease Control and Prevention. Lead poisoning associated with imported candy and powdered food coloring - california and Michigan. MMWR (Morb Mortal Wkly Rep) 1998;47(48). Available at: https://www.cdc.gov/mmwr/preview/mmwrhtml/00055939.htm. Accessed December 10, 2025.

54. Centers for Disease Control and Prevention. Demographics (Reported Tuberculosis in the United States, 2023). 2024. Available at: https://www.cdc.gov/tb-surveillance-report-2023/summary/demographics.html#:~:text=Key%20findings-,Origin%20of%20birth,non%2DU.S.%E2%80%93born%20persons. Accessed December 11, 2025.
55. Serván-Mori E, Garcia-Diaz R, Meneses-Navarro S, et al. Inequities in the continuum of maternal care in Mexico: trends before and after COVID-19. Int J Equity Health 2025;24(1). https://doi.org/10.1186/s12939-025-02470-x.
56. García-Romero CS, Guzmán C, Martínez-Ibarra A, et al. Viral hepatitis in pregnant Mexican women: its impact in mother–child binomial health and the strategies for its eradication. Pathogens 2024;13(8). https://doi.org/10.3390/pathogens13080651.
57. Smith A, Sabidó M, Camey E, et al. Lessons learned from integrating simultaneous triple point-of-care screening for syphilis, hepatitis B, and HIV in prenatal services through rural outreach teams in Guatemala. Int J Gynecol Obstet 2015;130(S1):S70–2.
58. Hennesy-Fiske M, Carcamo C. In Texas' Rio Grande Valley, a seemingly endless surge of immigrants. Los Angeles Times; 2014. Available at: https://www.latimes.com/nation/la-na-texas-border-chaos-20140614-story.html. Accessed December 11, 2025.
59. Galvan A. Migrants dropped off at bus stations in Arizona. WTOP News 2014. Available at: https://wtop.com/news/2014/05/migrants-dropped-off-at-bus-stations-in-arizona/. Accessed December 11, 2025.
60. U.S. Customs and Border Protection. Southwest land border encounters. U.S. Department of Homeland Security; 2025. Available at: https://www.cbp.gov/newsroom/stats/southwest-land-border-encounters. Accessed December 11, 2025.
61. Sanchez S. 10th anniversary of Humanitarian Respite Center coincides with new asylum rules. Border Report. 2024. Available at: https://www.borderreport.com/news/top-stories/10th-anniversary-of-humanitarian-respite-center-coincides-with-new-asylum-rules/. Accessed December 11, 2025.
62. Administration for Children and Families. Unaccompanied Refugee Minors (URM) Program. Office of refugee settlement. 2025. Available at: https://acf.gov/orr/programs/refugees/urm. Accessed December 11, 2025.
63. Centers for Disease Control and Prevention. Electronic disease notification System. CDC immigrant and refugee health. 2024. Available at: https://www.cdc.gov/immigrant-refugee-health/php/case-reporting-edn/index.html. Accessed December 11, 2025.
64. Government of Canada, immigration R and CC. Groups of five. Government of Canada. 2025. Available at: https://www.canada.ca/en/immigration-refugees-citizenship/services/refugees/sponsor-refugee/private-sponsorship-program/groups-five.html. Accessed December 11, 2025.
65. U.S. Immigration and Customs Enforcement. ICE enforcement and removal operations statistics. U.S. Department of homeland security. Available at: https://www.ice.gov/statistics. Accessed December 15, 2025.
66. Pan American Health Organization. Health in the Americas+ country profile: mexico. Pan American Health Organization/World Health Organization; 2024. Available at: https://hia.paho.org/en/country-profiles/mexico#digital. Accessed December 1, 2025.
67. Block MA, Morales-Vasquez M, Reyes H. Health systems in action (HSiA) insights: mexico 2024. North American observatory on health systems and policies. 2025.

Available at: https://eurohealthobservatory.who.int/publications/health-systems-in-action-insights/health-systems-in-action-2024-mexico. Accessed December 1, 2025.

68. Wassink JT. Out of sight and uninsured: access to healthcare among US-Born minors in Mexico. J Immigr Minor Health 2020;22(3):448–55.
69. Amuendo-Dorantes C, Juarez L. Health Care and Education Access of transnational children in Mexico. Demography 2022;549(2).
70. Ayoub-Rodriguez L, Fredricks K, Griffin M. The health of immigrant children on the border. Acad Pediatr 2024;24(5):44–5. Elsevier Inc.
71. Barajas-Gonzalez RG, Ayón C, Brabeck K, et al. An ecological expansion of the adverse childhood experiences (ACEs) framework to include threat and deprivation associated with U.S. immigration policies and enforcement practices: an examination of the latinx immigrant experience. Soc Sci Med 2021; 282:114126.
72. Borja S, Berger Cardoso J, de la Cruz PI, et al. Health insurance access among US citizen children in Mexico: national and transborder policy implications. Health Aff 2021;40(7):1066–74.
73. Castilla-Peon MF, Rendón PL, Gonzalez-Garcia N. The leading causes of death in the US and Mexico's pediatric population are related to violence: a note on secondary analyses of registered deaths from 2000 to 2022. Front Public Health 2024;12. https://doi.org/10.3389/fpubh.2024.1428691.
74. Zayas LH, Garcia Isaza A, Fuentes-Balderrama J, et al. Well-being and contexts of development of U.S. citizen children in Mexico following parental deportation or voluntary relocation. Am J Orthopsychiatry 2024;94(2):123–38.
75. Alegría M, O'Malley IS, Smith R, et al. Addressing health inequities for children in immigrant families: psychologists as leaders and links across systems. Am Psychol 2023;78(2):173–85.
76. Hlass LL. The paradox of immigrant children's rights. Texas Law Review Online 2025;104:142–54.
77. Moya E., Coronado I. and Mumme S., A call to action: reestablishment of the US-Mexico border Health Commission, *Health Affairs Forefront*, 2021, Available at: https://msmagazine.com/2021/08/03/united-state-mexico-border-health-commission/ (Accessed 11 June 2026).
78. Smith CE. "Children's Equity Law" in the Age of Parents' rights. Kansas Law Review 2022;71:533–46.
79. U.S. Department of Health & Human Services. Children's Health Insurance Program. Centers for Medicare & Medicaid Services (CMS); 2025. Available at: https://www.healthcare.gov/medicaid-chip/childrens-health-insurance-program/. Accessed December 11, 2025.
80. Assistant Secretary for Public Affairs (ASPA). About the Affordable Care Act. U.S. Department of Health and Human Services; 2022. Available at: https://www.hhs.gov/healthcare/about-the-aca/index.html. Accessed December 11, 2025.
81. Rosenberg J, Shabanova V, McCollum S, et al. Insurance and health care outcomes in regions where undocumented children are Medicaid-eligible. Pediatrics 2022;150(3):E20220570334.
82. Flores G, Lesley B. Children and US federal Policy on health and health care: seen but not heard. JAMA Pediatr 2014;168(12):1155–63.
83. Flores G. Language barriers to health care in the United States. N Engl J Med 2006;355(3):229–31.

84. Martinez-Donate AP, Ejebe I, Zhang X, et al. Access to health care among Mexican migrants and immigrants: a comparison across migration phases. J Health Care Poor Underserved 2017;28(4):1314–26.
85. Aristizabal P, Thornburg CD, Young J. At the border: a call to action for health equity for children with leukemia. Cancer 2023;129(8):1159–61.
86. Lindgren L, Fredricks K. A multi-level approach to promoting the health rights of immigrant children in the United States. Health & Human Rights 2024;26(2): 133–6.

Humanitarian Crises

Trainee Perspectives

Nabiha Subzwari, MPH[a,*], Sunwoo Lee, MPH[b],
Jordan O'Brien, MPH[a], Ugomma Korie, MPH[c], Maria Beg, MPH[d],
Rachel Novick, MPH[a], Yusra Ahmed, MPH[d],
Chetan Sree Muppavarapu, MPH[a]

KEYWORDS

- Humanitarian crisis/crises • Public health education
- Academic ecological sustainability • Displaced persons • Resilience • Legal literacy
- Higher education access

KEY POINTS

- The key to understanding humanitarian crises is collective action from public health professionals through educational innovation.
- The novel conceptual synthesis of the *academic ecological sustainability* framework emphasizes strengthening academic education itself and its accountability to each discipline, including public health.
- Institutions must be held accountable for designing equitable frameworks that facilitate academic and social mobility, supporting displaced individuals who face barriers to higher education.
- Reflecting on our unique journeys to the public health field builds resilience in the face of unprecedented challenges.
- Public health education should integrate legal literacy and collaborative resilience frameworks to enable trainees to use public health law as instruments of equity.

INTRODUCTION

The term *humanitarian crisis* is viewed in a myriad of ways: conflict-driven displacement, war, human rights violations, and pandemics among others. The Rohingya

[a] Department of Epidemiology, Columbia University Mailman School of Public Health, 722 W 168th Street, New York, NY 10032, USA; [b] Department of Sociomedical Sciences, Columbia University Mailman School of Public Health, 722 W 168th Street, New York, NY 10032, USA; [c] Department of Health Policy and Management, Columbia University Mailman School of Public Health, 722 W 168th Street, New York, NY 10032, USA; [d] Department of Population and Family Health, Columbia University Mailman School of Public Health, 722 W 168th Street, New York, NY 10032, USA
* Corresponding author.
E-mail address: ns3890@cumc.columbia.edu

Pediatr Clin N Am 73 (2026) 1117–1128
https://doi.org/10.1016/j.pcl.2026.05.010 **pediatric.theclinics.com**

Abbreviations	
CEPH	Council on Education for Public Health
IDPs	internally displaced persons
IOM	International Organization for Migration
UNHCR	United Nations High Commissioner for Refugees

refugee crisis, coronavirus disease 2019 pandemic, Russia-Ukraine war, Sudan crisis, and Gaza war are some of the many prominent examples that represent the span of humanitarian crises. Despite their different origins, these global events collectively demonstrate the increasingly frequent challenges that functionally burden humanitarian systems. In fact, the United Nations High Commissioner for Refugees (UNHCR) reported a globally estimated 123.2 million people experienced forced displacement due to a myriad of humanitarian crises at the end of 2024, a 6% increase from the end of 2023 by 7 million people.[1] Another unifying point in the aforementioned crises are their respective contextual complexities, which positions public health to intervene as an interdisciplinary field. Although initially subsumed under medicine, public health has been building its own unique identity within the health sciences. The domain of humanitarian crises reflects public health's immense breadth to summon different perspectives in understanding its pressing challenges, yet the persisting drawbacks of public health's identity are also represented in the work of humanitarian crises. To address the multifaceted areas of improvement, education ought to be the first area for the field to envision how to strengthen preparation for humanitarian work among emerging public health professionals.

As second year trainees and one recent graduate of an MPH program, we the article authors have grown to become competent public health leaders. Whether as a future pediatrician, radiologist, professor, or field practitioner—we are confident in tackling some of the most pressing public health challenges because of an effectively designed MPH program. Even so, we recognize glaring gaps in specific substantive areas that require more attention for all MPH candidates. Prior to each MPH student taking their required coursework, our program's MPH Core is a compulsory part of the degree program because of its comprehensive exposure to all pillars of public health: epidemiology, biostatistics, health policy, and health promotion. Beyond a human rights module and foundational lectures on humanitarian health in a global health module, we believe there is insufficient coverage to at least provide all public health students with the necessary framework to make sense of humanitarian crises. Especially to support aspiring humanitarian system professionals, public health schools/programs can benefit from expanding its unmet potential to enhance action in humanitarian crises. If combined with a collective willingness to reform academic and social institutions, an improved educational approach would bridge the gap between substantive/skills-based training and perspectives-based learning for public health trainees.

With education as the central theme of our article, we discuss some of the elements we believe to be critical to the growth of public health schools/programs. Said elements are represented by the following overarching questions that guide the article's structure: (i) how can public health education achieve *pedagogical success* in teaching the sophistications of humanitarian crises without getting lost in translation?, (ii) how can the global community establish and advance life-altering opportunities for *displaced persons* through education?, and (iii) how can public health navigate through the contextual fluidity of *resilience* in training its emerging leaders?

EDUCATIONAL PREPAREDNESS FOR ADDRESSING HUMANITARIAN CRISES

As the frequency and complexity of humanitarian crises increase—driven by conflict, displacement, climate change, and infectious disease—so too does the need for public health professionals prepared to respond effectively in these settings. In response, schools and programs of public health have begun to develop curricula and training models that equip future practitioners with the skills and competencies necessary to work in fragile and emergency contexts.

The Council on Education for Public Health (CEPH), the accrediting body for public health education in the United States, requires programs to meet standards related to institutional mission, governance, curriculum, and student outcomes. For MPH programs, students must gain foundational knowledge in public health history and values, research methods, systems thinking, and key health determinants, and demonstrate mastery of 22 competencies ranging from evidence-based practice to leadership, communication, policy, and concentration-specific skills.[2] In October 2016, CEPH adopted revised accreditation criteria that shifted from a traditional knowledge-based curriculum to competency-based education, emphasizing application of learning. The updated standards introduced the Applied Practice Experience, requiring students to produce real-world deliverables in a field setting, and the Integrative Learning Experience, a culminating project demonstrating synthesis of core and concentration-specific competencies. These changes responded to evolving workforce needs, expectations for public accountability, and a broader movement in higher education toward outcome-based learning.[3]

The 2016 CEPH revision was not developed in isolation. In fact, it was preceded by and influenced by major curricular reform efforts at several leading schools of public health. Columbia University's Mailman School of Public Health launched an ambitious overhaul of its MPH curriculum in 2012, with the goal of preparing students to meet the complex, interdisciplinary challenges of modern public health practice. Mailman's new curriculum emphasized integrated systems thinking, applied learning, and team-based problem-solving. It was also one of the first to embed competency-based education at scale, moving beyond siloed disciplinary instruction in favor of a cohesive, cross-cutting framework.[4] This bold redesign became an important reference point in national discussions about MPH education and helped pave the way for CEPH's 2016 overhaul.

Similar innovations were underway at other institutions. At the UNC Gillings School of Global Public Health, faculty introduced an interdisciplinary Applied Implementation Science program before CEPH's update, integrating implementation science with systems thinking, quality improvement, and design thinking to provide practical tools for addressing complex, real-world problems. Developed to meet the demands of *Public Health 3.0*, the curriculum emphasized preparing practitioners, not just researchers, for effective action in dynamic, multisector environments.[5] The University of South Florida's College of Public Health also restructured its MPH core using the Intervention Mapping framework, a theory—an evidence-based approach to curriculum design that incorporated experiential learning, flipped classrooms, and stakeholder engagement to strengthen competency development and prepare graduates for practice-based challenges.[6]

One area where competency-based training has been especially critical is in preparing students for work in humanitarian emergencies. Many MPH programs now offer specialized certificates, practical, and applied experiences to train public health professionals for response and recovery in crisis settings. These programs build skills in emergency preparedness, outbreak response, logistics, and the ethical dimensions of humanitarian work.

At Columbia Mailman, the Public Health and Humanitarian Action certificate trains students to work effectively in acute and complex emergencies. Students develop competencies in needs assessment, monitoring and evaluation, evidence synthesis, and ethical decision-making in humanitarian settings. The curriculum emphasizes critical thinking and communication skills, along with the ability to integrate quantitative and qualitative data to inform policy and programmatic decisions. A central feature of the certificate is the required 8 to 10 week field practicum in a fragile, low-income setting, where students gain first-hand experience responding to public health challenges in crisis-affected populations.

The Center for Humanitarian Emergencies at Emory University has similarly established a robust training platform through the Rollins School of Public Health, in collaboration with the Centers for Disease Control and Prevention's Emergency Response and Recovery Branch. The Graduate Certificate in Humanitarian Emergencies includes core and elective coursework, an Applied Practice Experience, an Integrative Learning Experience, and required volunteer service. It is one of the few certificate programs in the United States focused exclusively on humanitarian response and is highly competitive, admitting a limited number of students each year. The Center also offers a fellowship program for midcareer professionals from low-income and middle-income countries affected by conflict, aimed at building local capacity for humanitarian leadership.[7]

Together, these examples illustrate how public health education is evolving to meet the demands of an increasingly complex world. Through curriculum reform and competency-based training, MPH programs are better preparing students not only to respond to current global health challenges but to lead in uncertain, rapidly changing environments. The current state of training in humanitarian crises is best reflected in the following statement:

> *"The lack of a standardized curriculum and competency framework will remain an issue for the credibility and quality of humanitarian training. A recent survey has shown that the majority of recruiters in humanitarian organizations would favor experience over qualifications, a practice that raises questions about humanitarian respondents' accountability, but it may also reflect the lack of trust in the academic sector to satisfy the evolving needs in the field."*[8]

Though public health education has made great strides, it is far from sufficient to meet the demands of the 21st century's public health challenges. Given the introduction of humanitarian health into North American and European schools of public health in the late 1990s,[9] there is a clear pedagogical gap in how emerging public health professionals are being trained to work in nuanced situations. Beyond the methods of improving humanitarian health curricula, it is just as crucial to achieve the highest possible levels of pedagogical cohesion across different academic institutions and programs of public health. Even with the continued existence of accreditation bodies like CEPH in the United States and evaluation-based research that highlights the strengths of program(s) and interrogates its limitations, public health education can be elevated further through research-practice harmonization among field professionals and social acceptance: *academic ecological sustainability*.

Research-practice harmonization can be achieved by holding scholars and practitioners mutually accountable to inform each other's respective work; in other words, researchers should consider how their work can meaningfully benefit communities, while practitioners should ground their approaches in evidence-based research. We define *academic ecological sustainability* as a framework that cultivates interprofessional education and complex systems thinking, grounded in the responsibility to adapt to a discipline's evolving challenges. Public health thrives when it is recognized as a nuanced system comprising a multitude of intertwining academic disciplines. For instance, there is a difference between simply understanding air pollution and understanding environmental injustice with respect to air pollution; the former requires the sciences (biology, chemistry, and physics), whereas the latter requires a wider substantive knowledge base (politics, economics, culture, and so on). While knowledge and skills must be taught, education systems cannot reach their potential without having a dynamic relationship with other entities crucial to public health (eg, community-based organizations, government agencies, the general public). This vision was discussed in a 2010 publication to the Lancet by Julio Frenk and colleagues through the term *interdependence*, describing its importance to achieve the following educational transformations: *from isolated to harmonized education and health systems, from stand-alone institutions to networks/alliances/consortia, and from inward-looking institutional preoccupations to harnessing global flows of educational content/teaching resources/innovations*.[9] Of course, such an ambitious outlook on innovating public health education does not come easily. It calls for large-scale reform of academic and social institutions. Not to mention, because an individual's perspective is shaped by their upbringing and early education, we must be conscientious and respectful of the many contexts driving the profound network that is public health. Furthermore, public health as a field should regularly engage in a mutualistic relationship with the general public on the direction of practice and research, while also gaining and maintaining the public's trust organically; after all, public health professionals enter the field with a commitment to the populations they care most about. Although there will never be a clear answer to globalizing public health education, it would be well worth the investment of training professionals to tackle humanitarian crises and other pressing public health challenges.

Education will always hold onto its global reputation as the most vital asset for humanity, in how it provides an arsenal of valuable skills and experiences. Even with the improvements made to address its many imperfections over the years, public health education will benefit from upgrading its adaptability to contexts of all kinds. In the case of humanitarian health, curricula must continue to grow into an authentic reflection of what it means to work in the field. Alongside these characteristics, it is paramount to consider how structural factors shape the limitations of education and how the professionals—emerging and established—perceive the future direction of public health education, both of which will be explored in the remainder of this article.

IMPORTANCE, CHALLENGES, AND TRAINEE PERSPECTIVES

In humanitarian work, the terminology used for people forced to flee their homes carries significant weight. Major organizations define *refugee* and *displaced people* with different scopes, which can shape both policy and practice. The UNHCR adheres to the 1951 Refugee Convention's strict definition of a refugee: someone who has crossed an international border due to a well-founded fear of persecution (for reasons such as race, religion, nationality, social group, or political opinion) and cannot safely return home.[10,11] In contrast, UN agencies and the International Organization for Migration often use broader terms like *displaced persons*, encompassing *all* people forced from their homes by conflict, generalized violence, human rights violations or disasters—whether they fled abroad or remained within their own country.[12] US government sources (eg, US Citizenship and Immigration Services) mirror the Convention-based refugee definition, requiring that a person be outside their country and fear persecution on specific grounds.[13] At the same time, US policy distinguishes internally displaced persons (IDPs) as those uprooted within their own borders, who do not benefit from the legal refugee status and its protections.[14] This highlights a key caveat: the label *refugee* by itself is limited, excluding millions of IDPs and others who don't meet the narrow legal criteria. Indeed, unlike refugees, IDPs remain under their national government's protection and lack the special international status and aid that refugee designation confers.[15] Accordingly, for this section we will use the inclusive term *displaced people* to encompass everyone forced from their homes—refugees, asylum seekers, and internally displaced persons—regardless of legal status or whether they crossed an international border.

> *"Education is the most powerful weapon which we can use to prepare our youth for their role as leaders of tomorrow".*
>
> —*Nelson Mandela*[16]

The policies, structures, and systems that characterize the world around us have been largely defined by individuals whose privileged attainment of higher education has credited their decision-making authority. But what happens when the systems we exist in fail to create opportunities for marginalized communities to advance?

In 2023, the UN Refugee Agency (UNHCR) reported that global enrollment in tertiary education was merely 7% for refugees—a fraction of the global average among non-refugees standing at 42%.[17] This urgently calls for investments in facilitators of higher education attainment for displaced people and communities who are not duly represented in higher levels of power in decision-making. The intellect, perspectives, and incomparable way of viewing the world that displaced persons embody are far-reaching and cannot be overstated. Education is not a luxury but a necessity for these communities.

Graduate-level education is not sought after, let alone necessary, for every individual to unlock their full potential as they define it. But for those to whom higher education serves as that necessary space to honor academic curiosity, to evolve in community, and to set the foundation for the intersection of learned knowledge and personal experience—the lack of access to it is destructive. Not only is it true for the individual but also inextricably so for their families, communities, and nations at large. For displaced students, higher education equates to opportunities for shared prosperity for their nations, host communities, and our global community. Students are able to build a plethora of knowledge and skills for self-reliance, resilience, and socioeconomic advancement. To invest in scholars who have experienced forced displacement is to invest in peace, stability, and human potential. In a world where hostility and warfare are increasingly prevalent, it's more important now than ever to build systems where refugees are recognized *as they are*—resilient individuals with immense potential.

Displaced people from humanitarian settings face significant barriers in accessing higher education. These barriers encompass structural, economic, cultural, and psychological dimensions that compound existing vulnerabilities. Displaced individuals are not a homogeneous group, and factors such as age, gender, prior educational experiences, and caregiving responsibilities further influence their ability to pursue higher education. Moreover, displaced individuals often face difficulties in obtaining official recognition for prior educational qualifications due to lost or inaccessible documentation. Psychological distress, stemming from displacement and instability, also negatively impacts academic pursuits.[18]

Institutions of higher education often fail to provide tailored support to help displaced students navigate these complexities. For example, while higher education enhances cultural and social capital for displaced people by fostering specialized knowledge and skills, returning to such communities is not always an option. Instead, they may face stigmatization or discrimination based on their identity, even after demonstrating academic success.[19] Many universities continue to rely on admissions procedures that exclude those whose schooling has been interrupted by conflict or displacement. Even when displaced students successfully enroll, they frequently encounter institutional cultures that overlook their specific needs, such as trauma-informed counseling, flexible study options for those with caregiving or employment responsibilities, or structured guidance on academic expectations in a new cultural context. As a result, displaced students often experience institutional abandonment, where they are admitted into universities but left to navigate complex administrative systems, language demands, and financial pressures on their own.[19]

Access to higher education does not necessarily translate into meaningful inclusion. While higher education is often framed as a tool for empowerment, the experiences of displaced students reveal that academic success does not shield them from social stigmatization and identity-based discrimination. Their displaced status can subject them to suspicion from peers, faculty, and administrators, who may perceive them as politically sensitive or socially vulnerable bodies rather than full academic participants. Some displaced students even report feeling pressure to suppress or distance themselves from aspects of their identity to gain social acceptance within academic spaces.[19] For those who hope to use their degrees to return and contribute to their home communities, political persecution or ongoing conflict often prevents return. Students gain educational capital but remain immobile socio-politically, trapped by restrictive immigration systems and institutional barriers. Thus, without intentional and structural support from universities, higher education can reproduce, rather than challenge, inequalities faced by displaced people.

A growing authoritarian political climate intensifies these challenges, as seen in the unjust detainment of Mohsen Mahdawi, a Palestinian student at Columbia University, who grew up in a West Bank refugee camp in Palestine.[20] Mahdawi's experience highlights how displaced students are disproportionately vulnerable to shifts in political and administrative policies, even when they hold proper documentation.[19] Such political scrutiny weaponizes their identities and jeopardizes their security, further diminishing their access to education. As authoritarianism encroaches on academic autonomy, universities must critically reflect on their responsibilities to scholars and students, particularly those from displaced backgrounds. Institutions have a responsibility to create safe environments for intellectual exploration and advocate for policies that support the autonomy of academia.[19] Universities must develop frameworks that address the specific needs of displaced students, including robust legal and psychological support, as well as inclusive and equitable access to education. In doing so, they affirm their role as spaces of empowerment and resistance against political violence and marginalization.

In our graduate public health programs, immediate issues that often jeopardize student stability include time pressures, visa uncertainties, funding constraints, and academic performance. Institutions, meanwhile, focus on setting curricula, credit systems, documentation policies, and risk protocols. Between these realities lies a crucial gap—the space where students' lived experiences, particularly those shaped by displacement, conflict, or migration, meet the rigid frameworks of academia.

Our classrooms are geopolitically diverse: students come from across regions affected by war, economic upheaval, and climate displacement, bringing perspectives that could deepen collective understanding of global health inequities. Yet the structure of our programs—oriented toward deadlines and measurable outputs—can leave little room for processing or integrating these lived insights. The emotional content of learning, including the weight of personal histories and the vulnerability of navigating unfamiliar systems, often remains unspoken. When that human context is overlooked, much of the deeper learning about displaced people—and about ourselves as future practitioners—risks being lost.

The deepest learning comes in conversation with peers—through short, guided debriefs with faculty, supervisors, or peer facilitators after placements (practicum or internship fieldwork in community organizations, clinics, or agencies), cross-cohort rounds that bring together students across years and disciplines, and *case talk* based on anonymized scenarios from that fieldwork. These exchanges help connect theory to lived realities, including the cultural and emotional dimensions of working with displaced communities. Yet they are often incidental and easy to miss, especially for students balancing work, caregiving, or immigration obligations. Simple moves help: schedule brief debriefs after each placement, hold periodic cross-cohort or community case rounds, and support compensated near-peer mentorship that includes trainees from displaced backgrounds.

We can name the factors that shape displaced people's access to higher education—immigration status, gaps in documentation, interrupted schooling, funding eligibility, work restrictions, language access, and trauma—yet we struggle to carry them into daily choices. Syllabi acknowledge these realities, but evaluation rarely requires us to apply them. Aligning assessment with practice helps: evaluate case decisions that center entry and persistence—admissions and credit-transfer judgments when records are missing, financial-aid choices under work-authorization limits, attendance and placement requirements that intersect with court dates or caregiving. Pair this with credit for community-engaged advising and brief reflections that link coursework to how campus policies open or close doors. These shifts signal that competence includes improving pathways into higher education for displaced people—not as an add-on, but as the work.

Public health improves when displaced people can enter, persist, and lead in higher education. Aligning admissions, credit recognition, funding, advising, scheduling, language access, and privacy practices with the realities of displacement lowers daily friction and keeps doors open. We see progress in small, steady changes—clearer information, flexible pathways that do not depend on perfect documents, and recognition of community-based work. When institutions design for inclusion and students are supported to learn in context, training aligns with what communities need—and the benefits extend well beyond campus.

BUILDING RESILIENCE IN FUTURE PUBLIC HEALTH LEADERS

Our call for improving the system stems from lived experiences. Our generation has been shaped by power's uneven hand which has taught us who power protects, and who it ought to serve. We were raised with school lockdowns while young children had access to weapons. We come from families of color, who face a greater risk of police violence and incarceration. We live in New York City, where countless people face housing insecurity and death by overheating. We are immigrants and international students, who now face a greater risk of deportation. And, we are the *social media generation* who, through our screens, witnesses daily who defines the phrase humanitarian crisis and who cares enough to do—or to *not* do—something about it. Our generation has been uniquely positioned to not just grow up frustrated with these power imbalances, but to translate our frustration into actionable items to build a safer, more equitable world.

The visibility of these injustices not only led, but pushed us on the path toward becoming public health professionals. And while we all will recite the same "Public

Health Oath", thus committing ourselves to a career of protecting the health of all people, our diverse stories and unique set of attributes will distinguish us as professionals in the field and allow us to uniquely contribute to the ideals of public health. Our article's authors, for example, exemplify this notion.

Nabiha

Growing up in post 9/11 America, Nabiha witnessed how racism and Islamaphobia permeated institutions that influence health. Public health offered her a framework to connect advocacy with analysis—helping her to understand how upstream social forces shape individual and community outcomes.

Sunwoo

Growing up in New York City, Sunwoo witnessed how environment and opportunity influence chronic disease. His path through biostatistics and epidemiology reflects a desire to translate data into justice, advancing equitable cardiovascular health through research.

Jordan

Raised in a predominately white town, Jordan first learned about health disparities during college. Realizing her future role as a physician must go beyond individual care, she pursued public health to better understand and dismantle systemic inequities.

Ugomma

A second-generation Nigerian-American, Ugomma was raised to view education as a form of empowerment. Her pursuit of public health stems from a mission to improve equity within educational and global health systems alike.

Maria

In her small hometown in India, Maria saw patients not only face medical neglect but a theft of dignity. Public health became her path to design interventions that restore access and dignity to those ignored.

Rachel

Inspired by the One Health movement, Rachel became interested in the intersections of human, animal, and environmental health. Guided by the idea that *science does not operate in a vacuum*, she seeks to address health disparities through an interdisciplinary lens and is pursuing a career in epidemiology to advance this work.

Yusra

Raised in a working-class immigrant household, Yusra saw how language and systemic bias shape access to care. She chose public health to advance equity for immigrant communities through community based research and prevention programs rooted in dignity and self-determination.

Chetan

During his medical rotations in India, Chetan observed inequities among patients from diverse socioeconomic backgrounds. These experiences inspired him to pursue public health, seeking the tools to understand and address those disparities.

As seen through these brief narratives, the backgrounds, motivations, and aspirations of these public health trainees are all uniquely different. Yet their similarity lies in their central mission to improve the health of communities and advance the public's knowledge of health through collaboration and teamwork.

However well-intentioned, isolated initiatives cannot dismantle the legal frameworks that entrench injustice. Racist statutes, unequal access to care, and legislative neglect persist because efforts remain fragmented and under-resourced. Revitalizing public health practice, therefore, requires cultivating 2 interdependent competencies among emerging professionals: Legal literacy to identify, challenge, and reform discriminatory policies; Community-built resilience to sustain collective advocacy over the long term.

Our lived experiences underscore that policy decisions fundamentally determine health outcomes. Integrating legal literacy into public health curricula equips practitioners with mastery of statutory interpretation and intergovernmental authority—skills essential for holding decision-makers accountable for lead-contaminated water, substandard housing codes, or restrictive immigration health policies. We define legal literacy as the practitioner's ability to understand, interpret, and leverage laws and policies to advance public health goals. This is not about creating lawyers, but about empowering advocates to move from identifying a problem to knowing the precise legal mechanisms for its solution. For example, when confronting a lead water crisis, a legally literate professional would do more than document blood lead levels; they would be equipped to identify the violated provisions of the Safe Drinking Water Act, navigate the complex interplay of state and local enforcement authority, and draft compelling public testimony to hold the correct agencies accountable. Moreover, balancing individual rights with population health imperatives informs debates on vaccination mandates, harm-reduction services, and other critical interventions. As Michael Sparer of Columbia University's Mailman School of Public Health observes, fluency in public health law transforms abstract statutes into instruments of equity, enabling rights-based, sustainable measures for vulnerable communities.

Yet sustained engagement with entrenched systems exacts a heavy toll. In the absence of formal support networks, practitioners confront isolation and burnout. We therefore reconceptualize resilience as a collective endeavor: community-built resilience rooted in solidarity and shared purpose. In a field confronting systemic trauma, resilience is a shared resource, not a personal responsibility. Structured platforms—peer-mentoring circles, interdisciplinary workshops, and student-run journals—bring together epidemiologists, legal scholars, political scientists, and sociologists. These networks foster innovation while providing the social infrastructure vital for maintaining transformative work within resource-constrained environments.

Persistent barriers—chronic underfunding, workforce attrition, and political opposition—continue to limit public health's impact. Nonetheless, the expansion of pandemic-era investments and renewed emphasis on health system strengthening reaffirm the field's indispensable role. By uniting legal expertise with collaborative resilience frameworks, the next generation of practitioners will be poised to convert critical insights into evidence-based policies and institutional reforms that advance sustainable health equity.

SUMMARY

In a time where public health faces administrative threats amid human rights crises escalating nationally and internationally, readjusting public health education is more urgent now than ever before. We, as public health trainees, advocate for a realignment of public health education with current-day humanitarian realities, as this will better prepare emerging leaders to engage thoughtfully and effectively in such settings.

Achieving competencies in public health education focused on the response to humanitarian crises and the training of competent health professionals, especially those individuals who themselves have been displaced, will require steadfast resiliency. We believe that efforts at achieving this goal are well worth the investment. From the appraisal of the use of seatbelts to avert injuries, vaccinations to deter infectious disease spread, a framework of health equity, integration of lived experience, and valuing work on the front lines of crises and pandemics are the essential elements in the formation and training of 21st century public health professionals.

The academic ecological sustainability framework we have proposed offers a pathway forward. By holding scholars and practitioners mutually accountable to inform each other's work, and by cultivating interprofessional education grounded in complex systems thinking, we can bridge the persistent gap between theoretic knowledge and field-responsive practice. This framework, with its core emphasis on adaptability and mutual accountability, naturally necessitates and supports the integration of legal literacy with collaborative resilience frameworks. Legal expertise enables emerging practitioners to identify and challenge discriminatory policies through mastery of statutory interpretation and regulatory analysis, while community-built resilience networks provide the collective infrastructure necessary to sustain this transformative work overtime. Together, these elements operationalize academic ecological sustainability by forging the dynamic, accountable relationships between academia, practice, and community that are essential for transforming public health education from isolated coursework into harmonized, evidence-based action.

Ultimately, the trajectories we have mapped do more than expose asymmetrical power dynamics—they constitute a critical epistemology demanding structurally competent public health pedagogy. Realizing academic ecological sustainability requires moving beyond theoretic acknowledgment to concrete curricular integration: embedding specific skill sets like statutory interpretation, regulatory analysis, legal advocacy into core courses, and complementing them with required, for-credit practica in interdisciplinary collaboration and moral distress management. This praxis-oriented model equips emerging practitioners with the analytical skills to challenge inequitable policies and the collective infrastructure to sustain transformative work. Achieving a more equitable distribution of power, therefore, requires more than individual heroism; it demands a unified field, grounded in empirical evidence and collaborative action, that is purposefully built through a revitalized and courageous curriculum.

DISCLOSURE

The authors declare that they have no relevant financial relationships with ineligible companies or personal relationships that could have appeared to influence the work reported in this article.

REFERENCES

1. UNHCR. Global trends report 2024 | UNHCR. UNHCR. 2024. Available at: https://www.unhcr.org/global-trends-report-2024. Accessed July 13, 2025.
2. Council on Education for Public Health. Accreditation criteria for schools of public health and public health programs. 2021. Available at: https://media.ceph.org/documents/2021.Criteria.pdf. Accessed July 13, 2025.
3. King L. New MPH curriculum in the United States: report on successes and challenges. Eur J Publ Health 2020;30(Supplement_5). https://doi.org/10.1093/eurpub/ckaa165.024.

4. Begg MD, Galea S, Bayer R, et al. MPH education for the 21st century: design of Columbia University's new public health curriculum. Am J Publ Health 2014; 104(1):30–6.
5. Ramaswamy R, Mosnier J, Reed K, et al. Building capacity for Public Health 3.0: introducing implementation science into an MPH curriculum. Implement Sci 2019; 14(1). https://doi.org/10.1186/s13012-019-0866-6.
6. Corvin JA, DeBate R, Wolfe-Quintero K, et al. Application of the intervention mapping framework to develop an integrated twenty-first century core curriculum—part three: curriculum implementation and evaluation. Front Public Health 2017; 5. https://doi.org/10.3389/fpubh.2017.00285.
7. Evans DP, Anderson M, Shahpar C, et al. Innovation in graduate education for health professionals in humanitarian emergencies. Prehospital Disaster Med 2016;31(5):532–8.
8. Awsan B, Trentin M, Hubloue I, et al. Humanitarian health education and training state-of-the-art: a scoping review. Front Public Health 2024;12. https://doi.org/10.3389/fpubh.2024.1343867.
9. Frenk J, Chen L, Bhutta ZA, et al. Health professionals for a new century: transforming education to strengthen health systems in an interdependent world. Lancet 2020;376(9756):1923–58.
10. UNHCR. Refugees. Available at: https://www.unhcr.org/us/about-unhcr/who-we-protect/refugees. Accessed October 20, 2025.
11. UNHCR. The 1951 refugee convention. Available at: https://www.unhcr.org/about-unhcr/overview/1951-refugee-convention. Accessed October 20, 2025.
12. International Organization for Migration. Forced migration or displacement data. Migration data portal. Available at: https://www.migrationdataportal.org/themes/forced-migration-or-displacement. Accessed October 20, 2025.
13. U.S. citizenship and immigration services. *Refugees*. Available at: https://www.uscis.gov/humanitarian/refugees-and-asylum/refugees. Accessed October 20, 2025.
14. Office of the High Commissioner for Human Rights. About internally displaced persons. Available at: https://www.ohchr.org/en/special-procedures/sr-internally-displaced-persons/about-internally-displaced-persons. Accessed October 20, 2025.
15. UNHCR. Internally displaced people. Available at: https://www.unhcr.org/us/about-unhcr/who-we-protect/internally-displaced-people. Accessed October 20, 2025.
16. Raw video: Nelson mandela visits Madison park HS in roxbury in 1990. 2013. Available at: https://www.youtube.com/watch?v=b66c6OkMZGw. Accessed October 20, 2025.
17. UNHCR. Higher education and skills. UNHCR; 2025. Available at: https://www.unhcr.org/what-we-do/build-better-futures/education/higher-education-and-skills. Accessed October 20, 2025.
18. Mazzero C. Higher education in displacement: empowering pathway or double-edged institution? Insights from Belarusian students' experiences. J Refug Stud 2025;38(4):feaf014.
19. Berg J. Higher education for refugees: relevance, challenges, and open research questions. SN Soc Sci 2023;3(10):177.
20. Betts A. Mohsen Mahdawi, Palestinian green-card holder and Columbia student, detained by Ice. Guardian. 2025. Available at: https://www.theguardian.com/us-news/2025/apr/14/mohsen-mahdawi-palestinian-detained-ice. Accessed October 20, 2025.

United States Postal Service

Statement of Ownership, Management and Circulation
(All Periodicals Publications Except Requester Publications)

1. Publication Title: PEDIATRIC CLINICS OF NORTH AMERICA	2. Publication Number: 4 2 4 - 6 6	3. Filing Date: 08/28/2026
4. Issue Frequency: FEB, APR, JUN, AUG, OCT, DEC	5. Number of Issues Published Annually: 6	6. Annual Subscription Price: $311.00

7. Complete Mailing Address of Known Office of Publication (Not printer) (Street, city, county, state, and ZIP+4)
Addr 1: Elsevier INC
Addr 2: 230 Park Ave Ste 800
City, State ZIP: New York NY 10169
Contact Person: Mohana Priya Damodharan
Telephone: 91-44-4299-4077

8. Complete Mailing Address of Headquarters or General Business Office of Publisher (Not Printer)
Addr 1: Elsevier INC
Addr 2: 230 Park Ave Ste 800
City, State ZIP: New York NY 10169

9. Full Names and Complete Mailing Addresses of Publisher, Editor and Managing Editor (do not leave blank)

Publisher (Name and complete mailing address)
Name: Dolores Meloni, ELSEVIER INC.
Addr 1: 1600 JOHN F KENNEDY BLVD. SUITE 1600
Addr 2:
City, State ZIP: PHILADELPHIA, PA 19103-2899

Editor (Name and complete mailing address)
Name: KERRY HOLLAND, ELSEVIER INC.
Addr 1: 1600 JOHN F KENNEDY BLVD. SUITE 1600
Addr 2:
City, State ZIP: PHILADELPHIA, PA 19103-2899

Managing Editor (Name and complete mailing address)
Name: PATRICK MANLEY, ELSEVIER INC.
Addr 1: 1600 JOHN F KENNEDY BLVD. SUITE 1600
Addr 2:
City, State ZIP: PHILADELPHIA, PA 19103-2899

10. Owner (Do not leave blank. If the publication is owned by a corporation, give the name and address of the corporation immediately followed by the names and addresses of all stockholders owning or holding 1 Percent or more of the total amount of stock. If not owned by a corporation, give the names and addresses of all the individual owners. If owned by a partnership or other unincorporated firm, give it's name and address as well as those of each individual owner. If the publication is published by a nonprofit organization, give it's name and address.)

Full Name	Complete Mailing Address
WHOLLY OWNED SUBSIDIARY OF REED/ELSEVIER,	1600 JOHN F KENNEDY BLVD. SUITE 1600
US HOLDINGS	PHILADELPHIA, PA 19103-2899

11. Known Bondholders, Mortgagees and Other Security Holders Owning or Holding 1 Percent or more of Total Amount of Bonds, Mortgages, or Other Securities. If none, check box → None

Full Name	Complete Mailing Address
NA	

12. Tax Status (For completion by nonprofit organizations authorized to mail at nonprofit rates) (Check one)
The purpose, function, and nonprofit status of this organization and the exempt status for federal income tax purposes:
[X] Has Not changed During Preceding 12 Months
[ ] Has Changed During Preceding 12 Months (Publisher must submit explanation of change with this statement below)

PS Form 3526, July 2014

13. Publication Title: PEDIATRIC CLINICS OF NORTH AMERICA

14. Issue Date for Circulation Data Below: October 2026

15. Extent and Nature of Circulation			Average No. Copies Each Issue During Preceding 12 Months	No. Copies of Single Issue Published Nearest to filing Date
a. Total Number of Copies (Net press run)			209	199
b. Paid and/or Requested Circulation	(1)	Mailed Outside-County Paid Subscriptions Stated on PS Form 3541 (Include paid distribution above nominal rate, advertiser's proof copies, and exchange copies)	111	112
	(2)	Mailed In-County Paid Subscriptions Stated on PS Form 3541 (Include paid distribution above nominal rate, advertiser's proof copies, and exchange copies)	0	0
	(3)	Paid Distribution Outside the Mails Including Sales Through Dealers and Carriers, Street Vendors, Counter Sales ,and Other Paid Distribution Ouside USPS	83	76
	(4)	Paid Distribution by Other Classes of Mail Through the USPS (e.g. First-Class Mail)	10	6
c. Total Paid Distribution [Sum of 15b. (1), (2), (3), and (4)]			204	194
d. Free or Nominal Rate Distribution (By Mail and Outside the Mail)	(1)	Free or Nominal Rate Outside-County Copies Included on PS Form 3541	4	4
	(2)	Free or Nominal In-County Copies Included on PS Form 3541	0	0
	(3)	Free or Nominal Rate Copies Mailed at Other Classes Through the USPS (e.g. First-Class Mail)	0	0
	(4)	Free or Nominal Rate Distribution Outside the Mail (Carriers or other means)	1	1
e. Total Free or Nominal Rate Distribution (Sum of 15d. (1), (2), (3) and (4))			5	5
f. Total Distribution (Sum of 15c. and 15e.)			209	199
g. Copies not Distributed (See Instructions to Publishers #4 (page #3))			0	0
h. Total (Sum of 15f. and g.)			209	199
i. Percent Paid (15c. Divided by 15f. Times 100)			97.61%	97.49%

* if you are claiming electronic copies, go to line 16 on page 3. If you are not claiming electronic copies, skip to line 17 on page 3.

16. Electronic copy Circulation		
If present, check box		
a. Paid Electronic Copies		
b. Total Paid Print Copies (Line 15c) + Paid Electronic Copies (Line 16a)	204	194
c. Total Print Distribution (Line 15F) + Paid Electronic Copies (Line 16a)	209	199
d. Percentage Paid (Both Print & Electronic Copies (16b divided bt 16c x 100)	97.61%	97.49%

[X] I certify that 50% of all my distribution copies (electronic and Print) are paid above a nominal price

17. Publication of Statement of Ownership
[X] Publication required. Will be printed in the October 2026 issue of this publication. [ ] Publication not required

18. Signature and Title of Editor, Publisher, Business Manager, or Owner: Mohana Priya Damodharan
Title: Distribution Controller
Date: 8/28/2026

I certify that all information furnished on this form is true and complete. I understand that anyone who furnishes false or misleading information on this form or who omits material or information requested on the form may be subject to criminal sanctions (including fines and imprisonment) and/or civil sanctions (including civil penalties)

PS Form 3526, July 2014

9780443428876